COUN
2020
Richard Constance

Springer Series on Rehabilitation

Myron G. Eisenberg, PhD, Series Editor
Veterans Affairs Medical Center, Hampton, VA

Thomas E. Backer, PhD, Consulting Editor
Human Interaction Research Institute, Los Angeles, CA

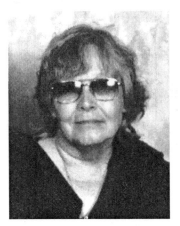

Carolyn Vash, PhD, is a psychologist whose current professional interests span theoretical and philosophical psychology, humanistic psychology, psychology of the arts, and the psychology of religion. She conducts a limited consulting practice based in Altadena, California but devotes most of her time to writing. She has previously worked as a rehabilitation psychologist, administrator, researcher, and educator. In addition to the first edition of *Psychology of Disability*, she has had two other books published by Springer Publishing Company. Their titles were *The Burnt-Out Administrator* (1980) and *Personality and Adversity* (1994). Her next book examines the nature of consciousness through lenses provided by the most ancient of wisdom teachings and the most recent conceptions of complexity science.

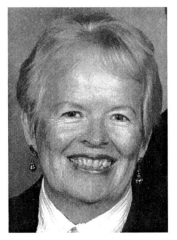

Nancy Crewe, PhD, is a rehabilitation psychologist and professor at Michigan State University where she coordinates the master's degree program in rehabilitation counseling. Prior to taking that position she spent 16 years as a faculty member and clinician in the Department of Physical Medicine and Rehabilitation at the University of Minnesota. Her research interests have revolved around psychological and social aspects of spinal cord injury. She won the American Rehabilitation Counseling Association's 1997 Research Award for *Life Stories of People With Long-Term Spinal Cord Injury*. Previous books include *Employment After Spinal Cord Injury* (1978), written with G. T. Athelstan and A. S. Bower, and *Independent Living for Physically Disabled People* (1983), edited with Irving K. Zola. Current interests include narrative psychology, spirituality and disability, and complexity science.

Psychology of Disability

Second Edition

Carolyn L. Vash, PhD
Nancy M. Crewe, PhD

 Springer Publishing Company

Springer Publishing Company, Inc.
536 Broadway
New York, NY 10012-3955

Acquisitions Editor: Sheri W. Sussman
Production Editor: Sara Yoo
Cover design by Joanne Honigman

04 05 06 07 08/5 4 3 2

Library of Congress Cataloging-in-Publication Data

Vash, Carolyn L.
    Psychology of disability / Carolyn L. Vash, Nancy M. Crewe.—2nd ed.
      p. cm.—(Springer series on rehabilitation)
    Includes bibliographical references and index.
    ISBN 0-8261-3342-8
    1. People with disabilities—Psychology.   2. People with disabilities—
Rehabilitation.   I. Crewe, Nancy M. II. Title. III. Series.
HV3011.V37 2004
362.4'048'019—dc21   2003052980

Printed in the United States of America by Integrated Book Technology.

Contents

Foreword

What a gift this second edition of *Psychology of Disability* is! Such wisdom, such clarity, such practicality. What a gift to have the opportunity to experience the partnership of Carolyn Vash and Nancy Crewe, each a recognized leader in the field of rehabilitation of persons with physical disabilities. Each woman has decades of valuable and practical experience in the counseling psychology and vocational rehabilitation arenas, giving them personal experience with thousands of individuals who have faced the challenges of surviving the draconian financial web of social legislation, individuals who have coped with the psychosocial issues of relationships in a society that does not openly embrace those with disabilities, and individuals who have found satisfaction and contentment from life in the family, the workplace, and community.

Life for people with disabilities has changed dramatically since 1945 when the United States was flooded with individuals injured in WWII and those who had survived the polio epidemics of the 1940s and 1950s. This influx of people challenged the notion that individuals with impairments should not expect to participate in society fully and publicly and should be content to remain at home, cared for by family. Thus the fields of medical and vocational rehabilitation evolved and gained great credibility in the 1960s through major infusions of federal funds for state departments of vocational rehabilitation, rehabilitation research and training centers in major medical schools, and training programs for psychologists and vocational rehabilitation counselors in universities. In this era, the professionals were viewed as the fount of all wisdom regarding disability, but unfortunately this "wisdom" was sometimes nothing more than ivory-tower philosophical speculation, especially when it came to the process of adjusting psychologically to disability. Although most professionals were very well intentioned and sincerely desired to help, their personal knowledge of the disability process was limited to textbooks and offices. In the hospitals, many physicians took a "father knows best" attitude, but despite helpful medical knowledge, this paternalistic attitude grated. Thus, the disability rights movement arose in the early 1970s in order to give people with disabilities a greater voice in their own rehabilitation planning and service delivery system. Eventually, federal and state governmental policies shifted to include those with disabilities in the overall right to have equal opportunity in the community and at work, and with regard to health care services.

It is helpful to place the changes in the lives of those with disabilities in the context of the changes occurring in American society. In the 1950s and even early 1960s, America was a country in which the interests and attitudes of the White, Anglo-Saxon, Protestant—and, we should add, male—group dominated. However, in the last forty years, this country has evolved into a celebration of multicultural diversity so that people with disabilities are one of many groups expecting full participation in society. But this book becomes an opportunity not only to celebrate our multicultural diversity, but also to celebrate our unity. Each chapter addresses issues that are relevant to *everyone*. People with disabilities have the same needs, hopes, and dreams as the readers of this book. And this book addresses issues that are crucial to all of our lives and presents some of the challenges that a person with disability may face which the reader may or may not face. The abiding message is that we are all part of the family of man, all welcome, and that the ways in which we are the same are vastly greater than the ways in which we are different. The beauty of this book is in its essential humanity.

Both Drs. Vash and Crewe began their careers in the 1960s, somewhat prior to the advent of the disability rights movement, and thus they have had the opportunity to observe and participate in the almost dramatic changes at the societal level leading to the inclusion of people with disabilities in all phases of community life. Furthermore, each of them has had a profound impact on the attitudes of two generations of rehabilitation professionals through their research, publications, lectures, and involvement in policy oriented conferences and reports. Thus, this book represents a most beautiful integration of their decades of professional and personal experience and the wisdom that accrues with such seniority.

Roberta B. Trieschmann, PhD

Preface
to the Second Edition

Two eventful decades have passed since the printing of the first edition of this book. The disability rights movement has grown and come of age. Its achievements include taking a key role in the creation and passage of stunning legislation, particularly the Americans with Disabilities Act. Although attitudinal and social barriers remain, people with disabilities have more opportunities and greater basis for optimism than they did a generation ago.

Technology has developed remarkably and presented new opportunities for overcoming functional limitations. Legislation has made illegal the kinds of overt discrimination that used to be commonplace. Health care systems have evolved, offering improved medical and rehabilitation care but also creating economic barriers that limit access for uninsured people, including many with disabilities. In contrast to our rapidly changing society, human nature changes slowly. The writings of David, Socrates, and Shakespeare reveal thoughts and feelings that are immediately understandable to twenty-first century readers.

Consistent with this observation, differing degrees of change were necessary in the parts of the book that deal with human emotions, thoughts, and behaviors and the parts that discuss the environment in which people live. One of the ways in which the world has changed is in the language that we use. Terminology has evolved from words like crippled to handicapped to disabled. "Person first" terminology is currently most widely accepted because it is seen to focus on the whole person rather than on the disability as his or her defining characteristic. On the other hand, some disability activists are calling for a return to the earlier custom of referring to a disabled person. They maintain that it accurately represents their identification with the disability community and their disability pride. We still prefer the person first approach and have generally used it throughout the book, but not slavishly. Both rationales have merit, and both are presently acceptable styles.

Another change involves the burgeoning body of research related to the psychology of disability. Several significant journals are focused on disability research, and other journals occasionally include relevant articles. Further, the Internet provides both direct access to quantities of information and ready entrée to material published in traditional formats. The second edition has taken advantage of these expanded resources and put additional emphasis on research citations.

The book still represents an effort to share the authors' decades of personal and professional experiences with disability. The first author has lived for some 50 years as a severely disabled individual, and the second author is experiencing disability as a concomitant of aging. Both authors have been enriched by careers as rehabilitation psychologists, educators, and researchers.

Acknowledgments

As with any significant project, many people contributed directly and indirectly with ideas, criticism, and support to the development of this book. Our thanks and love especially go to family members: Dick Vash; Jack and Betty Pond; Laurel, Bill, and Ruby Faith Cibik; Janet Johnson; and John Moe.

Among the colleagues who have provided insight or a motivational boost at opportune moments are Jodi Saunders, James Krause, Virginia Thielsen, Roberta Trieschmann, Michael Leahy, Rhonda Egidio, Darlene Groomes, John Victory, and John Kosciulek. Other influential colleagues, past and present, include Irving Kenneth Zola, Denise Tate, Gary Athelstan, Garland Meadows, Rick Baisden, Michael Andary, Margaret Fankhauser, Donald Stanton, Beatrice Wright, Ann Hakkila, Robert Fabiano, and Rochelle Habeck.

The first edition of this book acknowledged a number of individuals who had contributed its development. Because their influence continues to live in the current edition, we express continuing appreciation to Jacqueline Sanchez, Herbert Rigoni, Barbara Waxman, Diana De Bro, Robert and Patricia Hadley, Gregory Kimberlin, Sanford Bernstein, John Millen, Jerry Kuns, Maria French, Edward Roberts, Elizabeth Pan, Thomas Backer, Barbara Morrione, Harry Grace, Bryan Kemp, Edward Workman, Tony Hickey, Pam Kauss, and Danleigh Spievak.

Further, to each of the individuals with disabilities who have contributed to our research, clinical understanding, and personal lives we send our thanks.

Introduction

It has been said that everyone is like all of the other people in the world in some ways, like those in similar groups in some ways, and like no other person who has ever lived in some ways (Leong, 1996). Dangers inhere in acknowledging the validity of the concept "the psychology of disability," since, in the past, it has led to unhelpful exaggerations of the perceived differences between people with disabilities and those without. The fact is, human beings are more alike than different, regardless of variances in their physical bodies, sensory capacities, or intellectual abilities. To illustrate, a disabled person is said to experience a sense of loss over the functional abilities that an illness or injury has destroyed. Similarly, a nondisabled person may experience a sense of loss over something she or he once had and now has lost. The stimulus is different, but the sense of loss, the fear that life will be painful or meaningless without the lost element, are virtually the same. Viewed in this light, the psychology of disability is little different from the psychology of being human.

The definition of the psychology of disability underlying the material in this book is considered here to be largely, though not entirely, the study of how human organisms respond to a set of stimulus conditions associated with disability. Stated somewhat differently, it is a study of *normative responses from* (psychologically) *normal organisms to abnormal stimuli.*

Some of these abnormal stimuli are biological, such as being paralyzed. Some are environmental, such as inaccessible entrances. Others are social, such as having a salesperson ask your companion, not you, what size you wear. Not being able to get a job is an economic example. Some stimuli are obvious, such as a restroom door you can't get through, while others are subtle, like people not using the work "handicapped" when you are around. Some are pleasant, such as being allowed to enter an airplane first. Some are unpleasant, such as not being able to use the restroom on a long flight. Pages could be filled with such examples, which in itself illustrates the unusual stimulus situation the disabled person is in: a continual flow of perceptions and experiences that cannot be validated by the majority of people around one. Thus, isolation and lack of consensus for one's ideas and feelings are added to the list of unusual stimulus conditions. And so it goes.

Following from this, the psychology of disability becomes bifurcated as an applied science. One branch is a rather typical applied behavioral science, embodied in a group of professionals who use the findings of research and clinical experience to help people with disabilities cope with, adapt to, and adjust to other unusual stimuli. The other branch is embodied in an activist movement by a group of people determined to alter the stimulus conditions because the world needs "treatment" more than the people with disabilities.

This latter branch emerged slowly after World War II, when medical science found ways to save wounded soldiers who then returned, significantly disabled, to a society that felt it owed them something. Acknowledging a debt and paying it are two different things, however, and little progress was made. The civil rights movement pointed the way, with special impetus flowing from the 1965 Watts riots. A segment of the African American population in south central Los Angeles engaged in violent, self-destructive behavior for six days; somehow, one of the results of it was that blacks all over the country, other racial minorities, women, people with disabilities, and multitudes of other groups who had accepted powerlessness and half-filled cups all of their lives began to scream. They saw more clearly that society, even an indebted one, is not going to fix itself for you. The folks with the problem must come up with the solution. They also rediscovered the Constitution. Everyone had known all along that African Americans were deprived regularly of their constitutional rights, but whoever thought that people with disabilities were? The "expectation explosion" became a chain reaction, and "consciousness raising" tried to ensure that everyone's expectations were as high as they should be.

Prior to this paradigm shift, virtually all of the emphasis in rehabilitation was on modifying the "patient" to fit into the world as it was. Patients were modified by medicine, surgery, physical therapy, occupational therapy, psychotherapy, vocational counseling, social casework, prosthetic and orthotic devices, education, training, and much, much more. Family homes were remodeled, occasionally at public expense, but to expect all housing to be built to be accessible to people with disabilities would have been viewed as an idealistic delusion. The motto was, "If a round peg doesn't fit in a square hole, you square the peg, you don't ream out the hole."

Some changes have taken root. The "other half" of the psychology of disability has become the *politics of disability*. This is only right; it's not good for people, psychologically speaking, to be deprived of their constitutional rights. If the applied psychology of disability is to be a helpful discipline, then it must tend to the business of altering destructive stimulus conditions, as well as modifying disabled individuals and their responses.

Scope and Purpose

The Psychology of Disability is intended to serve as a textbook or collateral reading source for students engaged in the study of the psychological aspects of disability, as well as a general resource for rehabilitation professionals in the full spectrum of allied health and vocational service disciplines. The material is presented in two parts, which might be labeled "What it's like to be disabled" and "what people who are inclined to help can do."

Part I, "The Disability Experience," is an effort to admit the reader into sundry corners of the experiential worlds of people with disabilities. It is a phenomenological accounting of the ways in which disabled people confront and are confronted by the world and of how they go about the business of living under the sometimes peculiar circumstances disability can generate. It attempts to present the psychological experience from the perspectives of people who have disabilities; the inner states and processes, the interpersonal situations and interactions, and the behavioral mechanisms and patterns that emerge. The eight chapters of Part I chronicle both the objective and subjective experiences associated with being a disabled person in a handicapping world and how these affect the basic life functions of surviving, living, working, playing, and—for some at least—transcending both the disability and the more troubling aspects of the world.

Part II, "Interventions," is a response to the problems and sources of psychological pain that are exposed by the discussions in Part I. It describes some major ways in which changes can be wrought; some are designed to improve the world, and others are intended to help disabled individuals react constructively to the conditions life has proffered. Interventions aimed at changing the world traditionally were not thought of as psychological services, but they may have a profound effect on the psychological well-being of an individual. Transcending disability is much easier if basic survival and quality of life issues have been addressed by the society, so Chapter 5 deals with disability-relevant legislation and policy. The remaining five chapters are devoted to intervention strategies used by psychologically trained professionals (for example, psychologists, rehabilitation counselors, social workers, psychiatrists, speech pathologists), other rehabilitation professionals (for example, nurses, occupational therapists, physical therapists, physicians), peer providers (for example, peer counselors), and social/behavioral scientists. Four of these chapters deal with ways to help disabled people improve the quality of their lives by working on themselves (as opposed to changing the world). The last deals with the future, touching on some of the current and critical issues for people with disabilities in America. These include the growing interest in racial and ethnic diversity, aging, and technology. The chapter ends with an exploration of spirituality and disability.

Unavoidably, the choice of subject matter and manner of presentation reflect the authors' belief systems regarding what the psychology of disability is all about, thus determining the issues considered important enough to include, the programs viewed as successful, and the policy decisions suggested. Moreover, the authors' personal and professional experiences have been preponderantly weighted in the area of physical disabilities; therefore, the selected issues and case examples may reflect this experiential loading despite conscious efforts to the contrary.

The Issues

The commonality of experience among people with different types of disabilities is great because all of them share the processes of being devalued as a result of having a disability and learning to accept all that disablement entails. It may be too sweeping a statement, but devaluation and acceptance seem to constitute the underlying cause and inherent solution to most of the specific psychological problems associated with disability. The form of disability, however, does shape the manifest problems, so it is necessary to examine the specific ways in which various impairments impact people's lives. For example, deafness or even blindness may impede a person's participation in a conversation, whereas severe physical disability might prevent one from attending the gathering at all.

Probing further, although sensory, motor, and internal disabilities have significantly different impacts, they all reflect bodily dysfunctions, as opposed to impaired mental processes. With disabilities such as these, one can adopt rather comfortably the definition stated earlier: the psychology of disability is the study of normative responses from psychologically normal organisms to abnormal stimuli. Naturally, there are exceptions; people who could not be considered "psychologically normal" become disabled, too, and occasionally the disablement proves to be the stress that pushes a vulnerable individual into neurosis or psychosis. More to the point, many people have disabilities that are explicitly psychological in nature, such as mental retardation or mental illness. While it would not be reasonable to assert that they are "psychologically normal organisms," it is still true that many of the psychological problems experienced are not due to the mental disabilities per se, but to such abnormal stimuli as being devalued in the eyes of others. In this light, it is important to focus on abnormalities in stimulus situations before ascribing abnormality to the psyches of disabled individuals, even when the disability is mental in nature. Although the "letter" of the definition must be altered somewhat to accommodate this portion of the disabled population, the "spirit" of the definition is equally applicable.

Devaluation and acceptance: these are considered the pivotal variables in adjusting to life when it is complicated by disability. Let us look at each in more detail.

Devaluation

Following close behind outright oppression in terms of psychologically damaging consequences is devaluation, that is, being regarded as a lesser being, inferior, not very capable, not very useful, possibly burdensome, unaesthetic, and, generally, one down. People with disabilities consistently experience devaluation in the eyes of others, and their own. This is true regardless of the nature of the disability, whether it impairs physical, sensory, or mental functioning. The phenomenon was illustrated powerfully at a rehabilitation conference held in California a number of years ago. Dr. William Rader—psychiatrist, psychodramatist, and public performer par excellence—began an arousing display of the tragic, even deadly, effects of communication misfires between helpers and helpees with a simple routine. He addressed the audience, alternately standing up and then sitting in a wheelchair, all the while challenging them to deny that their perceptions of his competence fluctuated as he stood and sat, stood and sat. There was much discussion afterward, and virtually all in attendance, from able-bodied to very severely disabled, acknowledged that their views of his competence *had* changed, had alternated dizzyingly as he stood and sat; that he had appeared more credible, more worthy of attention when he stood. It was an emotionally draining experience for many. It was a confrontation of prejudice they had ignored or denied for a long time. Why such an impact from recognizing that one does, indeed, devalue people with disabilities? Can it be changed? Probably not, unless it is first acknowledged and examined in every aspect.

The first line of inquiry addresses whether such prejudice is biologically based. Does the human species instinctively shun damaged organisms because their perpetuation could threaten the survival of the species? The anthropological observation that numerous primitive tribes leave aged or injured members to die because efforts to save them would endanger larger numbers is familiar to many. Is it possible that biological mechanisms which once operated for species protection have not caught up with an affluent and technologically advanced civilization that has rendered them anachronistic? No one knows.

The second line of inquiry is psychosocial, but the content is similar. People tend to shun, be prejudiced against, or devalue individuals who are different. This is more so if the difference occurs at the low end of the distribution, that is, if the individual has less of something than most people have. But people who are too beautiful or too brilliant or too rich, or extraordinarily kind come in for their share of suspicion and punishment as well. This phenomenon may have biological substrates also, since it appears to have been "learned" by almost every culture on earth. Can people learn to tolerate a wider range of differences? How?

The third line of inquiry is politicoeconomic. In an affluent, technologically advanced society, saving lives and improving the quality of life for those saved but left damaged is not going to threaten the survival of the species. It can, however, reduce the sum total of goods available for the rest. Despite substantial advances in the past 25 years, people with disabilities, especially severe ones, are still viewed as a group of "takers" who don't put much back into the system, into the family, the community, or the larger society.

Considering materialistic values only, this may be a valid notion. If severely disabled individuals lack the inner resources or miss the strokes of fortune leading to jobs paying enough to support high-cost needs, then the issue is not whether the public pays, but how. Should there be a tax-supported welfare system or should the person be subsidized through an employer who, in turn, passes the cost on to the public in increased prices for goods and services? In terms of the long-run impact on the purses of the people, there may be little difference. In terms of the psychological well-being of the disabled people affected, the difference may be great.

Even in pragmatic terms, people with disabilities may contribute by serving as the impetus for technological innovations that then are adopted and benefit the population at large. One of the amusing objections offered to providing accommodations to a worker with a disability is that "if he gets it, everyone will want one." And if everyone should get it (e.g., an ergonomically designed chair or more flexible working hours), and if morale and productivity improve as a result, where is the harm?

If one looks beyond the material to spiritual values, the issue becomes meaningless. If one has faith, or at least adopts the belief, that the purpose of life is spiritual development rather than materialistic acquisition, then sharing of goods with those unable to produce their own is not inconsistent with enlightened self-interest. The reason for this is an associated faith that we are all parts of the same universal spirit, wherein selfishness and unselfishness become, paradoxically, the same. Just as one must "selfishly" pursue one's own development—and sometimes deny others—if one is to become a truly beneficial influence for others, so must one also pursue the removal of hindrances to others' development, because to do otherwise is ultimately to impair one's own. There is no reason to believe that people with disabilities put less into this system than anyone else.

Over the years relatively little investment has been made in the provision of psychological services to people with disabilities. In addition to the public's frugality, disabled individuals may be motivated to handle adjustment issues on their own. A great deal of help and dependency are accepted because there is no other choice consonant with survival. To need still further help, implying emotional as well as physical dependency, is unacceptable, so the need is denied. Beyond this, the social sanctions against getting psychological or psychiatric help interfere with asking, even when the need is recognized.

In addition, it is not easy to relate psychological services to savings of public dollars. Physical restoration can demonstrably reduce the lifelong medical costs for which the public pays. Vocational rehabilitation can reduce welfare costs and get some tax money coming into the system as well. Since physical restoration and vocational rehabilitation can produce those benefits, who is going to worry about *feelings*?

Again, such a position is shortsighted. Apart from humanistic concerns about quality of life, it is possible that sufficient attention to such soft data of rehabilitation— from the earliest moments post-onset through the entire life process—could further reduce medical, welfare, and related costs to a degree barely conceived of today. People who feel badly about themselves generate needs that must be served. Unfortunately, it too often happens after the person is in such deep psychological trouble that the effects are being felt by others as well.

Acceptance of Disability

In the earlier days of the rehabilitation movement, there was a great deal of talk about the importance of "accepting one's disability." This sometimes meant the absence of the defense mechanism "denial." At other times, it simply meant acknowledging one's loss without feeling rotten about it. Acceptance was good. People were never supposed to *like* their disabilities, however, because that was considered worse than denial. Profits reaped were labeled "secondary gain" and secondary gain was a no-no. This required the disabled person to know exactly where the line between acceptance and enjoyment lay, and to be eternally vigilant not to cross over. Acceptance was biting the bullet and smiling at the same time, and about equally easy.

By the late 1950s it was becoming unfashionable to talk about accepting disability. The literature explained to anyone gauche enough to use such language that it did not make sense to expect a person to accept disablement and that the professionals of a prior era had "laid a bum trip" on disabled people. No one should be enjoined to accept something that meant settling for second-rate hopes and goals. "Adapting to" and "coping with" became the preferred terminology.

Actually, it was this thinking that led, in part, to the advocacy revolution. Some realistic soul saw that counseling would not solve the problem if, at the end of it, disabled people still could not get from one point to another because there were stairs or no accessible buses in between. Life still would not be very much fun because the world was not a very reasonable place to live. Thus began the shift of emphasis from modification of the person to modification of the world; the new recommendations were for removing the stairs and the discriminatory hiring practices instead of counseling disabled people to stop liking upstairs restaurants and start liking the few jobs they would be allowed to do.

Now, early in the 21st century, a long-elusive but critically important distinction is finally becoming clear. If the disability cannot be changed, then it must be accepted as must any other reality, pleasant or unpleasant, if the person is to survive and grow. What need *not* be accepted is the unnecessary handicapping imposed on disabled people by a poorly designed or unaccommodating world or by their own failures to accept what is and go on from there. These are the causes of second-rate dreams, and they should be summarily rejected.

This volume is not a compendium of indisputable facts. It is an overview of the authors' observations on the experiences of people with disabilities and of individuals who try to help them with the harder parts. It is hoped that it will provide a useful base of information to students and practitioners in the wide range of rehabilitation disciplines wherein understanding of the psychological aspects of disability is integral to the work.

I

The Disability Experience

1

The Person

Reactions to Disablement

Some people are born with disabilities. They grow gradually into the recognition that they are different from most other people in ways that are negatively evaluated. Some things that everyone else can do, they cannot. The realization of having been shortchanged comes slowly; it is their parents who may experience the sudden shock. Other people become disabled after a lifetime—whether brief or long—of being more or less like everyone else. It may happen in a catastrophic moment, or it may take days, weeks, months, or years of illness to develop.

The reactions to the facts of disablement depend in part on when and how it happens and in part on a host of other factors to be explored in this initial chapter. The long-range response patterns, variously referred to as "adjusting to," "coping with," or "accepting" disability, will be dealt with in later chapters devoted to specific areas of human functioning. Here, the focus will be on the more immediate emotional and behavioral reactions of people who find themselves disabled, and on the array of personal characteristics and situations that determine the types and intensities of their reactions to the lack or loss of capabilities ordinarily taken for granted.

Just as "when and how it happens" contribute to determining a person's reactions to disablement, so also do such widely ranging factors as the type of disability, its severity, and its stability, the person's sex, inner resources, temperament, self-image, and self-esteem, the presence of family support, income, the available technology, and government funding trends. This sampling of causal factors associated with reactions to disablement illustrates four general classes of reaction determinants: (1) those emanating from the disability itself, (2) those linked to the person who becomes disabled, (3) those present in the person's immediate environment, and (4) those that are part of the larger cultural context.

Although Chapter 2 deals explicitly with the external forces impinging on people with disabilities, it is impossible to totally separate "the person" from "the world." To illustrate, George Hohmann, a rehabilitation psychologist who learned about spinal cord injury first hand, points out that spinal cord injury simply isn't as depressing today as it was decades ago when he was injured (Hohmann, personal communication). The reasons he cites are medical and technological advances, increased federal funding for needed programs, and the passage of protective civil rights legislation that have come about in the intervening years.

Thus, many different variables influence the types and intensity of reactions to disablement, and all of these variables interact with one another to create still greater complexity. To begin to understand what happens, let us look at what several people have had to say about their own reactions to disability.

Mike is mildly mentally retarded. He works in a rehabilitation facility as a custodian, and has reading skills comparable to the average second grader. His social skills are remarkable; he is poised and at ease and has a special gift for mediating other people's arguments. He speaks unhesitatingly about being a "slow learner" and how it felt when he first recognized that fact.

> The kids around home made fun of me because I couldn't catch on to things like they did. At first I cried, then I just stayed by myself. My folks put me in a special school where all the kids were like me. I was one of the smartest ones. I helped the kids who were slower than me. I really hated those kids that laughed at me. I still don't think people should laugh at slow learners. We're people like everyone else.

Mike's "folks" were actually his grandparents. His parents had sought to have him institutionalized when he was three, so the grandparents offered to take him. They were among the concerned citizens who established the facility in which he now works.

Maria was born with cerebral palsy. She was the first child of a ten-year marriage and highly prized by her parents. She believes her family's upper-class status in a Central American country, coupled with strong (Catholic) religious ties, served to facilitate their acceptance of, and dedication to, a disabled child. They moved to the United States when she was eight to avail themselves of better services for her.

For the first thirteen years of her life, she was taught to believe that she was "as good as anyone else and could do anything she wanted to do." This gave her the self-confidence to disregard the taunting of other children, to whom she attributed ignorance. She learned to walk, albeit awkwardly and at a fast pace to keep her balance, and learned to speak understandably to most listeners. She suffered such traumas as being placed in a school program for retarded youngsters until her intellectual gifts were recognized. In the main, however, she was a happy and energetic youngster who felt good about herself.

She says she can speak knowledgeably about both birth disorder and later-life disablement because at the age of thirteen, she fell and broke her hip. Thenceforth, she was unable to walk independently and, in her words:

All of the teachings of my first thirteen years were undone. My parents couldn't understand why I couldn't walk anymore (and it was only a few years ago that a doctor explained it to me) and they accused me of being lazy and ungrateful. I realized that I wasn't really a human being to them, I was a project that had been set back. Then, when a teacher encouraged me to go to college and I told them, I found that they had never believed all those things they had told me about being able to do anything I wanted to. They didn't believe I could do anything, really... not drive, and certainly not go to college.

Today, Maria is a happy and effective schoolteacher, the only severely disabled teacher to be hired after onset by a large city school system. She says those early years of confidence helped her combat the doubts and rejections she experienced later on, even though they were in one sense "undone." She believes having cerebral palsy forced her to mature quickly and to be less vulnerable to many of the emotional terrors that plague teenagers and young adults. She acknowledges that

People with my disability don't find it easy to get dates, and you can't be as bold as other women or you'll scare men off. Maybe I'll find someone and maybe I won't. Either way, I know and like who I am and, for the first time in my life, I now have good friends who accept me. Later on, I may adopt an older child with a disability, whether I'm married or not.

She believes there is a status hierarchy of disabilities in which polio and spinal cord injury are at the top and mental retardation and cerebral palsy are at the bottom. She considers this less a function of time of onset than the nature of the impairments; however, she laughingly recalls claiming that her disability resulted from "falling down and breaking my hip" for several years after that happened.

Dana, who got polio at the age of sixteen, was present when Maria described her experiences. She agreed that her disability was freer from stigma than Maria's, but quipped that any advantage was overshadowed by Maria's greater maturity. She especially marveled at how "together" Maria appears to be with respect to her impaired status on the marriage market. Essentially triplegic, with considerable weakness in her "good" arm, Dana indicated this was her most painful area of reaction to disability.

She, too, experienced singular acceptance within her (very scholarly) family and also within a wide circle of friends. Having planned since junior high school to get an advanced degree, she had little more than the usual doubts about her ability to "make it" in her chosen career. However, she recalled a long and torturous process of dealing with angry disappointment and consciousness-consuming fears about being "damaged merchandise on the marriage market." Of this she says:

> Mother always assumed I would get a PhD in something because it was "the thing to do." But she also conveyed that the most important thing in life was to be a good wife and mother. A PhD could be a cushion to fall back on in case you were widowed or divorced, but it wasn't a matter of trade training. When the doctor told us I would be permanently paralyzed, one of her first attempts to reassure me was, "Well, honey, think of it this way; you'll never have to wash dishes and your hands will always be lovely and smooth." I read the message, "Hopefully, you'll still be attractive enough to get a good husband."
>
> As soon as I could be up in a wheelchair, she started pushing me downtown to buy new clothes to fit my thinner frame. She would excitedly repeat appreciative comments she overheard from passing males. I now think they may have been apocryphal, but I believed them then and her strategy worked. I felt confident that, wheelchair or no, I was a pretty young girl who could expect to go on having lots of dates, and somehow believing it made it so. I determined never to do anything I couldn't look graceful doing, and I was off on a new career of proving to myself and the world that despite being in a wheelchair, I was still desirable.
>
> That neurotic adventure consumed a large part of the next sixteen years of my life. In my spare time, I got the expected PhD and developed a successful career, but most of my consciousness was going into countless lovers and a couple of husbands. When my second marriage imploded, I went to a shrink and started getting the whole silly script rewritten.
>
> I've now been happily married to my third husband for over ten years, the PhD is in "cushion" status, and my husband forced me to learn to cook and wash the dishes. I make Maria look as graceful as a ballerina when I start working in the kitchen. Sometimes, when I'm struggling to lift a heavy pot or something, I think back on the days when I wouldn't do anything that might look awkward. The irony is, it took so much craziness to come full circle. My present lifestyle is just about what mother had in mind. It makes you wonder about destiny.

Jamal has a different set of concerns that he believes are more difficult than those faced by either Dana or Maria. This muscular, macho, 35-year-old man was a policeman in a large city when he began to notice that his body was behaving strangely at times. Once he tripped and fell when he was chasing a fugitive, and he had a difficult time getting back up. Another time he dropped his revolver. He tried to put these and other incidents out of his mind, but they haunted him. He went to the doctor and was told that he was just suffering from stress. He was given an antianxiety prescription, but it did little good.

I kept complaining about these weird experiences, and they put me into the psych ward! I was there for almost three weeks. Even I was beginning to think that I was crazy. Several months later I got a new doctor, and he told me that I had multiple sclerosis. I didn't know whether to laugh or to cry. Mostly I was relieved. At least I knew what was going on in my body.

For a while Jamal's condition seemed to improve, but then the symptoms flared up again, leaving him uncertain about what to expect from week to week. Even during good times his speech is slightly slurred, and his gait is unsteady, and during a couple of bad flare-ups he has needed a wheelchair to get around. He has been transferred to a desk job in his precinct, something that grates on his ego. He is especially distressed by the effect that his symptoms have had on his dating life. Once he enjoyed parties, dances, and meeting new women. Now they find excuses to move on after brief conversations. He adds, "I wonder if I've missed my chance to fall in love and settle down with someone who could give me a family? Even if I could find someone who would have me like I am, how long would I be able to support her like a real man should?"

Harris, who has been deaf since an explosion occurred near him in Korea, speaks of different kinds of reactions from those described by Maria, Dana, and Jamal, all of whom have motor disabilities. He described the loneliness of being "left out" even when physically present in a group and his anger at being ignored when a conversation partner seeks the easier path of talking with the interpreter instead of him. He described his disbelief, years earlier, when he worked for the first time as a deaf person in the produce section of a supermarket. A customer, calling to him repeatedly from behind, grew increasingly frustrated and angry at getting no response. Harris first became aware that his attention was being sought when he was hit in the back of the head by a pound of hamburger, which the customer had lobbed at him. Boredom also is a problem when he travels and doesn't have his work or other pursuits available to absorb his consciousness. He says hearing people don't appreciate how much they amuse themselves by simply listening to the ambient sounds.

Reaction to loss can take many forms, and so can loss itself. Earl's story illustrates this. Earl spent his twenties becoming blind. Although he always had done strenuous physical work, he was exceedingly bright and says he was able to adjust to college and a professional career with relative ease. He had been totally blind for seven years when his vision was significantly restored by surgery. He was delighted, of course, but totally unprepared for the adjustment agonies in store. He put it this way:

I had become a superblindman. Everyone marveled at how well I could manage every aspect of my life. My traveling skills were so good that a lot of people joked that I was faking it. They couldn't imagine how a blind man could get around so well, even without a cane. Then, all of a sudden, I was just an average guy again; no big deal, nothing super about me. I'd lost my special status and there was no support coming from anywhere for what I was going through. When I tried to tell people how I felt, they would shut me up, saying, "I don't want to hear this. You're spoiling my fantasies about the wonderful thing that has happened to you." Obviously, I don't want to be blind again, but I'd like a little understanding that what's happened to me isn't totally the magical happy ending without any adjustment problems of its own. It's not pleasant having people regard you as some kind of nut.

Mary knew that problem well. She had a "nervous breakdown" when she was twenty-three years old and for the next four years she was hospitalized intermittently about half of the time. She no longer considers herself mentally ill, but believes she carries with her a residual lifelong disability. She says:

I am not sick now, but I will always be very vulnerable to stress, and I have to pay attention to that so I don't end up getting sick again. I've learned to do that pretty well. The harder part is dealing with the way other people treat you when they know that you've had a mental problem in the past. Some of them act scared, and some just discredit you like your opinions and judgment can't be trusted any more. I am in a group living situation, not a halfway house run by institutional types who run your life for you, just a group of four people who got acquainted when we were all patients at the same hospital. We know we need each other's support to stay out of the hospital, and with it we can. We're all working, but none of our employers knows we've been in a mental hospital. If you lie about it and get caught, you can get fired. But if you don't lie about it, you'll never get hired in the first place. The anxiety of being found out is what's really disabling.

Mary's fear dates from an earlier time when employers actually could ask about an applicant's disability history and fire them without recourse if a concealed condition were discovered. The ADA has made such practices illegal, yet many people still fear indirect retaliation that would be long and costly to prove.

Mei-Ling was a beautiful 19-year-old dancer, just launching her career in television, when she sustained a severe head injury in an automobile collision. Her adjustment challenges included cognitive problems in addition to physical ones. Two months in coma were followed by months of medical and rehabilitative care. Once her graceful body had been her greatest source of pride. When she was discharged to home she was still using a wheelchair for mobility. Dogged determination and ongoing therapy led to her first unsteady steps behind a walker. Eventually she exchanged the walker for a cane and then discarded the cane, walking with an uneven but serviceable gait. Her cognitive abilities also improved in response to therapy and accommodation.

I decided after all this time in the hospital that I had to have a change of scenery and get back to seeing some people my age besides therapists. Everybody was skeptical, but I convinced them to let me try one course at the local junior college. It was a lot harder than I expected. I would sit in the classroom, trying to take notes. The words just poured in, and I would forget the beginning of the sentences before the instructor got to the end. I would have to read the assignments over and over. It took me twice as long as the other students to take tests, too. Fortunately, when I talked with the professors, most of them were willing to let me take untimed exams in a quiet, separate room. I got through one class and then the next and the next. In seven years I had my bachelor's degree in social work. As if that weren't enough, I decided to tackle graduate school! I still have problems with memory and with speed. I think the hardest assignment I've ever had to do was learning how to do research on the internet. It seemed so foreign and confusing at first, but I found a partner to help me through the first paper, and now I'm pretty good on the computer.

My parents got divorced a few months after my accident. Sometimes I wonder if the stress they all went through played a part in bringing that about. I felt guilty for a while, but they assured me that it was not my fault. They have both been there for me all along, and I can't imagine how I could have accomplished these things without their support. I've been frustrated sometimes by the attitudes of people in my classes. Supposedly they are preparing to work with people who have disabilities, but they all did everything but hide under the desks to avoid being my partner on team projects. I guess they thought I would drag their grade down. I would have been terribly lonely if I hadn't met Jack, my fiance. We will be married next June. He admires the way that I've fought back from this injury, and I love him more than I can tell you.

Frank had his second stroke when he was sixty-three. He was an old sixty-three, having had a first stroke and a heart attack three and five years earlier. His hearing was very poor in one ear, and he had to use a magnifying glass to read the newspaper. Both strokes affected the left side of his body and spared his speech, which he used mainly to say, "Poor Papa." Self-pity had been a way of life since he was forty. Having been a successful, young, small-town banker, he never recovered, psychologically or economically, after his bank failed. Now, living in an extended-family household with his wife, a divorced daughter, a divorced son, and a granddaughter, he settled, uncomplainingly, for the occasional attention they paid him and showed no inclination to broaden his activities beyond watching ball games on television and muttering, "Poor Papa." He died two years later, following a second heart attack, leaving a guilt-laden, grief-stricken family. His gentle nature was deeply loved, but he had been easy to ignore.

As these vignettes illustrate, disablement has the power to elicit the full range of human emotions, from fear, anger, and sorrow to relief and even joy. Almost universally experienced are anxiety about survival and episodes of rage. Some people rage against themselves, their own incompetence to do what everyone else takes for granted; others rage against the universe for being unjust. Some turn their rage against other people for failing to help. While the spectrum of human emotions may be limited, the ways of manifesting or expressing emotions are virtually infinite. Also reflecting enormous variation from one person to another are the specific triggers of emotionality. What hurts or angers one may seem inconsequential to another. As with human variation generally, the question of determination arises: what causes whom to react, and how?

The ensuing pages will refer to the foregoing vignettes, and to other "case examples" as well, in the course of delineating factors that determine (1) how, and how intensely, different individuals feel about their disabled status, and (2) how their feelings affect a wide range of their behavior.

Determiners: The Nature of the Disability

This chapter began with the observation that both time and type of disability onset influence how the person reacts. In addition, other influences relating to the nature of the disability are the types of functions that are impaired, the severity and visibility of the disability, its stability over time, and the presence (or absence) of pain.

Time of Onset

As Maria suggests, self-concept may be influenced by whether a disability was present from birth or happened later to a previously "normal" individual. To her, having been born disabled seemed somehow less respectable than to have acquired a disability adventitiously later on. Although such feelings appear to be fairly common among people with disabilities, the matter is seldom discussed unless it makes a functional difference—as in deafness and, to a lesser degree, blindness. Never to have seen objects in space puts a congenitally blind person at a learning disadvantage compared with those who have visual memories, and the far greater difficulty in learning to speak intelligibly for people who were deaf before language acquisition is well-known.

One's stage of life when adventitious disablement occurs influences the kinds of reactions that will be experienced. This is so partly because it affects the way one is perceived and reacted to by others and partly because different developmental tasks are interrupted during different life stages. The person who becomes disabled in infancy or childhood may, like the person born with a disability, be subjected to isolation, unusual childrearing practices (such as overprotection or rejection), and separation from the mainstream in family life, play, and education. The person who becomes disabled later on may not have to face these same issues, but will have different ones to confront.

Dana's story illustrates one way of reacting to having been "nipped in the bud" just as the wonders and pleasures of womanhood were becoming realities. Earl, who became disabled after completing the developmental task of establishing himself vocationally, found he had to do it all over again. Frank was well into the "decline" stage of his life when he experienced disability; he no longer had the motivational resources necessary to react in any but a passive way. Research done with people who have sustained spinal cord injury (Krause & Crewe, 1991) generally indicate that those who become disabled as young adults adjust more effectively to life changes than do people who are older at the time of onset, but this is only one of many factors that affect any given person.

Type of Onset

The experience of a close brush with death may be a powerful influence on a person's life, and many disabled people feel they cheated the grim reaper by surviving their disabling accidents or illnesses. It seems strange that so little attention has been paid to this issue within rehabilitation circles, especially in view of the importance assigned to the topics of death and dying in both the popular and professional presses in recent years. The claims of some disabled people that they were "given up for dead" tend to be discounted as melodramatic bids for attention, and no further probing is done to learn how an actual or perceived near-death experience might influence their emotions, values, beliefs, and behavior.

The reaction to nearly dying, or believing that one has nearly died, is complexly interwoven with such other variables as religiosity and self-concept. Dana, for example, reported that for years she felt guilty for having survived to be a burden.

I felt I had been slated to die but somehow tricked the great scythe wielder and lived to be a damn drag on a number of people. A lot of my achievement trip was feeling I had to earn and re-earn my right to a place on the planet. What looked like ambition was actually paying penance for not having been gracious enough to just die.

A very different reaction was shared by Lillian, who is paraplegic as a result of spinal meningitis. A devout Mormon, Lillian related that the sense of having been spared led to an intensification of her faith and purpose, which was especially helpful to her when she was abandoned by her husband following disablement.

A year after experiencing a cardiac arrest, Emma was still reliving the terror and frustration of hearing herself pronounced dead and being unable to signal otherwise. She says that nearly every time she is confronted by her memory losses or impaired coordination and strength she recalls the operating table comments and consensus that, "It's just as well, she'd be a vegetable if she lived anyway." She says she sometimes thinks she fooled them and at other times thinks they were right.

The type of onset also is associated with greater and lesser degrees of placing blame for the disabling outcome. Accidents, in which an official designation of responsibility is made, are simply the most obvious case. To believe that a permanent disability resulted from a momentary, foolish act of one's own may strongly affect reaction to the disability itself at least until the feelings of self-blame are resolved. Blaming someone else may have an even stronger impact. Keith, who lost a leg when the motorcycle he was riding collided with a truck, became consumed with hatred toward the truck driver, especially after the courts found him not at fault. Fred, shot in the spine accidentally by his younger brother, believes both of their lives would have been better if their parents had permitted him to express the anger he felt. Kathy remembers wondering childishly why her parents wouldn't do whatever they were supposed to do to make her get better when she had polio as a child. They had always done so when she was sick before.

There are no formulae to describe how a sudden versus prolonged onset or a self- versus other-induced injury generally will affect reactions to disability. Some researchers have found that people who were judged to bear some responsibility for the onset of their spinal cord injury seemed to achieve more positive psychological adjustment over time than did people who were innocent victims (Athelstan & Crewe, 1979). They hypothesized that it would be more difficult for someone whose life had been drastically changed through no fault of their own to maintain an internal locus of control—in other words, to believe that their own efforts would determine what they received from life. Other investigators have looked at the relationship between the individual's own attribution of self-blame or other-blame and the likelihood of depression. The findings have been very mixed, with some indication that early after the onset of disability attributions of self-blame may be positively correlated with coping (Bulman & Wortman, 1977). Others indicate that self-blame initially may be unrelated to adjustment, but after a period of time, it may correlate with greater depression (Reidy & Caplan, 1994). Inevitably, the matter of responsibility or blame for the onset of disability will be only one of many factors that help to shape a person's response. Keith, to cite an extreme example, had been previously diagnosed a "paranoid personality." Another person would not necessarily react as he did.

Functions Impaired

The body-mind system affected is the most central issue and almost too obvious to mention. In spite of the commonalities across all types of disablement, it is nonetheless clear that losing your eyesight, your hearing, or your ability to move is going to generate different reactions because each creates different problems. Impaired mental functioning or energy reserves create different problems still. This can be illustrated, in part, by what happened at a party at the first author's home when a fuse blew and all of the lights went out. Among the 200 guests were a number of people who use wheelchairs, are deaf, or are blind. The wheelchair users tried to dodge effectively when walking party-goers stumbled over their chairs and fell into their laps. The deaf guests definitely were not amused when their only means of communication was cut off. Those who were blind simply chuckled and asked, "So what's the problem?"

Typically, when nondisabled people are asked what disability they most dread, the majority respond, "Blindness." This reaction may be one reason why legislation for blind people in nearly all countries seems to be ahead of that for people with other disabilities. Even as adults, it seems, we are most afraid of the dark. People with motor-system impairments tend to respond as nondisabled people do; no matter how severely immobilized they might be, the concordance is that blindness would be worse. Blind and deaf people offer different opinions, however. Blind people, who have "been there," are much less apt to think that blindness is the worst disability that can happen. From a different perspective, deaf people often declare that blindness would be preferable to their disability and note ruefully that nondeaf people have little appreciation for the implications of being unable to hear. At the same time, many deaf individuals now proudly identify themselves as part of Deaf culture and reject the idea that deafness is a disability at all. They maintain that they have a communication difference, much as a person who speaks a different language would have within the culture.

Wright (1983) maintains that the "insider" (the person who has the disability) almost invariably sees his or her disability as less troublesome than outsiders presume it to be. Empathy is wonderful, but projecting ourselves into a position that we have never actually experienced, and making assumptions that lead us to incorrect conclusions, are not wonderful.

Beyond these general observations, most of the impact of the impaired function is tied to characteristics of the disabled individual. For example, an "auditory" person—one who learns better from lectures than from a text and loves music better than the visual arts—is likely to be far more devastated by the loss of hearing than a "visual" person with the opposite pattern. Also, the individual's unique combination of assets and disabilities will affect the impact of a given disability. Rajeev is a middle-aged man who became tetraplegic in an automobile crash approximately 20 years ago. What he considers to be his *real* disability, however, had its onset about five years ago. He was in the hospital, being treated for pneumonia and had an allergic reaction to penicillin. As a result he became deaf. In the years following his spinal cord injury he found much of the joy in daily life came from conversations with friends and from listening to music. Now, hearing loss has prevented those activities, and frustration has turned into depression. His life is now limited to home and personal care assistants.

An additional aspect worthy of mention here is the extent to which a disability interferes with physical attractiveness. It is well-known to psychologists and lay persons alike that physical beauty is a very functional attribute to possess. People attribute all sorts of positive traits, including high intelligence and friendliness, to physically attractive people (Berscheid & Walster, 1974). Sensitivity to its lack or loss sometimes can exceed the pain felt about the more obviously functional impediments disability creates. Aesthetic displeasure with oneself also may be compounded by the reactions of others when disfigurement or deformity is extreme.

Severity of Disability

It has become a truism among rehabilitation professionals that there is not a one-to-one relationship between severity of disability and the intensity of reaction (or quality of adjustment) to it. One person can assimilate total paralysis with fair equanimity, while another is devastated by the loss of a finger. They have their reasons, and some of them will be explored in a later section (see Determiners: The Person); however, varying degrees of severity do create different kinds of situations for disabled people to respond to, somewhat independently of personal dynamics. A young woman with one partially paralyzed leg will not experience the fear associated with the realization of total dependency on others for survival; and the totally paralyzed person will not experience the embarrassment of being swung impetuously onto a dance floor by a handsome stranger. Similarly, a mildly retarded person will not know what it is like to be so severely damaged that life is an incomprehensible blur, and the profoundly retarded person will (presumably) escape the pain that comes from awareness of unwelcome limitations to learning ability. One study (Huebner & Thomas, 1995) suggested that there may be a U-shaped relationship between adjustment and severity of disability, with individuals having the mildest or the most severe disabilities encountering the most difficulty. Perhaps either kind of situation is equally difficult in its own way.

Visibility of Disability

Closely related to the issue of severity is the visibility to others of the functional impairment. The young woman with the mild disability of a partially paralyzed leg was put in an embarrassing situation because her disability was not visible to her would-be dance partner. Jamal, too, illustrated the issue of visibility when he noted that women seem interested in him until he speaks or gets up to walk. Invisible disabilities can be very difficult, interpersonally, simply because you appear to be what you are not. Ken, a husky-looking, barrel-chested man, related that he is often asked to help when something heavy is being moved. However, his barrel chest is a result of emphysema and he must reply, "I'm sorry, I can't." He says he is tired of explaining because "They always act like they think I'm just lazy and making excuses anyway . . . they can't figure anyone who looks so strong could really be too weak to lift one end of a couch."

Stability of the Disability

Ken's condition exemplifies another aspect of the disability itself, one that influences reactions: the extent to which it changes over time. Emphysema is known to have a downward course leading to a hastened death. It also fluctuates, now better, now worse, as it moves along that path. The same is true for numerous other conditions affecting virtually every body system. This creates a very different situation from that experienced by the person with, say, a spinal cord injury, wherein the disablement occurs rapidly, improvements take place and reach a plateau, and then stability is reached.

Not all progressive disorders reduce longevity. For example, retinal detachment is a degenerative condition that has run its course when the individual becomes totally blind; no threat to life or other body systems is entailed. During the degenerative phase, the person merely has to wonder how long the residual vision will hold out. Multiple sclerosis, on the other hand, has more pervasive implications, including a less predictable and therefore potentially more unnerving end to anticipate. Reactions to such disabilities are shaped by these realities and by what the affected people tell themselves about their projected futures.

An important point in either case is that people with progressive disabilities are dealing with more than residual disablement; they confront an active disease process plus whatever residual disablement follows in its wake. Also a potent stimulus to reaction, cessation of symptoms and remissions sometimes occur, encouraging hope for containment or cure. When neither is forthcoming, a new round of disappointment, fear, anger, or other reactions may take place.

Pain

Arthritis is a progressive condition prototypic of the last nature-of-disability factor being considered here. A cardinal symptom is pain. Joint stiffness and deformity are surely undesirable, but pain tends to usurp consciousness, depending on its degree, whenever it is present. Progressive disorders are not the only ones to have associated pain; people with such stabilized conditions as spinal cord injuries and amputations have their share of pain as well. Whatever the stimulus, when pain occurs, it is certain to influence a person's feelings and behavior. It is hard to be jolly, creative, or maybe even civil, when you hurt but some can learn to do so. Chronic low back pain is another common disabling condition. As with arthritis, grinding daily pain can take its toll on energy and concentration. In addition, because the condition is typically invisible, people must deal with questions about whether the pain is "real" or "all in their head." Family members who are initially sympathetic may become discouraged or critical of the person who becomes uncongenial or unproductive, leading to a downward spiral in adjustment.

The extent to which pain is prepotent over other stimuli in capturing consciousness depends largely on the extent to which such learning has occurred. This reflects individual differences among people, which leads to the next topic for discussion.

Determiners: The Person

Emotional and behavioral reactions to disablement also depend importantly on characteristics of the people who become disabled. What remaining resources do they have for developing effective and gratifying lifestyles? For those whose disabilities occur adventitiously, what activities and behavior patterns are interrupted by disablement, and how central are these to their happiness? What kinds of temperaments do they have? What is the spiritual or philosophical base in their lives? What personality traits do they have that will influence the type and intensity of their reactions to disablement? Specific aspects of such determiners as these will be explored next.

Sex

Perhaps the most obvious personal variable affecting reaction to disablement is the individual's sex. It is important to stress at the outset that being male or female does not necessarily imply better or worse reactions, only different ones. Jamal pointed out a sex-related difference that he considered crucial: the expectation that a man will be the family breadwinner and that society is more accepting of a passive, dependent lifestyle for women than for men. He believes, therefore, that when disablement forces such a lifestyle upon someone, it is less disruptive of self-concept for women than men. This, he holds, is true even if the woman had not been a passive or dependent person before, simply because she will be punished less by society for assuming those traits after disablement.

Karen, a disabled feminist whose work centers around sexual counseling for disabled women, acknowledged (ruefully) that such a viewpoint has validity, but countered that the advantage is virtually destroyed by the far greater demand placed on women to be beautiful, physically perfect specimens in face and figure. She points out that, by definition, disabled women cannot hope to meet this social ideal.

In ways such as these the two sexes have somewhat different burdens to bear and their reactions will vary accordingly.

Activities Affected

The story about the executive secretary who lost both legs and went right back to doing her job, compared with the violinist who lost his little finger and was destroyed forever as a concert performer, may be the oldest cliché in the rehabilitation business. Clichés come about, however, because there is repeatable truth in them, and this hackneyed tale conveys an important fact. The impact of disablement is largely contingent on the extent to which it interferes with what you are doing.

Earl was operating a ranch when he began losing his eyesight. When Dana contracted polio, she was rehearsing for a modern-dance exhibition. Both valued and engaged in vigorous activities that no longer would be possible for them, and they reacted with grief. Dana mourned for many years the loss of her prime outlet for physical energy and creative expression. Olivia, on the other hand, was a stenographer whose hobbies were chess and gem-cutting before she lost both legs in an accident, and none of these activities was significantly affected. Although she assuredly reacted to her loss with considerable emotion, her ability to resume previously rewarding activities helped to mitigate a prolonged reaction of grief.

A rare but not unique occurrence is illustrated by Stephen. This seventeen-year-old had been a "behavior problem" throughout his school years, and much of his trouble was attributed to his father's disdain for his lack of athletic prowess. Following a spinal cord injury, Stephen seemed less troubled than before, as if he now had an acceptable reason for being unable to meet his father's expectations.

It is not only the actual, ongoing activities interrupted by disablement that influence a person's reactions. Activities never engaged in but held out as goals for the future may be equally powerful determinants.

Interests, Values, and Goals

An irony often pointed out is that people who sustain spinal cord injuries through adventurous, potentially dangerous activities are apt to be singularly intolerant of a sedentary life. If quiet pastimes turned them on, they wouldn't have chosen downhill skiing, surfing, auto racing, gang fighting, or armed robbery in the first place. It also is observed that people from cultures placing high value on physical or sexual prowess are more devastated by this disability than those whose traditions stress, say, scholarly pursuits. Whether one's goal is to climb the Matterhorn or break records set by Fanny Hill or Don

Juan, if it is quashed by disablement, the "loss" may be as painful as the forfeiture of extant activities. This applies not only to people with spinal cord injuries; similarly, interests, values, and goals can influence responses to the whole range of disabilities.

People with unifocal interests probably are going to react quite strongly to a disability that obliterates their expression, while people may adjust more easily if their interests range across several modalities: physical, intellectual, vigorous, rigorous, passive, active, and so forth. The chances are that the latter will have some interest areas that are spared. As the phenomenon of interest testing shows, however, people are not always aware of their interests, values, and potentially rewarding goals. Manifest interests at the time disablement occurs may reflect only a small part of the pattern of appreciations that could offer gratifying activity. The more varied this potential, the more protected is the individual from frustration and dejection over being disabled.

Dana, for example, had a variety of previously recognized intellectual interests to compensate her loss of dancing, at least in part. Others require a process of interest discovery to help them identify new directions and goals. Dana's value system, which already ranked scholasticism high, was ready to accommodate demanded changes; however, when an individual's values are invested almost totally in functions that are lost, the reactions to disablement and subsequent difficulties in learning to adjust are magnified accordingly.

Remaining Resources

The extent to which a person is devastated by the loss of function also is determined by what other resources for coping and enjoying are left. This can be illustrated by a conversation that took place between a disabled hospital patient and a similarly disabled staff member who had been held out by other staff as an example of what could be aspired to. After a very brief time together, the patient blurted, "Hell, if I had your brains and looks I wouldn't be depressed either!" In this instance, the staff member had had many more years to adjust to her disability; however, all else being equal, a quadriplegic with an IQ of 140 probably does have better prospects for the future than a quadriplegic with an IQ of 100. When capacities for physical activity are severely reduced, it helps to have the option of developing a "cerebral" kind of life. The staff member cited also had other resources that helped temper the intensity of her reactions; a naturally high level of energy, strong career motivations, a life history of emotional stability, numerous artistic talents, social poise, and considerable potential for leadership. All of these inner strengths can be used to build a secure and satisfying life. Recognizing the existence of such resources, and the alternatives they create, can do much to alleviate fears and other erosive emotions.

Some of the strengths just listed are employment resources, that is, capacities that can be developed to a level worthy of drawing a wage. Resources such as these will be considered in detail in Chapter 6. Others might be subsumed under a more general rubric of character resources, those qualities of personality or temperament that can influence reaction to disablement and subsequent adjustment in any realm of life.

Other Personality Variables

Interests, values, and most of the inner resources discussed previously are personality variables, and there are many additional ones that influence reaction to disablement. Depending on who defines the term and for what purpose, "personality" is imbued with a variety of meanings. Researchers define it operationally, writers define it literarily, and both groups do so idiosyncratically, to suit the purposes at hand. This book offers no exception. "Personality" is used here as an umbrella term, designating a constellation of interrelated constructs such as "personality traits" (factors), "behavioral patterns," "response tendencies," and "temperament." The use of the word "temperament" requires a little explaining, too, since it is not in high fashion today in either scientific or professional circles. We have a response tendency to use "temperament" whenever a connotation of biological determination exists. Emotionality and energy or activation level serve as examples.

Considerable research has been done to discover which personality traits are harbingers of good or poor adjustment to disability in the long run, but virtually none has examined their effect on more immediate emotional/behavioral reactivity. One problem is the need for preonset personality data in the study of such relationships, and it is seldom available. Nonetheless, these reactions are important because they set the climate in which adjustment efforts take place.

To give an illustrative sampling, such variables as flexibility, adaptability, maturity, and the polar opposites of these appear to influence reaction to change generally, and this includes changes imposed by disability. The relative strengths of an individual's needs also will influence reaction style. To cite a fairly obvious example, a person with high needs for succorance and little need to nurture others should experience less discomfiture over enforced dependency than a person with the opposite pattern. This does not imply an easier or more successful adjustment to disability; quite the opposite could be true if other factors failed to prevent the person from lapsing into passive acceptance of helplessness.

Countless other personality variables bearing prima facie relevance to style of reacting could be mentioned. A number of those measured by standard personality tests and research instruments will be discussed in Chapter 10 with respect to their impact on long-range adjustment. Here, we will consider just one last set of personality variables that seem to be particularly powerful determiners of disability-related reactions.

Spiritual and Philosophical Base

One's spiritual belief system and philosophy of life shape the meaning of disablement for each affected person; this, in turn, influences the ways in which one reacts. The person who views disablement as a punishment from God for past sins assuredly will feel differently about it than will a person who views it as a test or an opportunity for spiritual development. The person who sees it as a purely chance occurrence in a probabilistic universe will respond differently still. The "will to meaning" has been regarded as an important shaping force since Viktor Frankl wrote of his suffering in a Nazi concentration camp and the avenues through which he found salvation (Frankl, 1970).

A psychologist who contracted Guillain-Barre syndrome drew from Frankl's logotherapeutic concepts to describe her own experience, which she considered analogous to his world-famous ordeal. She writes:

> Seven months ago I was hospitalized with . . . Guillain-Barre syndrome. It was actually a great relief that was felt, rather than dismay at this diagnosis, just as the concentration camp victims felt relieved of their anticipatory anxiety when the hiding was over . . . I was told by a well-recognized neurologist . . . that mine was most certainly a case of hysteria . . . and that I needed many years of intense, in-depth psychoanalysis . . . I felt myself much too sophisticated to conjure up such an affliction . . . I knew my own system and knew that something was physically wrong . . .
>
> The paralysis [became] extensive . . . I was dependent on hospital staff for every need. A virtual prisoner in a metal-railed bed, lonely and isolated. Friends came initially as a matter of concern and, perhaps, curiosity. There were many at first, but the human condition prevailed. Like its counterpart in the animal world, the weakened member was left to its own demise while the fit continued with their own kind. (Hayman, 1975)

She points out that the categorical disease societies, such as the Multiple Sclerosis Foundation, adopt a posture not unlike that of Frankl's "medical ministry," facilitating acceptance of a permanently altered state by familiarizing people with their own attitudes and their freedom of choice. She quotes Frankl's statement, "Man is, and always remains, capable of resisting and braving even the worst conditions. To detach oneself from even the worst conditions is a uniquely human capability." She relates how she accomplished this in her own situation.

> I was detaching myself from the painfully lonely situation through humor, though at the time I called it hilarity! And, I must have succeeded in detaching myself from myself as well, since there was intense pain accompanying the destruction of the diseased nerves . . . Even though I was convinced that I would eventually walk, the uncertainty of how long it would take was a most depressing factor. Dr. Frankl refers to this phenomenon in terms of a "provisional existence of unknown limit," and charges it with being the most depressing influence of all . . .
>
> One day the tears of exasperation broke through in the presence of a very perceptive Sister . . . This wise lady sensed my need to look beyond myself at a critical moment of spiritual distress, or existential frustration, as the will to meaning in my life was most certainly being frustrated at this time. (Hayman, 1975)

Hayman takes care to separate spirituality from religiosity in her treatise, and this seems an important distinction. Acknowledging a spiritual aspect of life and having a life philosophy into which disablement can be meaningfully integrated appear rather consistently to ameliorate destructive reactions to disability. Specific religious beliefs may or may not prove helpful. For example, no cases are known to these authors wherein equating disability with divine punishment has aided an individual; the help has come when such a belief has been cast off. A belief that a disability is somehow part of God's purpose can be helpful, but belief in God is not requisite if the experience can be imbued with meaning or purpose in other terms. Diane, severely paralyzed and agnostic, illustrates this when she says:

> My disability has a purpose, but I don't consider it God's purpose; it is mine. My disability forced me to go to college and it's toughened up aspects of my personality that were a whole lot weaker than my legs and arms are now. No way do I like being paralyzed, but I do like a lot of the things that have come from it. Sometimes, when I start to get really mad at myself for being unable to do simple things, I think of that and simmer down.

A longitudinal study of people with spinal cord injuries found that most were able to identify both gains and losses that stemmed from their disability in the early years after onset and also two decades later. The most frequently cited gains involved personal growth, reflecting changes in values, priorities, and self-understanding. Other gains included new horizons and religious or spiritual insights (Crewe, 1996).

Determiners: The Environment

Reactions to disablement are determined not only by characteristics of the disabilities and the people who have them, but also by what is going on in the environment. Disability is neither an inherent characteristic of the person nor the environment, but is produced by their interaction. Both the immediate environment and the broader cultural context exert powerful influences on emotional and behavioral reactions to disability. Such immediate environmental variables as family acceptance and support, income, available community resources, and the presence or absence of loyal friends have a great deal to do with how a person feels about being disabled. Whether or not one is institutionalized and, if so, the characteristics of the institution are particularly potent determiners. For example, an almost totally paralyzed government administrator, the late Ed Roberts (1977) relates that "The affront, indignity, and impersonalness of mealtime situations in the hospital" had once triggered "a terrible rage that I could neither deal with myself, nor express for fear of reprisals. Mealtimes would leave me tired and defeated . . . I was deeply depressed and resolved repeatedly to die." He was 14 at the time. Fortunately he failed, and lived to be 59, heralded as "the father of independent living."

Whether or not your culture is characterized by a high degree of technology that could resolve (some of) your functional problems, sufficient funding of the programs you need and enforceable laws to protect your rights also will influence how you feel. It was the changing cultural context of which Hohmann spoke when he said that disability isn't as depressing now as it was thirty years ago (Hohmann, personal communication). Less tangible, but equally significant are the values and practices of the individual's cultural and ethnic group.

Since both types of environmental determinant will be explored in depth in the following chapter, they will only be mentioned here. This chapter will close with a poem chosen to highlight the fact that reaction to disability goes on as long as the person and the disability do. It doesn't stop at some point in time when the person has "adjusted," it simply changes with each step in the learning (adjustment) process. It was written by Dana after seventeen years of disability experience, on a lonely night after her second marriage had ended. She says that reading it the next morning was what prompted her to seek psychotherapy.

Requiem for Spring

One day, when she was thirty-three and had tasted some of the
    joys of life and several sorrows,
She pondered briefly, a matter of three days, and made a decision.
She would not destroy herself because she preferred to keep
    her weakness everyone else's assumption
And only her certain knowledge.

This decision firm, and, God knows, it had been twenty years
    in the making,
She looked up from the desk she had tidied while she thought
    and into the overgrowth of plantings that loomed above the
    windows, criss-crossing and falling.
Now, she said silently, what now?

It is not as if I had a choice, she reassured herself
    and quickly added that perhaps this was not true.
I still have a modicum of beauty and
    sufficient wit to appear intelligent.
No, Quasimodo loved only beautiful women and there is no choice
    and there is no hope.

Day before yesterday a great man died . . .
    today the flags are lowered . . .
    tomorrow workers get a day to mourn, rejoicing . . .
While I, relentlessly wishing, pitiable small thing,
    mourn the loss of passion. *

One day when she was sixteen and had tasted all of the joys
    of life and none of the sorrows,
She hesitated in her step and fell.
Sprawled across the dancing floors and propped against a
    fencepost in the corral,
Sitting woodenly watching elsewhere and elsewhere,
She smiled and nodded and convinced a number of people that
    pain was not pain.

At the age of eleven, it first occurred to her that
    death must be sweet.
Dark juvenile poems mark the way.
Miss Budd discouraged that sort of thing and so, two years later,
    did Miss Watson, who considered despair an inappropriate emotion,
Particularly during pubescence.

Liberated oceans drench me. Soon again they will rise from
 the sea and fall on me.
A tree sips from earth its anodyne while I, obsessed,
 protest my own apostasy.
Once a lover, now dispassionate, the dark affords no solace.
I have disavowed you darkness! is my cry.
No more the phantom comfort of the lonelier than I.

Ophelia, Ophelia, where have you been so long?
Off in the meadow, drinking wine,
Wandering, dreaming of an ancient song . . .
Sinking slowly into oblivion, having dreamed too long.

Dana's poem also points out an important caution; not everything labeled "reaction to disability" is precisely that. Dana reveals a dark side to her nature that predated her disability by at least five years. She says now that rehabilitation workers should not let their patients or clients "get by with making everything a disability issue," that she only began to unravel what was making her unhappy when she stopped blaming her disability for every unpleasant moment.

2

The World

People With Disabilities in a
Handicapping World

To be disabled is one thing. To be handicapped is quite another. Now that people with disabilities are coming out of the closet and proclaiming, "I am, therefore, I think," one of the things they think about is the effect of language on how they are perceived by others and how they perceive themselves. One camp abjures the term "disabled." They say it reminds them of a defunct automobile resting uselessly by the side of the road. Another camp abjures the word "handicapped." They say it reminds them of pitiful poster children looking up gratefully at benefactors dropping dimes into the can. Still another group signals thumbs down on both terms. "Inconvenienced" is their word. Others favor "impaired" or "physically challenged."

Sound familiar? Just when we had gotten it straight about "Black" and "Negro," along came people who insisted on "African." It's the same battle all over again; the reasons are the same and they are good ones. Words have the power to shape images of the referenced objects and their choice is important in building or breaking down stereotypes. A group is oppressed, hidden, stripped of power, and made to feel ashamed of the nature of its being. Then social conditions shift in a way that permits the lid of oppression to be lifted a bit. A few of the stronger members climb out and hold the lid aside so that more can follow. Before you know it, you have a "movement," and one of the first orders of business is negotiating acceptable language by which to identify the members when it becomes necessary.

The World Health Organization, which developed the International Code of Impairment, Disease, and Handicap (ICIDH) used these terms to convey distinctly different meanings. Impairment referred to conditions or diseases of the body or its organs. Disability referred to any functional limitations or restrictions in the ability to carry out activity resulting from an illness, injury, or birth defect. It is defined in terms of individual functioning and, assuming there is no longer an active disease process, is relatively unchanging for a given individual. Thus, it makes sense to speak of "a person with a disability."

Handicap refers to the interference experienced by a person with a disability in a restrictive environment. It is defined in terms of social consequences so it varies greatly, depending on what the person is trying to do and what opportunities the environment offers.

To illustrate, Carol is a person with a severe disability. About 70% of her muscles are paralyzed, and that is unchanging. But she is not always handicapped. Paralyzed muscles have little to do with thinking, talking, reading, writing, and listening, which are most of what she does in her work. On a dance floor, she is definitely handicapped. In the kitchen, her handicap varies from mild, when she makes a "whatever you've got, throw into the pot" stew—to severe, when she tries something that requires split-second timing, like a soufflé. Thus, while disabilities remain constant, handicaps appear and disappear, in varying degrees depending on what the person is trying to do.

Handicaps don't always come from disabilities. A big, burly college professor, whose worst disability is the farsightedness that often comes with middle age, commented one day that he is handicapped with respect to becoming a jockey. He mused, "That may seem a pretty trivial point, but what if I'd been born into a society where everyone else is jockey-sized and anyone who couldn't become one got put down?" People belonging to ethnic minorities are handicapped, not by disabilities, but by highly visible physical characteristics that are socially devalued. Observations such as these led to the title for the present chapter: People With Disabilities in a Handicapping World.

The new version of the World Health Organization system, the ICIDH-2, has maintained the general distinction between these concepts, but has moved to eliminate the labels applied to people, choosing instead to identify these categories: the body, activities, and participation.

The debate about terminology may never be fully resolved. In a syndicated newspaper column (Raspberry, 1989), Evan Kemp was quoted as observing that the terminology applied to any disadvantaged group will keep changing until the stigma applied to the group is removed and they become a truly equal part of society. In the meantime, there seems to be a general agreement within the disability community that "person first" language is most appropriate, so "a person with quadriplegia" is preferred to "a quadriplegic" and "a person with a disability" is preferred to "a disabled person." We regard these preferences as guidelines but not as rigid rules. Collective nouns such as "the disabled" or "epileptics" are also abjured because they obscure the people and imply that disability is their most important characteristic.

Much of the handicapping that people with disabilities experience is imposed by (1) the human-made parts of the physical environment, and (2) social customs, values, attitudes, and expectations. But not all of it is. Carol never will be able to climb a mountain and there is nothing anyone can do about that; however, it is unnecessary for her to be stymied by flights of stairs when ramps and elevators can serve the same purpose. Stairs are a part of the physical world, but their continuing existence in architectural design now that the problems they pose for a sizable segment of the population have been recognized is a function of social values and attitudes. It is these unnecessary handicapping effects of the human-made world that the activist branch of the applied psychology of disability is attempting to correct.

The world that disabled people must reckon with is composed, then, of two major aspects: physical objects and other people. The physical world is by far the less complicated. Conceptually, the topic of "other people" ranges from simple interactions between two human beings to the complex machinations of transnational organizations. Emotionally, it spans the cynicism of Jean Paul Sartre's "Hell is other people" and the beauty of John Donne's "No man is an island."

The remainder of this chapter will review environmental phenomena and events that interact directly or indirectly with people who have disabilities to determine their reactions and how little or how much they are handicapped in the various areas of life performance. To begin, consider the various external forces that impinge upon Sally, who has rheumatoid arthritis.

Getting Up and Off to Work. It takes Sally nearly two hours to get up, bathe, toilet, dress, groom, and eat breakfast each morning. It used to take her ten to fifteen minutes to button her blouse until she discovered a device that reduced it to three. There may be other assistive devices that she could profit from learning about.

Transportation. It was hard enough for her to find a job, but it turned out to be equally difficult to find a way to get there each morning. She can't drive, and although some accessible buses are available on main routes, she is unable to get to the bus stop during the snowy winters. Her community does have a dial-a-ride service, and this has been a great help. On the other hand, it does not allow for any spontaneous flexibility in her schedule; if she is delayed in the morning or needs to work late, she is in a bind.

The Workplace. Sally's building was made accessible when the company put in a ramp along a side entrance. It generally suffices, although on winter mornings she sometimes finds that the people who clear the parking lot have dumped a pile of snow at the foot of the ramp. She has asked for an electric door opener. The company has said they will consider it, but it is too expensive to install right now. The women's restroom on first floor has an accessible stall, but it is located at the other side of the building from her office. She was allowed to use the spacious restroom adjoining the executive's office, but she said she always felt so foolish going in there.

The Job Site. This was a miracle, which is why she put up with all the rest. Her counselor got a rehabilitation engineer to design a special desk for her so she could reach what she needed to operate independently. In the evening while waiting for her ride, she set everything up for the next day. Usually, someone stayed to help her.

More Transportation. A big day arrived. Sally was invited to attend an out-of-state meeting that could have an impact on her chances for promotion. She arranged for a ride to the airport, and made it through check-in uneventfully. The airline insisted on putting her wheelchair into the baggage compartment of the plane, however, and when she was reunited with it after the flight it had been damaged and required repair before it could be used.

Shopping. Sally has a friend who drives her and helps her with her shopping every Saturday. Imagine her surprise when she found a new barrier, designed to prevent the theft of shopping carts at the supermarket, which also kept her from entering. The barriers were removed after a few weeks. She is not sure whether this was because of the complaint she filed or because nondisabled shoppers objected to leaving their groceries unattended while they fetched their cars.

Recreation. Sally used to ice skate before her arthritis became too severe, and she loves the follies. She never used to go because of the accessibility problems. As soon as the auditorium announced their "renovations for the disabled," she got a group of friends interested in going with her. They sat together in the regular seating area. She sat alone in the area reserved for people who use wheelchairs.

Housing. She finally got an opportunity for advancement with another firm, which required her to move. She went into debt the first three months, paying an attendant to help her move until she could locate an accessible apartment in which she could live independently. She applied to a number of complexes that had advertised as having apartments available, but when she arrived she was told they had already been rented. She doubted that it was sheer coincidence that she arrived just "hours too late" on so many occasions.

These experiences could be depressing to even read about unless note is taken that such frustrating Catch 22s are signs of progress. A few years earlier, she might not have bothered to leave the house at all because she'd have known there would be little to expect. Enough progress has been made to make it realistic to try, and the Catch 22s are transitional phenomena that probably will disappear in time.

Sally was confronted by a series of barriers to living independently, working, and enjoying leisure time. Some of the barriers were physical, such as the stairs and inaccessible restrooms. Others were attitudinal, such as the airline policy that assumed disabled travelers don't know their own needs. Happily, her experiences included helps as well as hindrances: employers who were willing to hire her, friends who cared and would offer assistance, even the auditorium that accommodated her physical, if not her social, needs.

At the other end of the spectrum is the example of Juanita, who had worked for 20 years as an office manager for a physician who became her greatest friend and supporter. Two days before she died, Juanita, 56, put in a full day at the office. In recent years, when she was no longer able to sit in a chair, she worked from a special bed that had been installed in the office. She used a number of assistive devices to run the office efficiently. The doctor even provided a van that was specially adapted to transport Juanita and her equipment.

How people react and adjust to disability is partly determined by the mix of helps and hindrances they encounter in their lives. As pointed out in the previous chapter, environmental determiners of reaction to disability can be divided into two major types: those that are palpably present in the person's immediate environment and those that are interwoven more subtly into the larger cultural context. The former may vary sharply from one individual to another; the latter tend to be uniform for all individuals in a given time, culture, or subculture. In this chapter, environmental influences have been divided in still another way: those relating to the physical world and those relating to other people.

These distinctions are useful for comprehending the totality of interacting external influences that shape behavior; but, true to life, they do not remain in neat categories when in operation. The physical stairs cannot be separated from the architect who designed them, and the architect cannot be separated from years upon years of tradition in design.

With this disclaimer regarding the precision of categorization in mind, the ensuing pages will discuss first the environmental influences seen mainly as cultural determiners and therefore as exerting similar influence on all people with disabilities in a given time and place. Second, we will explore influences that are tied to individuals' personal situations and therefore reflect marked variations from one person to another.

The Societal Context

It may go without saying that the cultural context referred to in this volume is the United States of America at the beginning of the twenty-first century.

A few cross-cultural comparisons will be drawn, but, unless otherwise specified, the previous assumption can be made. The fact is, some of the most powerful influences on reactions and adjustment to disability may be pancultural, suggesting that they are, *au fond*, rooted in human nature. A large portion of the introductory chapter was devoted to what is considered the most potent negative influence of all: devaluation. There it was admitted that the genesis of devaluation, whether biological or culturally learned, is unknown. Being unable to discern which determiners are immutable aspects of human nature and which are potentially alterable products of human culture, all are arbitrarily assigned here to the "societal context."

A few isolated instances in which disabilities (or disabled individuals) have been revered rather than devalued can be cited. The best known example is epilepsy, regarded in earlier times as "the sacred disease." This elevated status was probably a result of the fact that epilepsy was very common among the ruling classes, and these rulers had little tolerance for being the brunt of devaluative statements. In addition, a few individuals scattered throughout history have been regarded as almost holy for reasons directly related to their disabilities. A current example is an artist from Japan who has mental retardation; his works are revered not only because of their superb quality but also because of the childlike innocent who produces them.

Exceptions aside, the rule is devaluation, and its form and degree are heavily influenced by the surrounding culture. Devaluation can be blatant or it can be subtle. The Nazis, to give a clear example of blatancy, killed disabled people. Other societies, for the greatest part, have been so subtle that their devaluative practices went unrecognized as such for generations, until the new breed of activists started pointing them out. In the United States, during the 19th and 20th centuries, laws provided for the involuntary sterilization of individuals with cognitive disabilities (Pfeiffer, 1999). Some people, including those with epilepsy, were prevented from marrying, and children were sometimes taken from parents with disabilities. The creation of separate, segregated educational and work systems provide prime examples in both the Eastern and Western hemispheres.

Devaluation may be tough, or it may be tender. Treating disabled people as pariahs and forcing them to sit outside the city gates to beg was a very tough stance to take. This attitude followed from a belief that "the afflicted" were sinners in the eyes of God and deserved to be punished. A more tender approach is to consider people with disabilities as unfortunates, not outcasts, and worthy of pity rather than contempt. Blatant or subtle, tough or tender, devaluation is devaluation and this is well understood by the objects of either attitude. Such awareness is illustrated by the comments of a woman with a severe disability who had just been introduced as a keynote speaker. Invited to speak because she has clearly made a success of her life, she acknowledged her introduction by saying, "I guess I will never stop being surprised to hear myself referred to as 'someone less fortunate than the rest of us.' "

Not only the form but the degree of devaluation is shaped by the prevailing philosophy of the culture. A dominant element of the Nazi philosophy was the principle of Aryan superiority, which leaves no room for damaged specimens, especially among Aryans. On the other hand, the principle of reincarnation, which is embraced by many cultures, allows for no misfortunes. An important element of the latter is that one chooses one's body, one's parents, one's total life situation for the purpose of "working out karma." Thus, one *chooses* to live in a disabled condition for reasons related to spiritual development; one is not the victim of a regrettable accident. A rehabilitation administrator who has come to embrace the principle of reincarnation commented one day that, as one result, when she meets a person who is mentally retarded she no longer feels the pangs of pity she once did. She doesn't think of herself as more fortunate than (and therefore superior to) an unfortunate (and therefore inferior) person. She relates as a peer, a colleague spirit, and finds herself asking, albeit quietly to herself, "Ho there . . . what are you working out this time? I wonder if you are at a higher level of development than I for having come to such a test."

Attitudinal Barriers

This widely used term says, in essence, that disabled people tend to be rejected by other people. The most forceful rejectors used to be other disabled people who didn't want to "identify," but the movement has changed that. Perhaps the commonest attitudinal barrier is the tendency to overgeneralize about what "they" are like, whether "they" can be helped, whether "they" can communicate directly with salesclerks or need nondisabled intermediaries, whether damaged bodies can coexist with undamaged minds and the reverse. Only rarely are attitudinal barriers manifested openly and directly, such as in expressions of distaste or avoidance of eye contact, conversation, touching, or even proximity. They are more apt to be manifested indirectly, in the form of exclusionary practices deemed "necessary" for the safety or convenience of people in general. The term "attitudinal barriers" combines, in a sense, the effects of devaluative attitudes and discriminatory behavior.

In order to understand why attitudinal barriers exist, it is necessary to consider what qualities are venerated by a culture and are found lacking in certain groups. Some of the issues selected for review appear to be specific to our culture; others are so pervasive across geography and history as to suggest that they emanate from human nature itself.

Overvaluation of Rational Intellect. Since the seventeenth-century beginnings of the age of reason, Western society has placed an increasingly high premium on the particular type of intellect referred to as logicodeductive, sequential, rational, or linear-thinking. Another type, which earlier in history was greatly prized, concomitantly came to be ignored or even derogated. "Women's intuition" was for long nearly the only reference made to the inductive, simultaneous, intuitive, or nonlinear thinking mode that was once considered *the* path to truth. It seemingly did not serve well in the growing physical sciences (and their mathematization) and, over the course of three centuries, was declared illegitimate and practically forgotten.

Partly as a function of societal dismay over where science and technology have led, and partly as a function of their very progress in the field of brain research, intuition is in the process of being relegitimized. Some researcher-theorists believe the two types of intellect can be assigned to the left (linear reasoning) and right (nonlinear thinking) hemispheres of the brain. As a direct result, intuition is gaining scientific respectability. As an indirect result, we are beginning to recognize that certain people, those intuitive souls who are lacking in logicodeductive reasoning ability, have been unnecessarily handicapped with respect to mental functioning simply because their kind of gift was disdained.

People labeled "mentally retarded" are sometimes gifted in terms of nonlinear, instantaneous data processing ability, and Mike appears to be one such person. His ability to penetrate immediately the obfuscations that generate and escalate misunderstandings between people is the talent that allows him to mediate others' arguments effectively. He does not reason through the haze in stepwise fashion; he appears to intuit at once what has gone wrong. His gift has become recognized in the light of recent attention to this other type of intellect, but it is important to note that it is rewarded only as an interesting oddity. This society as yet offers only the rarest opportunities for acknowledgment equivalent to that given sequential reasoning; specifically, there are few jobs that explicitly draw on such talents and pay living wages to individuals so gifted.

Overvaluation of Physique. Physical beauty and prowess are not only very highly prized in society, most cultures also set stereotyped, narrow bands of standards as to what "makes the grade." Here, today, men should be tall, tanned, and muscular, with copious character in their rugged faces. Women should have gigantic breasts but no fat anywhere else and a minimum of character lines to mar delicate, regular, facial features. Ideally, both should appear youthful regardless of their chronological age, but for women it is a must. Athletic prowess is a must for men and highly desirable for women, if not taken to extremes. Women have more latitude here; if she can't play a decent game of tennis, a woman is okay if she can dance or has the look of a "hard body." Such values are so deeply inculcated that merely to associate a product with youthful movement and beauty is to elevate its sales. We all want "the image" for ourselves. Most of us feel, in varying degrees, that we must at least approach it in order to be happy. But some of us don't. As Kathy pointed out, people with disabilities are almost automatically disqualified.

The counterculture of the sixties was a helpful ally in combatting this barrier in that it rejected the traditional standards and attempted to widen the range of acceptable physical attributes by (social) force. But according to well-publicized recent research, there is still a strong correlation between physical attractiveness and such hard-to-define but universally desired conditions as success, happiness, and life satisfaction. It doesn't help to label it shallow, irrelevant, inhumane, and undemocratic. It is a force to be reckoned with, and some ways for doing that will be discussed in Chapter 11.

Undervaluation of Spirituality. Just as modern society appears to have overstressed the importance of rational intellect and physique, at the same time it has reduced emphasis on matters of spirituality. These are natural outgrowths of the age of reason, with its advancing science, technology, and preeminent materialism. Descartes gave us the concept of mind-body duality in the seventeenth century, and we have been using and misusing it ever since. Somewhere along the line, the spiritual aspect of our being was mislaid. Like intuition, it is in the process of being rediscovered, and for essentially the same reasons. Again, a segment of the counterculture contributed substantially to initiating the shift.

People with disabilities are handicapped differently by a materialistic society than by a spiritually oriented one. A society which combined the technological advantages of the West with the spiritual values of the East might not handicap its disabled members so much. When you conceive of yourself as nothing more than mind and body, and one or both of those has been damaged irreparably, it doesn't leave you very much that is stable and intact. The balance changes, however, when credence is given to the spirit, which seems to be impervious to the onslaughts of disablement.

The degree to which a culture is materialistically oriented influences societal reactions to individuals with disabilities in a number of practical ways. Along with technological advancement, the levels of industrialization and affluence rise, yielding many benefits. Concomitantly, the ethic encapsulated by the phrase, "I am my brother's keeper" diminishes, to be replaced by a welfare system. When responsibilities formerly carried by the family and the church are shifted to the state, a businesslike atmosphere, rather than a loving climate, is created for recipients of care. This has both *good news* and *bad news* aspects. These and other cultural influences relating to style and level of social and technological development will be examined next.

Blaming the Victim. It is very difficult for humans to acknowledge how utterly capricious fate can be. Such an admission carries with it a disturbing awareness that we are not always in control of our own destinies. "If the fickle finger could point at them, it could someday point at me." To protect ourselves from the sense of impending vulnerability, we work things around in our minds to make misfortune the victim's own fault. "He must have brought it on himself. I'm not bringing anything like that on myself; therefore, I needn't worry, it won't happen to me."

A very popular form of blaming the victim is the attribution of masochism to people who are victimized by serial misfortune. We don't like to believe that fate could really be so unfair. We search for other explanations and find one that is sanctified by modern psychology: the urge toward self-destruction. However unexplainable that might be, it is preferable to giving up what Jules Masserman (1955) has called an essential, human delusion of invulnerability.

Like devaluation, the method of blaming the victim is sometimes blatant, sometimes subtle, sometimes tough, and sometimes tender. "I'm not surprised, she's always been accident prone!" "Arthritis occurs with people who are filled up with pent-up hostility." "He deserves it for trying to rob that store in the first place!" "Poor thing, if she'd just been able to think a little faster, the accident could have been avoided."

Unfortunately, after thus reassuring ourselves, we start looking askance at the "unfortunates." Nowhere is this seen so clearly as with disabled people who develop one complication after another or additional, unrelated disorders. Family, friends, and rehabilitation workers alike find themselves saying, "It can't just be happening; she (or he) must be doing something to cause all of this." Whether he or she is or isn't, fate is thereby dealing one more blow for him or her to react to.

Insistence on Mourning. We humans also have a tendency to assume that anyone who has lost something that we hold dear must be mourning its loss, be it physical prowess, money, power, or anything else. Allowing for the possibility of easy relinquishment seems to suggest that what we possess is unimportant. *Au fond,* it may be less what we possess than what we strive for that stimulates this insistence on mourning. When we dedicate our energies and consciousness to amassing wealth or building the body beautiful or gaining influence and power, we may not want to hear that someone else has discovered—in one way or another—that goals of these sort are not, after all, essential to happiness. What is the meaning of our struggles, then? To preserve the meaning we have ascribed to our own lives and efforts, we thus make the assumption of "sensible mourning." It is viewed as only sensible that a person would mourn, perhaps unremittingly, the loss of an essential ingredient of a satisfactory life.

This simply isn't always a valid assumption. Earl, for example, found that he mourned the loss of his disability, a process no one else could understand, more than he had mourned the loss of his vision. Stephen's disability also brought a compensatory trade-off in relieving him of the pain of failing in his father's eyes. That mitigated his mourning substantially. Even Dana, who mourned more expectably for a number of years, eventually surpassed mere reconciliation in an avowed embracement of all of her life experiences, including disability. Diehards may insist that this is "sweet lemon rationalization," but it does not seem sensible to believe that someone who has not experienced disability knows more about how it feels than someone who has.

Technological Level

In recent years, the United States Government has made a concerted effort to take mainland rehabilitation know-how to the islands in the Pacific. As a result, a number of rehabilitation experts have experienced directly the dramatic impact of cultural development on the lives of people with disabilities. Taking a spinal cord injury as an example, in Micronesia the concerns include getting the person into a canoe to reach a ship that can take him or her to a hospital in Hawaii, preventing pressure sores when he or she sleeps on a grass mat on a dirt floor, and finding a wheelchair that can withstand more than six months of the high humidity and rough terrain. One expert also observed that mainland values do not mesh well with life in Micronesia. She commented:

> The only real work there is gathering copra, which physically disabled people obviously can't do. But in order to be eligible for vocational rehabilitation funds to get the needed medical care, they are "punished" by being forced to go to work doing something . . . something that has no meaning in their frames of reference.

To those of us imbued with modern technological and materialistic standards, it would seem clearly preferable to be disabled in a culture with the technological means to circumvent many of the functional problems disability generates. Having grown used to the convenience and independence offered by motorized wheelchairs, powered lifts, electronic magnifiers, talking calculators, and portable computers, it would be hard to go back to a lifestyle bereft of these spin-offs from the aerospace industry. A story about motorized wheelchairs provides a striking example of how the application of technology can influence not only the ways individuals feel about having disabilities, but their efforts to adjust and build satisfying lives as well.

Years ago a number of rehabilitation hospitals had policies discouraging the use of motorized wheelchairs. It was reasoned that people with weak upper extremities would profit from the exercise of wheeling manual chairs. Lost in this trend were those with so much upper-extremity weakness that they could not propel manual chairs at all. Rather suddenly, a change in philosophy came about, and the "personality changes" observed in many affected individuals were remarkable. Several years later, Bob related how his new wheelchair affected him.

> I got polio when I was too young to remember. As long as I have known me, I've been almost totally paralyzed. I'd spent all my life at [hospital] until a couple of years ago. They didn't know what else to do with me. I went all the way through high school there, and everyone used to tell me, "You're so bright, you should go on to college," but I just couldn't imagine it. After I finished school, I just sat in the hallway all day and talked with whoever came by.
>
> When they first asked me if I'd like to have an electric wheelchair, I said, "No." It seemed freaky, somehow, and I was afraid I might lose control of it. But they kept after me and boy, what a change in my life! All of a sudden, for the first time, I could go wherever I wanted to whenever I wanted to . . . I didn't have to wait for a "gray lady" or escort service to push me. I went all over the hospital, down the street to where some shops were, and I finally enrolled in college. Somehow, being able to move around on my own, I could imagine doing it. I've done really well in school and just moved out into my own apartment.

It also turned out that the no-motorized-wheelchairs policy had been a disservice to people who could wheel their chairs, but with enormous energy expenditure. The hospital staff member cited earlier went through the same philosophical transition and relates that, after adopting the use of a motorized chair, she greatly increased her artistic and domestic activities because she at last had the energy to pursue them. A policy designed to maximize independence had proved to have the opposite effect.

The shadows of the anti-motorized-wheelchair bias still crop up in the attitudes of some individuals with spinal cord injuries who have developed carpal tunnel syndrome and shoulder pain after years of making their upper extremities function in place of their legs. Many still resist the shift to power equipment, however, because they fear that it will make them appear to be "more disabled."

Even more centrally influential on the quality of life for disabled people is the degree of industrialization and affluence that technological development permits. For example, new kinds of jobs are created, as technology advances, that do not require workers to move or manipulate physical objects—"thing jobs," in the terminology of *The Dictionary of Occupational Titles* (U.S. Department of Labor, 1991). "People (service) jobs" and "data jobs" come into being, jobs that workers unable to use their bodies as primary work resources are able to do. Moreover, an affluent culture can better afford to absorb the costs engendered by people with disabilities, restoring their functioning or supporting their additional needs when restoration is not possible.

Another benefit stemming from the proliferation of technology is that accommodations are now available that bring many vocational choices into the realm of possibility that otherwise might not have seemed feasible. For example, prior to the availability of personal computers, optical scanners, and the like, a blind person would have been ruled out of a job like accounting that required constant handling of papers and data.

On the problematical side, as the tempo of technological development increases, the rate at which jobs obsolesce is stepped up accordingly. This creates retraining needs among workers with or without disabilities, but narrowed options make such transitions more difficult for the latter.

Socioeconomic and Political Style

Relatively independent of their level of technological development, societies may diverge or change over time, in political philosophy and in socioeconomic style. The extent to which a society chooses to direct some of its resources toward the betterment of life for individuals with disabilities by creating/ enriching a welfare system, passing protective legislation, and channeling monies into service programs has a powerful impact on what it means to experience disability.

As an example, only a little over two decades ago, United States citizens so severely disabled as to require the help of a personal care assistant had only two options: to be cared for by family or friends, or to live in a maintenance-care institution. The alternative of being provided with funds to live as an independent adult did not exist. Today, independent living has become the norm as a result of legislation creating a system that takes account of both human and monetary needs. (Some of the ways in which this same system breaks down, from the functional and psychological viewpoints, will be examined in Chapter 3.)

All of these cultural influences on reaction and adjustment to disablement are relatively uniform for people who experience disability within the same society during a particular period of time. The following section will take these as givens and explore other environmental determiners that are more variable from one individual's situation to another's.

Cultural Influences

The preceding discussion addresses issues that apply, in general, to contemporary American society. At the same time, awareness has grown that this is a multicultural society, composed of varied racial and ethnic groups with diverse perspectives on life and disability. Recognition should also be given, then, to ethnic and cultural influences that are narrower than national characteristics and broader than a person's immediate environment. Swartz-Kulstad and Martin (1999) have likened society to a stew, in which people retain their distinct cultural heritage and are also flavored by the environment around them. Cultural forces help to shape an individual's values, interests, aspirations, communication patterns, and behaviors. They guide an individual in understanding the meaning of events, including the onset of disability, and help to prescribe how the individual and family should respond.

For the most part, the American rehabilitation system grew out of the paradigm of the dominant Euro-American culture, reflecting the values of individualism, independence, and the importance of gainful employment. In medical rehabilitation, great emphasis is placed upon functional independence in activities of daily living, and families are discouraged from doing things for a person that he or she might learn to do alone. For some cultural groups, standing by and watching a father or mother struggle to dress or eat without help is tantamount to extreme disrespect. Within the vocational rehabilitation arena, cultural differences may be reflected in such things as orientation to time and willingness to move from one's traditional residence in order to obtain training or work. Such conflicts could certainly impair the effectiveness of the rehabilitation system's work with an individual, thereby influencing his or her response to disability.

Swartz-Kulstad and Martin (1999) searched and analyzed more than 400 publications related to culture. Their qualitative analysis revealed five primary domains of culture and context, each with a number of subcategories. The findings suggest the many ways that culture affects individual perspectives. The first domain, ethnocultural orientation, reflects the extent to which one is involved in the culture of origin and in the dominant culture. Other elements in this domain include beliefs, values, norms, coping style, cognitive style, and traditions or ceremonies of the cultural group. Family environment, the second domain, involves both family relations and structure. The third domain, community environment, encompasses the community structure and support networks as well as norms and migration. The last two domains are communication style and language. Language facilitates the exchange of information between people, partly through the use of mutually understood words and partly through all of the nonverbal expression that occurs between them. Clearly, the potential for miscommunication is rife between a culturally naïve counselor and an individual from a different background.

Early efforts to remove the cultural blindfolds from rehabilitation practitioners often took a cookbook approach. Papers described the "typical" beliefs and behaviors of African Americans, Native Americans, Asian Americans, Latinos, and other groups. Perhaps it is useful to know that individuals of Asian heritage may be reluctant to describe their problems to strangers and may rely strongly on guidance from family elders. At the same time, such generalizations overlook great differences that may exist within any given ethnic group and perpetuate inaccurate stereotypes. An obvious problem involves lumping such diverse and huge cultures as Chinese, Korean, Japanese, Indian, Indonesian, Samoan, etc., into the category, "Asian." Even within one of these groups, significant disparities may reflect differences in socioeconomic status, degree of acculturation, and many other factors.

So how is it possible to acknowledge the influence that culture may have upon response to disability without falling into such traps? Some writers (Marshall, Johnson, & Johnson, 1996) have advocated developing a *transcultural* world view, one that welcomes and appreciates different perspectives as equally valuable, and that is open to varied solutions to issues. Rather than seeing the world in terms of dichotomies or fixed categories, counselors need to accept the existence of multiple realities and strive to understand the perspective that each individual brings. Coming back to our discussion of factors that affect an individual's response to disability, perhaps the most appropriate comment is that heritage plays a significant role in creating the filters through which a person views life experiences and that heritage must be explored if the individual is to be understood.

The Immediate Environment

A counselor specializing in the problems of people with very severe physical disabilities summed up his years of experience by expressing the opinion that:

The main problem with being disabled is being poor. If you were rich enough, you could buy all the fancy gadgets available to do what they can, and whatever was left, you could pay other people to do. I don't think being disabled would be so bad if I had a valet, a chauffeur, a personal secretary, a big, accessible home, a van with everything, and no worries about grubbing for a job.

This counselor has not experienced disability, and some of those who have may feel he is missing some important points, but he also is making one: how rich or how poor you are has considerable impact on how miserable disability can make you. Moreover, one of the problems with disability is that it tends to make or keep you poor. Available income may not be *the* problem associated with disability, but it is surely an important determiner of reactions and adjustment to it.

Family Influences

Income is but one aspect of the familial milieu surrounding a person with a disability. Other relevant variables relating to family structure and dynamics include the family's social standing and powerbase in the community, parental acceptance, spousal loyalty, and the proffering of practical and/or moral support. Having a family member who is skillful and assertive in mastering crisis, a name that is recognized by local agency personnel, or a relative who plays golf with the major employers in the community can alter materially the negative ramifications of most any disability. The effects of these and many other aspects of family capability and interaction will be examined in detail in Chapter 4.

The Influence of the Community

Just as one's position within the community makes a difference in the consequences of a disability, numerous aspects of the community itself influence the disability experience. Perhaps most basic are the community's size and location. A small town may offer a quality of human support that is lost in the big city, yet lack the sophisticated paraphernalia and services the latter provides. The differing demands made upon rehabilitation systems by rural and urban communities are felt most keenly by those in rural areas, since most service models are designed in and for the denser population centers with their relative wealth of medical, educational, psychosocial/vocational, and other resources.

The extent to which a given community has responded to protective legislation by eliminating mobility barriers, providing full inclusion for disabled youngsters in the public schools, and other such actions, also will have significant impact. So will the existence of voluntary service organizations and the service orientation of local churches. Does the transit authority have buses with lifts or at least a demand-response option for those unable to board standard buses? Does the responsible department of local government energetically enforce existing protective legislation? Is there someone with a significant disability among the ranks of elected officials? How far away is the nearest active center for independent living? The answers to all of these questions portend much concerning the quality of life for individuals with disabilities in a given community. These are the problem areas being attacked by the activists determined to alter the stimulus conditions "out there," all of which they view as stemming fundamentally from the attitudes and actions of "other people."

Institutionalization

Most people with disabilities have occasion to experience that unique kind of community known as "an institution." This may be limited to hospital stay during the acute treatment; or it may include additional time in a hospital for rehabilitation. For some, an institution becomes home for a major period of their lives.

However utopian an institutional setting might be, the inhabitants are not there by choice. Ordinarily, institutionalization is grudgingly accepted as an unavoidable necessity for accomplishing some other goal, such as rehabilitation. In point of fact, few, if any, institutions are utopian; by their very nature they tend to restrict the degree of freedom and violate the privacy of the people who dwell in them. Depending on specific institutional policies, procedures, and personnel, these effects may be minimized or magnified.

Erving Goffman (1961), in his well-known work *Asylums*, describes what he calls the "mortification process" wherein institutional residents are deprived not only of their privacy but of their power over themselves, usually for the convenience and efficiency of those running the institution. Rules that would be considered intolerable if imposed on noninstitutionalized citizens are enforced and accepted. That they are behaviorally accepted does not indicate an absence of psychologically damaging consequences. Yielding self-mastery, even for a time, may have long-lasting, negative effects. Staff in rehabilitation hospitals have become alerted to the irony that the patients most willing to cooperate with medical usurpation of crucial decision making about their lives during institutionalization may be the least well prepared to resume effective, assertive self-mastery when they return to the ordinary world.

Psychologically speaking, it may be the irony of all ironies that, in hospitals, the staff member most important to the patient is the one considered least important, if prestige, remuneration, and care in selection are any indicators. A long-term follow-up study (Kemp & Vash, 1971) reported that the vast majority of a sample of fifty spinal-cord injured individuals interviewed five to ten years after hospitalization, when asked to recall their "brightest memories associated with being in hospital," responded with recollections concerning particularly caring members of the nursing assistant staff. Obversely, their "grimmest recollections," in the main, concerned assistants who were cruel or demeaning. The more prestigious and highly paid staff were not once mentioned. It is the assistants who carry out the most intimate ministrations; it is they who are there at the end of the day when memories and doubts flood consciousness, and on the weekends when no visitors have appeared. Yet in many settings, these employees are still selected and paid in the same way as the housekeeping staff who take care of the physical plant.

Roberts' observations on the indignities to which he was subjected during mealtimes in an institution (see Chapter 1) suggest that some of the caregivers he experienced might have been better suited to building maintenance tasks. Using feeding as a potent example of the emotionally loaded interactions between attendants and patients, it is important to note that not all of the error results from uncaring or hostility-laden practices. Baby talk accompanying the feeding of an adult patient can have equally destructive effects. (Whether infantilization of this sort is also a form of hostility belongs to another book.)

Agencies

Contact with institutions doesn't end when one is no longer a resident of one. After returning to the community, people with disabilities often continue to interact with other types of "bureaucracies" or "agencies." These provide vitally important services and are appreciated for that reason, but the mortification process goes on. In order to receive the benefits allowing survival outside of a residential institution, disabled people still must tell all, hand over the reins, and oftentimes swallow much, possibly for a very long time. The widely publicized suicide of Lynn Thompson in 1978 galvanized the disabled community into a coalition determined to alter the laws and agency procedures that resulted in her conclusion that death would be preferable to the life she foresaw upon being forced to return to a residential institution. Chapter 3 will treat these and related subjects in more detail, and Part II will take the further step of exploring ways in which problems cited can be minimized.

Regional Differences

Just as legislative thrusts and government funding trends affect disabled people in relatively uniform ways, so may similar phenomena influence subgroups of people, as defined by their localities or in various other ways. Marked regional differences have been noted in the nature and effectiveness of national programs from one state or locality to another, but disabled people seldom have the choice to live where the services are best. One effort may be reflected in the tendency for motor-disabled people to migrate to California. This is not solely a result of more extensive health-related services, however; the Mediterranean climate and relatively accessible architectural style offer sufficient lure. The happenstances of geography, climate, and building style can have a significant impact on how one reacts to a disability. For example, having to cope with snow when you're blind or use crutches can take its toll on your safety, your independence, and your sense of humor.

As always, it is not just the physical facts that create or eliminate problems, but also how people respond to them. In the western states, for example, if your home doesn't "work" for you after you begin using a wheelchair, the chances are you simply will move into one that does. This is not so in New England and other parts of the eastern seaboard. The tradition of the family home is far more sacrosanct there than in the West, and a home that has served a family for several generations will not be relinquished lightly, however difficult it may be to get a wheelchair in and out, or up and down the stairs.

Exotica

One influence that affected a particular subgroup of disabled people positively for a number of years is worthy of mention because of its implications for future reform vis-à-vis environmental influences in adjusting to disability. This was the operating style of the National Foundation for Infantile Paralysis. The families of children (or adults) who contracted poliomyelitis were given the financial help they needed to deal with catastrophic illness, but they were not subjected to the mortification process that accompanies such government-administered aid as Supplemental Security Income. The program was "abused" in a way that consternated almost no one: because only polio patients were eligible, some physicians are thought to have intentionally misdiagnosed cases of Guillain-Barre or infectious neuronitis, which have very similar symptoms. It saddened rehabilitation workers to see patients with still other disabilities have nowhere to go for comparable help. Today, the generations of "polio kids" who are now adults can appreciate the Foundation that helped without imposing elaborate screening/monitoring systems that shatter the peace of mind financial aid should bring, by destroying dignity and privacy during a time of extreme emotional vulnerability.

3

Surviving

Living Independently

The previous two chapters have described and placed the disabled person in the context of a world composed of the physical environment and other people. This chapter will begin the process of examining what happens when that person tries to partake of the American ideal in a world wherein survival (life) and independence (liberty) are prerequisite to the pursuit of happiness. As shown in Chapter 2, that pursuit is seriously impeded for some, and life and liberty may be in continual jeopardy. What does this do to an individual, psychologically speaking? Before exploring answers to this question, let us examine several ways in which "survival" and "independence" are interpreted.

The dictionary defines "survive" as meaning "to remain alive or in existence, as after an event or the death of another." This definition clearly implies biological survival; however, in conversational practice, the word is used to mean much more. Survival of the ego is implied sometimes, or survival of a preferred lifestyle, economic base, normalcy, or feelings of well-being. Such is the essence of the commonly made distinction between "merely existing" as opposed to "really living." The word "survival" will be imbued with this broader meaning here. The fact is, biological survival issues are the rarest kind encountered as one moves past the acute stage of an illness or injury—usually a brief period—and on to the years and decades of living with a disability in the community.

"Independence" is a controversial term. "There's no such thing; we are all interdependent" is a familiar objection to the concept. Again turning to the dictionary, we find "independence" to mean "freedom from the influence, control, or determination of another or others." This is not a difficult definition to accept; what is often rejected is an added connotation of "ability to survive alone, without the aid of others or respect to their actions." Activists in the disability rights movement are endorsing the limits of the dictionary definition when they explain that independence, to them, does not imply being able to survive without the help of other people or assistive devices; it simply means freedom of decision-making and the power of self-determination. It would be impossible to write about this topic without using the term in both of these ways, since the embellished connotation is prevalent within rehabilitation circles. ("Independent" is used often as a synonym for "unassisted," such as in independent dressing or transfer activities.) It is expected, however, that the context will make clear the sense in which "independence" is meant.

The processes of surviving and living independently after the event of disablement can be viewed from infinite perspectives. The following is but one alternative way of conceptualizing what happens, without and within. Maximizing one's health and capabilities, mastering the physical world, interacting with other people, striving for normalization, and taking charge of one's life—all the while altering conditions affecting disabled people generally—will be discussed in turn.

Maximizing Health and Capabilities

At the most primitive level of existence, the ability to locomote to find food and shelter is the basic requirement for independent survival. However, as civilization creates interdependencies, communication with other individuals also becomes essential. Disabilities impair one or both of these capacities; rehabilitation attempts to replace or restore them. When a disability is present at birth or develops gradually over time, rehabilitation efforts begin whenever the individual, a parent, a physician, or some other observer notices the need or believes the time is ripe. When the onset is sudden, rehabilitation ordinarily begins immediately after the acute medical care has ended, regardless of the individual's readiness for such procedures. Newly disabled people may be transferred directly from an acute-care hospital to a longer-term rehabilitation center with no intervening period of returning to familiar surroundings. As a result, they seldom understand accurately what they need to learn during rehabilitation in order to return to their previous lifestyles or move on to improved ones. Many rehabilitation programs assume that the professionals know what must be learned—an assumption that may be flawed.

In the past, it was common for all of the newly disabled people in a given rehabilitation facility to be offered a standard ("shotgun") battery of rehabilitative services which proved later to have missed the mark because it was not individualized to each person's particular lifestyle and needs. This approach has been altered by changes in health care reimbursement systems. Now it is more typical for individuals to be offered a brief course of rehabilitation and then discharged back to the community as soon as they became medically stable. Many rehabilitationists expressed concern that in the absence of extended time for the process of adjustment to disability to occur, people who were quickly discharged would develop both physical and psychological secondary complications. Interestingly, research has not confirmed these predictions in terms of basic functional improvement among a sample of people with spinal cord injuries (Warschausky, Kay, & Kewman, 2001). Perhaps the reason is that Independent Living Centers have stepped in to provide community-based assistance to replace some of the professional services that previously occurred in the hospitals (Tate & Forchheimer, 1998).

Nevertheless, many critical needs are being insufficiently met for people with recent disabilities. It has been said that our *health care system* might more accurately be called an *illness management system,* and it is true that for many years little to no attention was given in rehabilitation to the importance of exercise, nutrition, behavior (health-affecting habits), and state of consciousness. Exercises focused more on strengthening weak muscles than on tuning general physiological functioning; diet was seldom stressed unless it was clearly responsible for disease symptoms, as in diabetes. Even now, rehabilitation programs rarely give more than cursory mention to the fact that eating habits must be dramatically altered when a person changes from a robust lifestyle to a sedentary one. Thousands of overweight wheelchair users attest to the need for consultation and intervention, while hospital canteens continue vending junk food to patients needing to make every calorie count, nutritionally. As a result, many people with disabilities are handicapped further by impaired general health or having their limited energy drained through poor nutrition, excess weight, poor habits of rest and exercise, and inattention to their own states of consciousness.

As part of its "Healthy People 2010" initiative, the Centers for Disease Control and Prevention (CDC) examined the health indicators of people with disabilities and set objectives for improvement over the decade. Their findings (CDC, 2001) indicated that many people with disabilities have preventable secondary health complications, some of which lead to early deaths (for example, from diabetes-related cardiovascular disease or kidney failure). They also found relatively low rates of formal patient education and low rates of treatment for mental illness. Further, they found that compared with people who do not have disabilities, those with disabilities have higher rates of chronic conditions, less health coverage, and lower rates of exercise and other recommended behaviors such as smoking cessation.

Fortunately, as national leaders are becoming attuned to these issues they are starting to support programs that should increasingly affect local services. For example, the CDC (1998) held a national conference on disability and health that included such topics as Creating a Public Health Focus on Disability, Barriers to Health Promotion for Women with Multiple Sclerosis, Peer Counseling for Pressure Sore Prevention, and Aging with a Disability: Early Onset of Unexpected Medical Problems. The National Institute on Disability and Rehabilitation Research (NIDRR) has funded centers on the study of aging and disability. It has also sponsored individual projects such as one involving a wellness program for women with polio (Tate, Forchheimer, & Roller, 1998) and another involving wellness workshops for people with spinal cord injury (Chiodo, Cole, Finkel, Jacobson, & Stockford, 2001).

The reasons for maximizing general health and functional capabilities relate to reckoning with the world. The less external help needed to accomplish day-to-day tasks, the more spontaneously and economically life can be lived. The next two sections will explore a sampling of issues that arise when people cannot achieve total independence with the aid of other individuals, the government, or assistive devices, even after health and functionality have been maximized.

Mastering the Physical World

The physical environment offers enormous obstacles to people who have motor or visual disabilities. Those with hearing or mental disabilities are somewhat less affected because their locomotion abilities are not so directly impaired. For them, mastery of the physical environment devolves upon communication capacities, to be addressed in a subsequent section.

The prime environmental mastery issue for motor-disabled people is accessibility, whereas safety is the major problem for people who are visually impaired. On the surface it might seem, then, that individuals with motor disabilities would be most vulnerable to angry emotions, whereas blind people would experience fear more frequently. To an extent this is true, but the matter is more complex. Inaccessibility has implications for survival. To illustrate, if you can't get into a building, you can't take a job there, and the prospect of endless unemployment can be frightening as well as annoying. At the same time, having to forego important or pleasurable activities because needed safety factors are lacking can engender ample irritation.

Accessibility and Safety

The commonest ways in which disabled people cope with the problems of inaccessible or unsafe facilities are by (1) minimizing their own handicaps by developing every feasible adaptive skill, and (2) keeping up the good fight to get remaining environmental barriers removed. Some physically disabled people are interested in the development of wheelchairs that climb stairs, but most prefer to see stairs disappear from architecture altogether. The passage of the Americans with Disabilities Act in 1990 marked a watershed in the battle for accessibility. Although it is not a panacea, it served to shift the burden of proof from the individual with a disability to the organization providing public goods or services. Accessibility of services is required unless the provider can prove that it would cause an undue hardship. External ramping for multistory buildings still is rare, but the idea no longer is treated as ludicrous. Good evacuation systems for disabled inhabitants of skyscrapers are rarer still, but feasible plans exist, and as one result of the "9-11 catastrophe" implementation may not be too far away. Here and there a bus system agrees to install visual street-name displays for deaf passengers, and more promise to do so in the future.

The University of California at Berkeley pioneered in the 1970s by offering courses on universal design as part of its regular architecture curriculum (Lifchez, 1987). Individuals with severe disabilities participated as consultants to the students who were designing public buildings, plazas, restaurants, and shopping areas. Designing buildings that are accessible to everyone is no longer an arcane science, yet there are still many examples of new construction that overlook basic requirements. Probably the most consistently inaccessible segment of our society is that of private housing. This is not covered by legislation, but it still seems ironic that even within gated communities that have been designed to attract retirees, homes that could be used by a wheelchair user are the rare exception. The concept of "visitability" is beginning to command a bit of attention within the disability community. It purports that new private housing also should be designed using universal standards that would enable people with disabilities to visit acquaintances at home. Although it seems unlikely that legislative mandates will be extended to private homes, with the growing numbers of older people in the population, perhaps buyers will begin to request accessible design features as a matter of common sense and visitability will become more commonplace.

The current era is one of fulminating improvements and opportunities for people with disabilities; however, this is bringing with it new varieties of exquisite frustrations. The crux of these is being lulled into expecting accessibility and safety and then suddenly, periodically, being confronted with their troublesome or dangerous absence. The deaths of blind and otherwise severely disabled people under such circumstances are reported regularly. Unpublicized are the untold numbers of "near misses" that leave individuals emotionally shattered for long periods of time.

A less dramatic but more typical example of what happens follows. Let's say you've grown accustomed to going, spontaneously, to restaurants without making prior calls to confirm accessibility. When you and your date discover five steps down after entering the restaurant, you are embarrassed and angry. The restaurant was built after statutes requiring accessibility were in effect, and the target of your anger is out of compliance with the law. Some dates might enjoy watching you confront management; others would be "turned off." You feel considerable pressure in judging what to do.

Periodic fear, embarrassment, and righteous indignation are improvements over chronic depression, but they, too, exact their tolls from a person's happiness. Many of today's disabled people could be termed an angry generation, expecting change to come faster than it ever does and seething inside when it doesn't. Then they must deal with the perplexing realization that even justified anger isn't very good for them, yet they need its impetus to sustain their demands for change.

Delays in achieving accessibility goals are perhaps tolerable, but the elimination of safety hazards is urgent, now that mainstreaming is exposing hundreds of thousands of formerly sheltered people to increasing risks. Hanging on to life is not a background variable for people with disabilities, especially when severe. People who have learned the hard way that "it can happen here" are frequently confronted by additional jeopardy. Moreover, it seems that as social or scientific advances eliminate one source of anxiety, another emerges to take its place. For example, less and less often now does a wheelchair user have to risk further injury by being hauled up a flight of stairs or sailing down an overly steep ramp. At the same time, energy shortage problems periodically produce the threat of brownouts, which would immobilize electrically-powered assistive devices and life-support or environmental-control systems—a threat that disrupts the inner peace of people who rely on them.

Assistive Devices

Occasional anxiety about the actual or potential breakdown of assistive devices is a small price to pay for the practical and psychological benefits being enjoyed by their users. Just as widespread usage of motorized wheelchairs by people with impaired upper extremities produced a quantum leap in their quality of life (and may have been a causal factor in the closely following advent of the consumer movement), so is the accelerating production and use of other assistive devices upgrading the quality of life for more and more severely disabled people.

Mac, who is totally blind, came of age in the turbulent sixties. He longed for a career in law and a chance to contribute to the changes that he hoped to see in society. Handling so much reading and paperwork seemed unrealistic, however, so he accepted his second choice of a career in counseling. In contrast, Reiko, who is 22 years old and also blind, had the freedom to enter law school last fall. Her computer translates text into either auditory or Braille output, and databased software as well as the internet have made independent research feasible for her. Carol, quadriparetic from polio, reports that an electrical lift that allows her to do unassisted toilet transfers has saved her a significant monthly output for attendant help. It also has changed the nature of her dreams. Before acquiring the lift, she says about 10% of her dreams had some anxiety-laden representation of her dependency on others for attending to toilet needs. Within two weeks after obtaining the lift, all such dream symbolism had disappeared. Perhaps unimportant in itself, the changed dreaming pattern reflects a highly important and deeply experienced reduction of disability-related anxiety.

Although Mac, Reiko, Carol, and many others eagerly embrace new assistive devices, numerous disabled people resist them for a variety of reasons. Some say they feel dehumanized by mechanical aids or that they are leery of hardware. Others express fears that they will "turn off" other people by appearing "freaky" or comical. Ned drew an analogy between a device suggested for him and Charlie Chaplin's feeding machine in the silent film classic *Modern Times*. Loved ones who "need to be needed" may resist, too. The process of accepting assistive devices runs parallel to the acceptance of disability, involving a gradual admittance to consciousness of the way things are that is coupled with sufficiently strong desires to do what you want to do.

As noted earlier, people with impaired hearing have their share of anxieties about the physical world, too. Warning signals are frequently auditory and thus pose safety problems, and many events are "inaccessible" because no visual readout or interpreter services are provided. However, most of the problems "out there" for deaf people might better be subsumed under the rubric "other people," since communication is the capability impaired.

Interacting With Other People

The term "communication" is used here in the most general way, encompassing all aspects of information exchange: the transmission and reception of speech, writing, and miscellaneous other auditory (for example, screeching tires) and visual (for example, "body English") data. Blind people have problems with reception of writing and other visual data; deaf people have a primary problem with reception of speech and other auditory data and sometimes a secondary problem with transmission of speech. Speech dysfunction also occurs with a number of neuromuscular disorders, and people with mental disabilities may have trouble with all aspects of communication due to failure to interpret data in consensus with others.

The communication problems of deaf people are yielding somewhat more slowly to technological intervention than those of people who are blind. Braille, audio tape, and optical or electronic devices have greatly reduced the need for personal services (readers, primarily) for visually impaired people. Closed captioning capacity is now built into virtually all new television sets, and new developments such as amplification loops for those with some hearing capacity and real time interpreting (where someone similar to a court reporter takes notes that appear on a screen) have been helpful to many people. Nevertheless, hearing impaired individuals often continue to need interpreters to convey any auditorily presented information. Signing is a tiring activity and ideally is done by pairs who alternate turns. Marta, a deaf administrator, says:

> It was hard for me to accept the notion that I'm worth having two whole human beings to accompany me to meetings. My feelings are still confused, frankly. One minute I'm overwhelmed with gratitude that my little corner of the universe is willing to make this investment, and the next minute I'm angry because it doesn't make more. More pressure should be put on schools to make sign language as much a part of the core curriculum as English, and more funding should be directed toward developing portable devices that will decode speech and turn it into a visual readout. These are the only kinds of solutions that will work in the long run. Two-for-one is okay as a stopgap, but it can't go on forever.

A critical problem area for hearing-impaired individuals involves the legal-judicial system. Innumerable instances have been reported of police mistreatment of deaf people for failing to comply with commands they didn't hear, and the rights of hearing-impaired people to have adequate interpreter services during court proceedings are only beginning to be recognized. Individuals thus affected express fear and rage over the threats of harm and injustice entailed in these situations. The disabled community has grown quite capable of asking, as a group, for changes needed by disabled citizens at large. At the same time, however, disabled individuals often find it difficult to solicit help for themselves.

Asking for Help

Peter Leech, a psychiatric social worker who participated in the establishment of the Center for Independent Living in Berkeley, California, captures the inward recognition of many disabled people when he describes an insight-provoking experience he had soon after returning to school following disablement. He was sitting outdoors on campus when it began to rain. Unable to propel his wheelchair at that time, he waited for a passerby whom he could ask for a push to shelter. Several people came and went, but he was unable to ask. He explains:

> I was getting drenched in the rain, but I still couldn't ask anyone to give me a push. Suddenly, it hit me that I was waiting for someone to make eye contact with me and then I could ask. Somehow, I couldn't reach out through the "dark" and force my presence on someone who hadn't acknowledged me . . . especially when I was looking for a favor. Then I said to myself, "This is ridiculous!" and the next person by got collared. I thought about it later and came to the conclusion that the reason people don't make eye contact with disabled people is that they got punished for doing it when they were little kids. "Don't stare at cripples, Johnny!" says some flustered mother as she yanks him away by the arm. So he obeys, and never looks at a cripple again. I encourage kids to look and ask questions . . . and try to reassure their moms when they lunge in to drag the kids away. Maybe when they grow up they'll be looking at someone like me when he needs help.

Another of Leech's observations bears upon the wider issue of other people's reactions to those with disabilities. It also validates, somewhat, the fears expressed by disabled people who are reluctant to use assistive devices. He notes that people tend to see and respond to the clutter of a wheelchair, crutches and braces, or other appliances in evidence before they see and respond to the individual using them. This places heavy demands on each disabled person to have so prepotent a personality or such astounding good looks as to neutralize this perceptual tendency. Such demands are seriously handicapping since very few people, disabled or nondisabled, can develop and maintain without enormous effort maximal attractiveness plus consummate poise, charm, and assertiveness.

Managing Expectations

The devaluative attitudes discussed in Chapter 2 can subtly infiltrate the experiences and outlook of people with disabilities, particularly those with lifelong conditions. Even if they are not consciously recognized, lowered expectations need to be fought if they are not to impose a ceiling on the individual's accomplishments.

Ali was diagnosed with cerebral palsy, several months after his birth. His parents, though shocked by this discovery, were determined to raise him just like his brothers, with the same expectations and responsibilities. Ali recalled, however, that his grandparents often tried to shelter him and to try to make up for some of the frustrations that he had to endure as a result of his slurred speech and awkward gait. One November, as they prepared to leave for their winter home in Arizona, they suggested that Ali accompany them for a few months. His parents responded with an unequivocal "no." Ali belonged in school—how else would he ever be prepared to take his place in the adult world?

School was a miserable experience for Ali as other students tended to tease or avoid him. Nevertheless, he got good grades, and was accepted at the state university upon graduation. Like many others with developmental disabilities he never obtained part-time jobs after school or during the summers. This proved to be a serious disadvantage when he reached college graduation. He had a degree in economics and finance, but the hundreds of resumes that he sent out brought almost no response.

One day my vocational rehabilitation counselor called and told me that he had found a position for me with a large milling and manufacturing company. I was so excited that I could hardly sleep that night. The next morning I put on my suit and went down for my interview. It turned out that the job involved running a machine that pasted labels on cereal boxes! It could have been done by someone with a sixth grade education, and the pay was ridiculous, too. I just told them to forget it.

Eventually Ali did obtain a position with a technology firm that utilized his degree and provided a pathway toward possible advancement.

Asserting Oneself

Certain of the problems just discussed are moving toward solution fairly rapidly, now that the people who "own" the disabilities are asserting themselves and demanding their rights rather than leaving this job to professional rehabilitators and other concerned advocates who are not themselves disabled. The need for assertiveness, leavened with irreproachable diplomacy, is nowhere more evident than in dealing with people whose positions of authority allow them to determine the directions and quality of others' lives. For example, knowing how to "interview" taciturn physicians to obtain medical information on which to base one's own decisions is a valuable survival skill; so is the ability to secure helpful cooperation from teachers when one is physically unable to fulfill course requirements in the ordinary ways.

Perhaps the most challenging test of interpersonal survival skill is the ability to extract from agencies help to which one is entitled, without stimulating resistance on the parts of agency workers.

Disabled people, especially those whose disabilities are severe, often rely on funds and services from public agencies to continue living normative lifestyles in the community. Failure to obtain either can mean institutionalization or being trapped in poverty. Some people get everything to which they are entitled and a little bit more; others fail to secure even the minimum for which they are eligible. The former may have propitious contacts, but success and failure are both determined significantly by personality variables. A severely disabled woman who skillfully avails herself of every existing benefit grinned and revealed:

> My mother always told me, "You can catch more flies with honey than with vinegar," and I'm here to tell you she was right. The most important thing to remember is that those workers are so drained by the teeming hordes of downtrodden souls they have to deal with daily that they have no tolerance for anger. If you can lighten it up with a little humor, you can get by with showing your exasperation, but it's better to keep your cool. You have to be well informed. The workers usually don't know as much about the rules and regulations as you do if you've been around for awhile, because their turnover is so high. Also, of course, they don't care as much . . . it's not their lives that hang in the balance. You have to know what you're talking about, be very firm, and, at the same time, make with the sunny disposition. If you can do all that, you at least have a chance of getting what you need and deserve. Course if you can do all that, chances are you have a great job somewhere and don't need any help!

This illustrates the wide range of knowledge, skills, and personal qualifications needed, and it does not bode well for the novice or the person with merely average poise, verbal fluency, cheerfulness, or ability to feign it. Few rehabilitation programs prepare their patients or clients for agency management, but consumer-run independent living programs have begun filling this gap for people who have discovered that their skills in this area are deficient. On the light side: the clients of a consumer-run independent living program in one of the western states were given a course in assertiveness training. Within a few weeks, the counselors in the local rehabilitation agency were asking their psychological consultant for assertiveness training to help them cope appropriately with these newly assertive clients.

The quality of assertiveness also is helpful in dealing with the general public. Salesclerks might tend to ignore a disabled shopper if permitted to do so, or strangers inclined to help may actually hinder. The ability to put people at ease when they fear their own words in conversation with a disabled person, or to firmly decline assistance while simultaneously showing genuine appreciation of the helping motive, are more than survival skills. They can radically elevate the quality of a disabled person's life.

Issues related to the most central interpersonal relationships in people's lives will be discussed extensively in subsequent chapters dealing with families, friends, lovers, and employers. Here we will consider just one group of individuals who are particularly important to survival for people with severe disabilities.

Personal Service Providers

Many people with severe disabilities find themselves in a situation ordinarily reserved for the relatively well-to-do. They must hire and supervise one or more personal employees. Instead of personal secretaries or domestic staff, their employees are attendants, readers, drivers, and interpreters. Problems arise for several reasons.

First, the selection and supervision of employees, especially when they provide intimate or crucial services such as personal assistants do, require employers to have various high-level skills and personal qualifications. Well-to-do individuals are more likely to have developed the skills, acumen, and assertiveness underlying success in these activities by the time they are necessary than are average people, often fairly young and inexperienced, who suddenly must employ personal assistants because of disabling conditions. Moreover, the employer-employee relationship is more delicately balanced because servants for the well-to-do constitute luxuries, whereas the personal employees of disabled people are essential to continuing survival. To illustrate, when an applicant with excessive power needs, or an alcohol problem, is not assessed accurately and is hired as an attendant, the employer is less free to terminate the worker peremptorily when unsatisfactory performance becomes evident. The "cost" will not be reckoned in terms of having to clean house or prepare meals until a replacement is found; it might be having no way to eat, get out of danger, get into bed, or go to the bathroom.

Second, well-to-do employers have a psychological advantage in gaining respect and compliance from personal employees, simply because the latter know the former are able to pay their salaries. Many disabled people are not; the employees know their salaries come from public or charitable sources and the balance of perceived power between the two is affected accordingly, to the disadvantage of the disabled employer. This makes the job of supervision even more taxing, especially for people who question their own self-worth in the first place. Mistreatment, unreliability, exploitation, defection without notice, subtle cruelties of withholding help, and countless other abuses are reported regularly. They occur when disabled employers don't know how to screen out the "bad apples" at the outset or how to create a rewarding job for those they do hire. It is absolutely essential that the jobs be made intrinsically rewarding because the public funds provided do not constitute a living wage. A society that transmits the message, "You're worth taking care of, but only by someone who will work for less than an adequate wage," is not clear in its values, and the consequences must be managed.

Finally, many disabled employers are so anxious about finding help quickly, before other aspects of their support systems fall apart, that they often say "yes" to the first person who applies. Then they don't know how, or are afraid, to fire unsatisfactory workers, so the abuse goes on. Awareness that one's survival is contingent on the good will of others sometimes leads to fearfulness about rejecting anyone at least explicitly. Unfortunately, what often happens is that the fearful individual's resentments emerge in indirect ways, leading to the very alienation that is feared.

Such problems are more prevalent with respect to personal assistants than the other classes of employees for disabled people. Interpreters for the deaf, for example, possess well-paid skills and make significant commitments to the type of work they do by developing those skills. Such is seldom true for assistants. Many feel trapped in their employment situations and would prefer other work if they could obtain it. This, in itself, strains the perhaps already impaired self-esteem of each party. Nonetheless, interpreters also can pose problems for their deaf employers; for example, some "take over" conversations and others distort meanings to serve their own ends. The critical difference can be summed up in this way: readers and drivers for blind and interpreters for deaf individuals are extremely important aids to independent living, but assistants for severely disabled people may be essential to their biological survival. The potential of such a dependency to affect both persons' lives is not always fully appreciated.

Thus, to survive, psychologically as well as physically, disabled people using personal service providers must develop skill in their selection and supervision. Many resources are available on the internet and in the form of consumer-written books to help people learn how to more successfully select and supervise assistants. In addition, in some parts of the country public agencies register and monitor personal assistants. However, impediments to good supervisory practice and harmonious coexistence, especially when live-in providers are required, arise as much from mood and self-concept problems as from skill deficits. Therefore, the material in Chapter 8 on transcending the erosive emotions associated with disability will be highly pertinent to this issue. Also relating significantly to the matters of self-esteem and feelings of well-being is the concept of normalization.

Striving for Normalization

The goal of the inner and outer struggles recounted so far is to live a more or less normal life in a more or less normal community and to break out of poverty and restrictive environments offering nothing to do and no one to do it with. It is to stay out of institutions and break into the mainstream of everything—school, work, politics, and love affairs. Disabled people now know that they have the right to participate, to give and receive, take risks like anyone else, and dramatically demonstrate when their requests or demands are not met.

Conflicting "Rights"

For the most part, "other people" are cooperative and helpful, expressing dismay over having been unaware in the past, and vowing to correct what they can in the future. At least this is true when the economic impact of implementing needed changes is either negligible or affects someone else.

When significant costs are entailed, however, resistance rises rapidly, often accompanied by the rhetoric of politicoeconomic conservatism. An illustrative example came from a field deputy of a very conservative state senator. In a telephone interview following an address he gave before an assembly of rehabilitation workers, he was informed that his remarks had outraged attendees, and he was asked to clarify. It was assumed that he had been seriously misinterpreted. He had not. In paraphrase, the following encapsulates his explanation.

> The State Architect has promulgated regulations requiring that 80% of a restaurant must be accessible to wheelchairs. This would impose costly changes on the owners of existing restaurants and it restricts the freedom of choice for those building new ones. If a businessman likes stairs in his restaurant, he should be free to have them. After all, if it weren't for the people with risk capital to build such businesses, none of us would have them to enjoy. The Senator believes that it is not right to use the law to promote one group's interest at the expense of another's, and this is what all these laws about architectural barriers in privately-owned buildings are attempting to do: promote the interests of disabled people at the expense of

businessmen's. Frankly, the world could get along better without disabled people
than it could without businessmen.

For those who may wonder: no, he did not see that a parallel exists between
the disabled population and ethnic minorities who successfully challenged
businesses' freedom of choice. The reason: "No one has ever hated disabled
people." Also, of course, it doesn't impinge on aesthetic preferences in
architectural style to accommodate ethnic minorities, nor are alteration costs
on existing facilities entailed.

Interestingly, members of the disabled community expressed hurt as much
as anger at these pronouncements. Sheltering assumes many forms and one
form that is resistant to extinction is protection from the fact that certain
sectors of society "couldn't care less." Many disabled people have been
beguiled by predominant contact with "other people" who are in sympathy
with the underdog; they are caught off guard by the disdain of those with
different value systems and motives. The blunt pronouncements of individuals
sharing this senator's views come as shocks, creating alarm and fear among
people who can only wonder what will become of their improving conditions
if such views become widespread. In a more personal way, it simply hurts
to be told, just as you're beginning to believe that perhaps you are as worthwhile as anyone else, that to some, you're worth far less than a businessman's
fancy for split-level restaurants.

This issue forms the basis of a controversy within the disabled community
over the advisability of encouraging the development of fully accessible,
service-rich housing arrangements explicitly for people with (usually severe) disabilities.

Independent Living Arrangements

Some people fear that the creation of independent living arrangement projects
will detract from the perceived responsibility of the total community to
eliminate mobility (and other) barriers from the world at large. They foresee
ghettoization of disabled people within accessible subcommunities and progressive lessening of movement between them and the mainstream of housing,
shopping, work, and recreation. Equality is considered unfathomable in micro-
cosm; and separate, even if equal, is abjured. Others would prefer to forego
the remote, future possibility of general access in favor of creating a more
immediate, accessible universe allowing unhindered living now. This camp
cites the opportunities such communities offer for economical sharing of

attendants and expensive equipment, as well as the preference of some to associate predominantly with others who share the disability experience.

This last turn of phrase reflects an important aspect of the emerging consciousness within the disabled community. In the past, many disabled people who wanted to make their marks on the world believed they should dissociate themselves from others with disabilities and thus avoid being stereotyped as "another of the unfortunate ones" by the nondisabled majority. More than this, they also felt that disabled people were inferior beings, and to be forced into their sole company was to be deprived of the privilege of consorting with interesting, worthwhile people. However, just as black became beautiful and led to the positive choices of some to live in segregated communities, a similar process has taken place among people with disabilities. In contrast with the past, valued camaraderie issuing from common experience is cited more often as the reason for preferring association with other disabled people than is discomfort or feeling inferior to those who are not.

Independent living arrangements can be as large and formal as a complex of several hundred accessible, fully equipped apartments that offer extensive personal services. They can be as small and informal as one disabled person living in an ordinary apartment and having an agreement with a neighbor to provide needed morning and evening attendant care. There is fledgling agreement in the disabled community that the full range of possibilities should be made available to allow for individual choice.

Taking Charge of One's Life

Legislative advocacy, by and for people who are blind, was fully operational by the 1930s. A comparable thrust for other disability groups could not be said to have existed before the 1960s. The last four decades have seen accelerating efforts among all disability groups to secure promised constitutional protection of their rights through the legal-judicial system and through public education in their communities.

The Organization of People With Disabilities

Most of the early advocacy efforts were made by disabled individuals fortunate enough to have broken into the establishment through familial, professional, or business channels. Gradually, other disabled people also became involved. Although they might not be working, they had the foresight, time, and motivation to press for needed changes. As some of the changes came about, still more disabled people were enabled to join the fight. The few, scattered social clubs for disabled members came to be complemented, occasionally absorbed, and, finally, vastly outnumbered by political action organizations wherein socialization and recreation constituted no more than secondary goals.

They recruited, expanded, hired paid staff, coalesced, and created chapters; in short, disabled people organized. They started finding each other and discovered that they were not alone. They started talking to each other and learned that other people with disabilities are okay, that they themselves weren't the only exceptions to a negative stereotype they'd accepted, and that all had valuable experience and information to share. Then they started taking action together and discovered that, indeed, in unity there is strength. Together, they have made significant progress toward reducing the full range of barriers to a quality existence—in the law, welfare, education, architecture, transportation, employment, housing, shopping, recreation, and much, much more. The strength issuing forth from an organized constituency has made possible still another phenomenon that is radically altering the very core of what it means to have a disability.

Independent Living as a Movement

The advent of the "independent living movement" may be the most dramatic happening in the history of rehabilitation. After centuries of being isolated, downtrodden, ignored, managed, manipulated, and "taken care of," the people who own the problem finally said that they'd "rather do it themselves." "You gave us your dimes; now give us our rights" was a trenchant expression of the new deal being sought.

Disabled activists have made their needs known to governing bodies at all levels of societal organization, and, little by little, efforts are made to see that somehow these needs are met at least somewhat better. The validity of the claim that those sharing the needs are uniquely qualified to plan ways of meeting them is recognized. As a result, consumer-dominated advisory boards to professionally-run agencies have become integral parts of standard operating procedure, and the consumers are advising whether invited to do so or not. More important, all across the country the reins of service provision are being turned over to the consumers themselves, through independent living programs operated by and for people with disabilities.

Growing pains among these programs have been severe and the reasons are familiar. Similar to what occurred in "poverty programs" for ethnic minority groups a few years earlier is the fact that staff frequently are catapulted into more responsible jobs than their absent or impoverished work histories have prepared them for. A severely disabled, recent college graduate who had never held a job before suddenly found himself employed as the executive director of an independent living center. He was totally unprepared to handle the administrative complexities of managing nearly twenty employees engaged in widely diverse forms of service and advocacy, and so he shortly alienated both his board of directors and his poorly selected employees. After recovering from the shock of being fired, he described himself, with rueful humor, as a case of "instant Peter Principle."

Also reminiscent of a phenomenon from the 1960s, nondisabled staff report feeling rejected and unappreciated simply because they are not members of the "in" group—the disabled majority. Some disabled people learn to make nondisabled colleagues feel accepted and valued contributors. An extremist contingent declines to do so, explicitly denouncing the involvement of nondisabled individuals in any phase of service provision beyond the allocating of necessary funds.

In spite of the problems, consumer-run programs have matured to offer previously unobtainable services to people with virtually every type of disability. Advocates intercede for clients trying to wind their ways through bureaucratic red tape and regulatory obstacles. Just knowing that someone is there to help or at least explain, understandably, the basis of a dispute with an agency, brings considerable relief to some people overwhelmed with frustration, helplessly believing they are getting the "run around." Some programs have peer counselors available to help severely disabled individuals locate, select, and supervise suitable assistants or help with locating the best a community offers in low-cost, accessible housing.

Thus it goes that disabled people struggle to survive and live independently in the community. To succeed in doing so is to have an opportunity to engage in the life functions explored in the next four chapters: loving, working, and playing. Because it appears to be most central to the core of a person's being, the matter of loving will be taken up next.

4

Loving

The Family

The great Western psychologist, Abraham Maslow, and the Eastern mystical writings from which he drew placed the needs of belonging and loving in about the middle of the hierarchy of human needs (Maslow & Mittleman, 1951). More basic are those for survival, safety, and security. More transcendent are those for self-actualization and spiritual awakening. The need to love and be loved, to generate and enjoy a sense of connectedness with other human beings, occupies the central range of Maslow's now famous "needs hierarchy."

Most of us had our first experiences with belonging, loving, and being loved in the context of our parental families. Later, similar urges would lead us to break away from those groups to form new families of our own (issues to be covered in Chapter 5). Love relationships with friends are also of great importance and will be discussed in Chapter 7. The present chapter is devoted to the ways in which disablement affects and interacts with family relationships and functioning. It will examine the reactions, resources, coping strategies, pitfalls, and special issues that arise.

Disability: A Family Affair

Just as illness or injury disrupts the physiological homeostasis of the affected individual, so they and their sequelae disrupt the homeostatic balance of the family unit. When disability occurs, the entire family begins an adaptive struggle to regain its equilibrium. In other words, although only one member of the family "owns" the disability, all family members are affected and, to some extent, handicapped by it. The birth of a disabled child, the discovery of a degenerative disease in a youth, the catastrophic injury of a parent, or any other disablement befalling any member of a family can have as far-reaching and intense an impact on the others as on the one who becomes disabled. All experience shock and fear over the event or recognition of disablement, and the pain and anxiety of wondering what the future implications will be. The disability of one may alter the lifestyles of family members as much or more than that of the disabled individual: schedules, duties, plans, and roles all change. All experience loss—of a fully functioning cog in the family wheel—which generates disappointment, frustration, and anger, as freedom and time for fun disappear. At base, the family members must learn to deal with the same dimensions as the disabled person: their own reactions, the physical world, and other people. Although guilt is an issue with which disabled people must often reckon, especially when responsibility for an accident or unmet obligations are at stake, it is an almost universal problem for the loved ones of a person who becomes disabled.

The Research and Training Center at George Washington University (Gonzalez, Steinglass, & Reiss, 1987; Reiss & Oliveri, 1987) studied ways family systems theory could help professionals better understand and better serve families in the rehabilitation process. For example, it is necessary not only to understand the family as a holistic system, but also to understand the coalitions or subsystems that exist. A mother may become overly tied to a child who has sustained a disability, devoting all of her time and energy to meeting the child's needs and demands. Feeling left out, the father may respond by developing an alliance with one of the siblings. Such coalitions may have a serious impact on a marital bond.

Another important concept is that of boundaries, the often unspoken rules about how family members relate to one another. Do they draw a firm line around who belongs in the family, keeping everyone else at arm's length? If so, they may find it difficult to accept help from others, even in times of crisis. How effectively can they adapt to change? On the one hand, they might be so rigid that changes caused by disability are hard to navigate. On the other hand, they might be so flexible that the family lacks routines and order, so everyone feels insecure. How close are the family members to one another? If everyone goes his or her own way, paying little attention to each other, the family is said to be *disengaged*. On the other hand, if they are so close that no one is allowed to make decisions or go anywhere without seeking permission from the others, the family is said to be *enmeshed*. Either extreme can be problematic for the individual with a disability. In one case he or she has little support; in the other, the expectations are stifling. Communication patterns also influence the way in which a family copes with disability. Some families are closed, seldom sharing their deepest feelings with each other. Other families shoot from the hip, saying anything that comes to mind. Again, either extreme can cause problems, hurt feelings or isolation. Understanding the resources that each family brings to the rehabilitation process as well as the points of vulnerability that may complicate it is critically important.

Guilt

To begin with the obvious and proceed to the more subtle, parents who produce children with birth defects experience guilt, shame, and embarrassment, as well as disappointment, sorrow, and anger that their offspring are imperfect. Genetic and behavioral antecedents that may have contributed to the defect are sought, and unless a clear hereditary cause is found in the father's lineage, it is usually the mother who suffers most in this way. The guilt may be adopted as one's own, or it may be foisted onto the shoulders of another by blaming the doctor, the hospital, or the grandparents for passing on a genetic defect manifested in a later generation. The struggle to absorb versus repulse guilt and blame may go on for a very long time. In some cultures, the feelings of guilt are so intense that a child with a visible disability is kept at home and hidden away.

When it is known that poor nutrition, drugs ingested during pregnancy, or other improper prenatal care have caused or contributed to a birth defect, the parents and especially the mother may face a particularly torturous battle to overcome the guilt engendered. In recent years we have learned more about the deleterious effects of alcohol, tobacco, and drugs on a developing fetus. Fetal alcohol syndrome produces a child with visible facial characteristics and irreversible behavioral and learning problems. Mothers whose behavior is directly responsible for producing disabilities in their children may experience feelings of intense guilt and may be chastised by others for the harm they have caused.

Self-blame for the disablement of a child is in no way limited to those whose children are born with disabilities. When older children become ill or injured, self-blame occurs, too. Recriminations over failures to observe signs that might have led to earlier diagnosis and better prognosis, or inadequacies of supervision that could have prevented accidents, are not exceptions but the rule.

When any family member becomes disabled an aspect of guilt arises from the ambivalent nature of love relationships, especially when lives are interdependent, as in a family. That is, past angry thoughts about the person who has become disabled are apt to be recalled, such as moments when one has muttered, I hope one of these days that rotten kid (parent) (spouse) gets his (hers)! Suddenly, he (she) has. We all engage in a little magical thinking and at least fleeting moments of guilty terror—"Oh my God, my wish came true!"—are common. The rational mind says, "Don't be silly, of course that had nothing to do with it," but the gut still churns.

As if the self-blame were not problem enough, it is also far too common that guilt is inculcated in family members by others. Even more unfortunate, it may be rehabilitation agency workers who, sometimes unwittingly and sometimes not so unwittingly, create this effect. Because of the enormous costs associated with catastrophic illness or injury, the family often is urged to assume as much as possible of the financial and caregiving burdens. However, when urged to carry an extent of the cost or aspects of care which seriously distress or overtax them, many feel ashamed and exposed when they refuse, or try and fail.

Family members who appear to be more (or equally) concerned over the impact of their loved one's disability on their own lives may be subtly or not so subtly punished for this in a variety of ways. Direct remonstrances may be given, to the effect that the disabled individual needs all the help and attention the family can muster with the clear implication that the latter should tuck away their own needs until the crisis is past. This overlooks the fact that the family is also in crisis and is in need of help, too.

The Family Is Not the Enemy

Much is said among the various professions working with disabled people about the problems posed by family members who "sabotage" their rehabilitative efforts. Rehabilitation providers work from a value system that may be only partly explicit—that it is important to work hard and achieve maximum independence in physical functioning, even if other priorities or relationships are sacrificed in the process. Families, especially those from cultures other than mainstream American ones, may be more concerned with showing respect for the age or position of the individual in the family than for achieving physical independence, so they may provide more help than the team deems appropriate. Criticism is sometimes harsh, as in the commonly heard phrase, "That parent (or spouse) will undo everything we've tried to accomplish during the week when we send the patient home for the weekend." Even when conscientious efforts are made to understand and help the family with its problems, an attitude is frequently evident that family members are obstacles to goal achievement with their disabled relative, rather than people who need and deserve help themselves. The following language from a brochure on family counseling, prepared by a person sincerely concerned with just this problem, still reveals the bias described.

The rehabilitation enterprise can be facilitated or impaired by the attitudes and behavior of the family within which a disabled person lives. Sometimes a rehabilitation worker's consultation with a client's family can help this family process become less of an obstacle and/or more of a help to the rehabilitation process.

This statement shows the writer's concern with the problem and mirrors it at the same time. The family does not just affect the rehabilitation enterprise, it is an integral part of it; the family is the client. In other words, just as rehabilitation professionals criticize medical specialists for focusing on the object of their specialty (bones, nerves, various organs) to the exclusion of "the whole person," so do they, themselves, tend to focus on the "patient" to the exclusion of the family of which he or she is a part. Psychologists are amused when surgeons regard psychodynamics as alien factors muddying up what would otherwise be a clean job, but their own narrowness of perspective is little different. As a result, far more people than will ever come to them as patients are left to fend for themselves in handling the shock, disappointments, disruptions, fears, and suddenly imposed requirements as they cope with a vast array of totally new stimuli and demands—if they are to go on loving, working, playing, and transcending whatever fate deals them. The hospitalized patient may be fairly well insulated from the difficult and frightening adjustments the family must make in order to stay economically and emotionally afloat.

Ironically, the failure to extend genuine empathy and the sense of professional responsibility to the whole family can result in overlooking ways in which family members can serve as rehabilitation allies. This was dramatically illustrated in the case of an educational consultant who sustained a head injury. The man's wife was viewed rather unabashedly as "an aggressive bitch" who was highly opinionated and who intended to "dump" the patient in a couple of years. An outside consultant who participated in a discharge planning conference listened to lengthy, emotional descriptions of the wife's interferences and unpleasant ways and pointed out that what he had heard was that she was a remarkably responsible, capable, aggressive person who wanted to and would move mountains to make her husband's life as pleasant and uncomplicated as possible before she divorced him; that she was willing to use her time and considerable skills as an airplane pilot, among other things, to help him get vocationally reestablished; that she wanted out of the marriage but was a highly principled person who had made a conscious decision to give him the next two years of her life; that she had trusted the staff enough to share that fact with them; and that, in short, she was "one hell of a resource that is being not only wasted but mistreated."

Rehabilitation workers often feel constrained from acknowledging negative feelings about their patients or clients; thus, dislikes, frustrations, and disappointments may be ejected from consciousness as inappropriate or unprofessional lapses from the ideal image for which they strive. Suppression of such natural feelings may serve to magnify any antipathies felt toward family members and reduce motivation to help them build the resources they need for coping. Moreover, the family may be scapegoated by frustrated rehabilitation workers just as readily as the latter are scapegoated by frustrated family members. The rehabilitation job is a difficult one, and when another member of the team, whether a professional, the disabled person, or a relative fails to perform in line with the wishes and expectations of the others, blame placing is likely to follow. Family members are particularly vulnerable because they are seldom integrated into the cohesive work group and are only sporadically present in the rehabilitation facility, at least during the professionals work hours. The disabled person is less likely to be scapegoated by the professionals, who sometimes feel they must rehabilitate people in spite of themselves if that appears necessary.

With or without support, the family must progress through essentially the same stages of adjustment as the person who is disabled. Clinical experience suggests that the family often proceeds more slowly in the adjustment process than does the individual with the disability. The individual is confronted with the effects of disability on a continuous basis, whereas the family may be able to hold onto hope for a longer period of time that things will return to the predisability status quo. Any such difference in perspective can be stressful for everyone involved in the rehabilitation process, and the team needs to be both patient and helpful in facilitating communication. The question arises: when tragedy strikes, who copes? Once again, the answer is: those with the right combination of resources.

Family Coping Resources

Family members need many of the same kinds of resources as the disabled person, plus a few that differ. The required inner resources fall roughly into four groups: emotional, intellectual, personality, and physical. Emotional stability is the prime requisite for coping with any catastrophic change, in order to neutralize adverse reactions and facilitate the adjustment process. A loving nature, the ability to accept "what is" and proceed from there, and belief in one's own power to influence the future are crucial aspects of the emotional armamentarium needed. Families with such characteristics of emotional stability can rebound from catastrophe whether or not their intellectual resources are high. Unquestionably, however, possession of good intellectual resources will further aid the coping process and permit a richer style of adjustment to be reached. The ability to grasp the medical and other facts of the situation, to foresee and prepare for problems that may arise in the future, and to creatively devise and implement solutions to them, plus a working knowledge of the outer resources that exist in the community are exceedingly important intellectual resources to draw upon, both in times of crisis and later when the crisis stage has passed.

Complexly interwoven with the emotional and intellectual resources are personality resources, such as assertiveness, persuasiveness, diplomacy, and emotional supportiveness. The combination of strengths in these three areas (emotional, intellectual, and personality resources) will determine such practical matters as the family's skill in social management, both in general and under conditions of unusual need and stress. Many families lack, under ordinary conditions, adequate skills for procuring goods and services, managing money, and other family management activities. When disability affects a member of the family, these skills may be taxed to the maximum.

The list of personality resources that bear upon coping with disability in a family is endless. Some are primarily important in dealing with practical exigencies (for example, assertiveness, persuasiveness, and diplomacy in dealing with agencies), and some relate to helping the disabled individual and other family members deal with the changes imposed on their lives (for example, emotional supportiveness). Although emotional and intellectual resources are paid considerable attention in the literature, comparatively little has been directed toward the role of personality or temperament factors. To cite again the traits of succorance and nurturance as illustrative, family adjustment will probably be easier all else being equal if it is a succorant individual who becomes disabled and a nurturant one who is thrust into the role of caregiver. The reverse situation would be expected to create far more dissonance.

An additional resource area that may be highly important for family members is that of their own physical strength. Good general health, stamina, endurance, and an ability to marshal extra strength in times of crisis are essential ingredients when one is called upon to continue doing all one has done in the past, plus take over the duties formerly assumed by the disabled family member, plus, in cases of severe disablement, provide physical care for that individual. Family members with high energy levels will be at a considerable advantage in coping with the sequelae of disability compared with those whose ordinary level of energy tends to be low or even average.

In addition to the varieties of inner resources just described, there are two major types of outer resources that can make a significant difference in how effectively and easily a family deals with disability. These two are money and contacts. Having the financial resources to procure needed medical, nursing, and attendant care, equipment and supplies, and other illness/disability-related goods and services without having to worry about impending bankruptcy or suffer the frustrations and anxieties associated with reliance on public agency funds can reduce greatly the stress entailed. Similarly, having contacts with people who can help solve the problems can reduce the psychic wear and tear of coping.

The concept that parents or other family members also can be "casualties" of either the disability or the system is an important one. It happens when bureaucratic obstacles create more stresses than an agency's services resolve and when the family's needs for practical and emotional support are ignored. Both are related to changes that have come about in family structure. In the extended-family household of a previous era, there usually were relatives available to perform many of the special services needed when a member of the household became disabled. The disappearance of the maiden aunt and other extended-family personages willing and able to fulfill these functions has created increased needs for public and private agencies and sundry practitioners to fill the gap. At the same time, as the extended family is being replaced by the nuclear-family household, socioeconomic changes have made it necessary or desirable for both spouses to work outside of the home. For one of the only two wage-earning adults in a household to remain at home to provide needed care could be an economic disaster for the family and psychologically devastating to the person forced to interrupt a valued career.

Given the increasing numbers of people with chronic illness and disabilities plus changes in health care services (for example, widespread lack of adequate health insurance, shorter lengths of stay in hospitals and rehabilitation units, etc.), family members are taking on many of the responsibilities that were once reserved for health professionals (Elliott, Shewchuk, & Richards, 2001). Research has quite consistently supported the assumption that people who serve as caregivers experience both tangible and emotional burdens that affect their quality of life (Marinelli & Dell Orto, 1999; Segal & Schall, 1996). Interestingly, psychological characteristics seem to be more significant than objective characteristics of the condition or the caregiver in predicting caregiver adjustment (Schulz & Quittner, 1998). Several researchers (Lawrence, Tennstedt, & Assmann, 1998) studied the relationship between the stressors that caregivers experience and their well-being. They found that when behavioral problems were present, the quality of the relationship suffered, causing caregivers to feel higher levels of captivity and depression. They also found that among families with a higher quality of relationship, increased disability was related to higher levels of perceived overload. Chwalisz (1996) developed a perceived stress model to try to explain the extent of burden that spouses experience in providing care to a partner with head injury. She found that perceived stress was the strongest predictor of perceived mental health. Problem-focused coping was associated with lower levels of stress, in contrast with emotion-focused strategies, which correlated with higher stress. Higher levels of social support also were associated with better mental health. Another study (Shewchuk, Richards, & Elliott, 1998) found that anxiety was strongly related to physical symptoms in caregivers. All of these findings suggest the importance of making counseling and support available to all of the family members, not just the individual with a disability.

Public policy may exacerbate the stresses on families when a person with a severe disability requires substantial assistance with activities of daily living. Some public financial assistance may be available, but often only if the caregiver is not a relative. A spouse, therefore, may not have the option of quitting a job outside the home to provide care because there is no way to make up the lost wages. Furthermore, if the spouse keeps working, the family income may disqualify them from receiving assistance to cover the cost of outside care. This can leave the partner in an exhausting double bind—working what approximates two full-time jobs. The authors know of situations in which spouses have chosen to divorce in order to obtain the benefits that would allow them to continue living together.

Progressive Disability: Impact on Family

When the disability is progressive, family coping resources are taxed to the maximum. An active disease process exists here, one that progressively is eroding tissue: bone, nerve, muscle, or other tissues. Many deteriorative conditions are characterized by remissions and exacerbations of symptoms and by the presence of pain. Often, there also is the specter of a downhill course and a hastened death to be reckoned with by the disabled individuals and their loved ones. These are the primary aspects that make individual and familial adjustment to a progressive disorder different, and potentially more difficult, than adjustment to a stabilized disability.

Parents of a child with a progressive disability are likely to experience great marital stress. A study of the impact of life-threatening illness on parents (Mastroyannopoulou, Stallard, Lewis, & Lenton, 1997) revealed high levels of psychological distress and significant effects on relationships and employment. Family communication also was affected, showing patterns of high conflict, low cohesion, and low levels of expressiveness. Other studies of parents with a head-injured son or daughter (Allen, Linn, Gutierrez, & Willer, 1994) also showed substantial levels of burden and marital strain, even among relationships that had survived several years after the trauma.

Living around someone who is in pain can be difficult for several reasons. The helplessness of knowing that someone you love is hurting and there is nothing you can do to relieve it is mentioned more often in literary than professional works, but it is not a fictional matter. The experience of helplessness, when control or power are desperately needed or wanted, has been shown to be one of the most destructive mood states known to humankind and to other animals as well. Curt Richter (Richter, 1958) found that laboratory animals (rats), convinced of their own helplessness in a swimming situation, literally committed suicide by plunging to the bottom of a water tank to drown. He likened his finding to the phenomenon of voodoo death (wherein individuals convinced of another's power to kill them may actually die on cue) and to the reluctance of modern surgeons to operate on patients who are excessively fearful or pessimistic about the outcome because their chances of dying on the table are known to be elevated.

The loved ones of people in pain face not only the stress associated with helplessness itself, they are in triple jeopardy. As noted earlier, people who hurt may not have jolly dispositions, or they may have unpredictable moments of volatile emotionality. This puts wear and tear on the loved ones, too, who may get indignant when a minor infraction is met with a major response. Then comes the guilt: I'd overreact, too, if I hurt all the time. Triple jeopardy exists because there is little support or understanding available for anyone but the one who is in pain. Those who self-protectively harden their hearts are apt to be perceived and treated as monsters.

Fatigue can be a major problem, too. If the disability involves changes in cognition, judgment, or sleep patterns, the caregiver may be awakened repeatedly throughout the night. Another special kind of stress occurs if the disability (such as HIV-AIDS) involves social stigma. Caregivers may be isolated from their usual sources of social support because of reluctance to talk with others about their loved-one's condition (Hanson, 2000), adding to the burden of their responsibilities.

Remissions and exacerbations can put the disabled person and all loved ones on an emotional roller-coaster. When a deteriorative condition plateaus or improves, hopes abound and often exceed reasonable expectations. With many progressive disorders, there may be day-to-day variations that will necessitate changing degrees of assistance from family members who, accordingly, never know what to expect with respect to caregiving responsibilities or demands for emotional support.

When a downhill course is predicted, the family is faced with the double prospect of increasing responsibility and the eventual loss of someone they count on and/or love. When stress is considered an important determinant of the disease, guilt arises again as an issue for the family to deal with. If they grow fearful that expression of their own emotions will add to the stress of the disabled individual, they may begin to suppress their cathartic needs lest they become the trigger to accelerated deterioration or a fatal, acute attack. This, obviously, will lead to increased tension and stress for all concerned.

Regardless of whether the disability is progressive or stable, certain pre-existing patterns of family interaction, or unmet needs on the part of family members, can create additional sources of strain. Not infrequently, a form of collusion develops between the disabled person needing help and a family member whose needs to provide it are partly neurotic.

The Neurotic Tie That Binds

Just as Stephen found that his disability "paid off" by removing him from the threat of negative evaluation by his athletically oriented father, so some families find equilibrium in a way that requires the continuance of the disabled member in a dependent, needful role. Somehow, having such a person in the family pays off. A recently divorced mother of a young man with cerebral palsy described one such situation with remarkable nondefensiveness and humor:

> For years, having Teddy around was a great way of avoiding the fact that Jack and I didn't have a damn thing in common except three kids. We could pretend that all of our anger, depression, or whatever we were showing related to him, not ourselves. It was kind of like the way some people use a television set: they're together in a room, so they feel quite comfortable that they're big on togetherness, but each is attending to something else. They don't have to relate to each other, and, if they did, they'd get in a fight because they basically can't stand each other. Teddy was our television set. We watched him together for hours on end and our only conversation was to pick apart the last program.
>
> I had planned on going back to work after getting two babies into school, but Jack didn't want me to. So I got pregnant again to have something to do. When number three turned out to have cerebral palsy, it was clear that I would never have any other career. Teddy made it legitimate for me to stay home without acknowledging that I was selling out to Jack just to keep from rocking the boat.

And he became the stability point of the family, as well as my reason for being. I was a professional C.P. mother and oh! how cleverly I bludgeoned Jack with that! Greatest weapon a woman ever had!

Then all of a sudden, Teddy wants to leave home. He wants to go away to finish college and he has a roommate lined up to help him out. And the roommate's a young woman! He doesn't need me anymore, not to take care of him, and not to be the only woman who'll ever love him. What in the hell am I going to talk to Jack about now?

The next two years were awful. I bounced from one encounter group to another, getting told off for being a possessive mother and using a disabled kid's life to meet my own needs on a regular basis. Jack thought encounter groups were dumb and when he finally said so, we had the fight that should have ended our marriage twenty years earlier. The last two years have been okay, though. Life for a 52-year-old divorcee isn't half as bad as I imagined.

The most unusual aspect of this story is the fact that the neurotic pattern was dissolved successfully, at least for the disabled man and his mother. Far more instances exist in which the regressive symbiosis is not resolved, and no party to it could describe it with the insight displayed here. She alludes to two major issues involved in familial exploitation of a disabled individual: (1) the need for a stabilizing influence to keep the family together or maintain a familiar, comfortable status quo; and (2) the provision of a *raison d'etre* for another family member who feels otherwise bereft of purpose and direction.

A third issue encountered is the need for a scapegoat to explain and absorb the hostility stemming from the family's general dissatisfaction with life. A grisly illustration of the extreme to which this can go is reflected in the case of a childhood burn victim who provided a "whipping boy" to his impoverished, angry, and disturbed family for many years. Nearly every evening at home ended with the severe drunkenness of his parents, two siblings, and two cousins who also occupied the large, deteriorating house. When they became drunk, they made vicious fun of his disfigurement, ordering him to bring more drinks for them so that he would have "some earthly purpose in life." When they were sober, they either ignored him or blamed him, in crisper speech, for the family's squalor. One evening when the group had been more abusive than usual, he systematically lured each inebriated individual into a different room of the house and bludgeoned them to death. After fifteen years in prison, he was released to work in a sheltered workshop, where he is considered a "highly religious, gentle, spiritual sort of person who almost surely would never harm another living being."

Most disabled people scapegoated by their families never strike back at the true objects of their hurt or hatred; they are more likely to take it out on others—or themselves—later on. Usually, the scapegoating is far more subtle than in this case; for that reason, it is more difficult to identify and resolve in either a socially acceptable or unacceptable way. The martyred caregiver who "sacrifices" a way of life to serve a disabled child, spouse, or parent is a frequent example. Kevin describes with unresolved bitterness his experience with this form of scapegoating:

> From the time I got injured, mother was right there to help me, and I am grateful for that. But some funny stuff went down that I still can't sort out completely. She always found ways to kind of remind me that she was sacrificing everything for me; and, somehow, the implication was there that she was "buying" me forever. She was never so crass as to say, "After all I've done for you . . . ," but she mentioned, from time to time, that she had given up the chance to remarry after my father died in order to take care of me, and that she had virtually given up any kind of social life for the same reason.
>
> The fact is, she had been widowed for fifteen years before I got hurt, and she only dated a couple of times as far as I know. She had also complained, as long as I can remember, that her social life was terrible because "Everything fun is for couples." I just gave her an excuse to grab onto; somehow, pretending that she had no husband and few friends because sacrificing for me made it more respectable to her.
>
> What still drives me crazy is that, now that I'm grown and have a home and family of my own, she feels I'm responsible for giving her life meaning. Half of the time I feel like, "Wow! I do! After all she did for me." The other half, I know I can't. Sometimes I get really angry and tell myself, "She made those choices and it's not fair for her to feel I should be signed, sealed, and delivered to her because she can't figure out other ways to make her life meaningful." Then I feel ashamed of being so cold . . . and around and around I go.

This last example illustrates all three of the issues cited: the need for a stabilizing influence to maintain the status quo, the need for a *raison d'etre*, and the need for a scapegoat to "explain" dissatisfaction and absorb anger whether directly or indirectly expressed. (A martyred air can be a more effective way to "get" somebody than hollering.) The feelings experienced by all concerned may never be confronted and acknowledged in ways leading to growth unless outside help is proffered. Kevin ventured the opinion that he had received sufficient emotional nourishment from his mother (in spite of the neurotic aspects of her giving) to allow him to grow up strong enough to break away and be an independent adult when the time came, whereas she had not fared so well.

> She needed help to get some balance in her life, if she was going to withstand what was in store for her. Someone who could see what she was doing to herself should have given her some counseling. Her so-called friends just kept reinforcing

her self-sacrifice trip by telling her how wonderful she was. She was, but she needed honest confrontation about where she'd end up if she didn't make some kind of life for herself that didn't revolve around me. I sensed it, but I had a vested interest in seeing her go on giving, giving, giving. Someone should have been there to protect her from me!

The mother is elderly now, and her mental processes are impaired. For her, it is probably too late, but clearly she is not the only one to suffer for her lack of help. Kevin has been left with a tangle of conflicting emotions that he is only beginning to sort out.

Age of Onset: Impact on the Family

When disablement occurs during childhood, both parents and siblings face numerous problems related to childrearing practices. A complicated process at best, such issues as the appropriate degree of protectiveness to offer become incalculably more difficult. A primary issue that influences all others is the extent to which parents can accept—emotionally and intellectually—the facts associated with a child's disability. Their acceptance (or lack of it) will be an important determinant of the reactions of other children in the family. Also, the match between the mother's and father's acceptance levels is important in determining how their relationship with each other will be affected and the type and consistency of messages they transmit to all of their children.

Many divorces have been attributed to differing levels of acceptance; sometimes this is manifested by jealousy or disenchantment when one parent is viewed by the other as turning all attention toward a disabled youngster and withdrawing it from the marriage partner or the other children. Erich Fromm postulated, in his popular work *The Art of Loving* (Fromm, 1956), that the mother's role is one of loving unconditionally, in order to provide a base of security for the growing child; and the father's role is to love conditionally, thus to motivate striving for socialization and betterment. The clinical observation that mothers frequently are more accepting of disabled children coincides with Fromm's hypothesis.

Acceptance is not a straightforward matter. It can become especially convoluted when intellectual acceptance exceeds emotional acceptance. This situation can generate double messages to all other family members, breeding confusion and distrust. The overt message may be one of loving concern, solicitude, or acknowledgment of "hard realities," yet be accompanied by covert expressions of anger, disappointment, or desperate longing to be out of the situation. As for the disabled children themselves, the quality of acceptance in a family is contingent on the members' self-esteem. Parents and siblings unsure of their own self-worth are likely to be more disturbed by the prospect of being objects of pity or disdain from their peers than are those who are more secure and self-confident. Some families also simply have higher degrees of tolerance for disruptions and perturbations than others; those low in tolerance will find acceptance more difficult.

Cultural characteristics also will play a part in parents' views about how to raise a child with a disability and what constitutes appropriate treatment and intervention (Danseco, 1997; Westbrook & Legge, 1993). The degree to which communal, as opposed to individualistic, values are emphasized in a culture will color the way that the family interprets the meaning of disability and the appropriate ways of coping with the situation.

Such factors as these play determining roles in the soundness of childrearing practices used with both disabled and nondisabled children. As cited earlier, the issue of protectiveness is one that is critically affected by the presence of a disability. At one extreme, overt rejections may lead to neglect or underprotectiveness, if not to institutionalization. The more frequently observed problem, however, is overprotection, excessive shelter, and disallowance of normal risk taking for the age level of the child—the "a scorched child fears the fire" reaction (Holmbeck et al., 2002). This tends to add increased dependency and experiential gaps to the list of handicaps the child one day must overcome and, in true vicious-circle fashion, creates additional burdens for the parents.

Overprotection can constrict the life choices available to the parents, especially to the mother, who is typically the chief caregiver. Many tangible responsibilities demand her time and attention, making it difficult for her to find time for herself and for work outside the home. The objective burdens of caregiving are not the only explanation for the effects on family life, however. A study of 50 mothers who had school-aged children with chronic disabilities (Wallander & Venters, 1995) found that the objective indices of the child's disability did not predict the mother's role restrictions. The things that did affect the mother's adjustment were her perceptions of the child's disability and the social support available to her.

Parents don't need any more burdens. If they have other children, they probably are facing problems of sibling jealousy because attention to the disabled child appears to be given at their expense. Just as a newborn baby sometimes is met by an older child's return to infantile behavior, so may siblings of disabled youngsters vie for parental time by exaggerating their own helplessness. When the child reaches school age, the parents face the problem of securing an adequate education, not an easy task regardless of whether the disability affects the child's ability to learn. (Educational issues will be treated in detail in Chapter 6.)

If disablement occurs after the individual reaches adulthood, it may be the marital family—a spouse and offspring of one's own—that will be most critically affected and visible to rehabilitation workers. The impact of disability on marriage relationships and parenting will be discussed next.

The Marital Family: Maintaining an Established Marriage

Disablement impacts differently on marriages that began before it occurred from those that begin afterward. In the former case, the disablement of a spouse may materially alter the basis of the partnership both parties made commitments to. In the latter, both have more realistic views of what to expect. In either case, spousal disability will critically influence family striving toward a homeostatic balance that facilitates the pursuit of happiness.

Herbert Rigoni, who directed the psychological services program at a major rehabilitation hospital for nearly a decade, indicates that a necessary, recurrent duty was to reassure spouses of recently disabled patients that it was "okay" for them to contemplate getting out of the marriages (personal communication). He points out that general population statistics show that a high proportion of marriages are failing at any given time; therefore, when a married person becomes disabled, a high probability exists that the marriage was in trouble already. Clearly, the additional stresses placed upon it by the sequelae of disability easily could be the "last straws."

As is true of shared tragedy in general, the disability experience sometimes strengthens the bonds of a relationship. This appears to be most likely, however, when the bonds were fairly strong in the first place. In other cases, the marriage bond may be tightened rather than strengthened, as when a dissatisfied partner feels, "Now I can't leave because he or she needs me." These are the cases to which Rigoni referred, and in which he attempted to help the individuals see that they had the freedom to go, so that staying could be a positive choice.

If a marriage survives the initial shock, the marital family will face essentially the same disruptions and adjustments described earlier in this chapter, and they will need to call on the same kinds of inner and outer resources. Their richness will determine whether the marriage will survive in the long run. In addition, the degree of genuine intimacy that existed in the predisability relationship is of paramount importance because, as several people quoted in this volume have repeated, "Disability is one hell of a test of love!"

Numerous observers have pointed out that a significant proportion of marriage relationships are reminiscent of "independent/parallel play." The term emanates from child psychology and describes very young children who play together at identical games—scooping sand, pounding blocks—but do not, in this process, relate in any meaningful way to each other. The stability of such marriages is founded on shared activity interests: sex, skiing, the theater, political activism, or whatever it may be. The partners may have fewer than average problems in "getting along" and may even be viewed as a model couple. Their harmony is only skin deep, however; it is a facade born of conflict avoidance through suppression and diversion of attention. The lack of genuine intimacy between them may remain unrecognized until disablement occurs. If there is no hope for resumption of shared activities, the marriage is likely to end.

This instance reflects the general principle that the survival of a marriage after disablement occurs depends largely on its prior solidity and the nature of the relationship. One important question is whether the couple was in the process of growing closer together or whether they already were growing apart. Regardless of the previous status of the marriage, however, the disability experience can create a dramatic disjuncture in the individual growth rates of the partners. For example, the disabled partner's emotional growth may accelerate or decelerate in comparison with the nondisabled partner. (The phenomenon of accelerated psychological growth among people with disabilities will be discussed further in Chapter 8.)

In addition to intimate and parallel play relationships, other possibilities exist. Symbiotic relationships are fairly frequent, and these are expectably thrown out of homeostatic balance when disability weakens or destroys the contribution of the affected partner. For example, the hostess wife may lose her value if a disability precludes continued entertaining and/or appearing to her husband's business associates to be an enviable "trophy wife." On the other hand, if sufficient latent resources are present, positive outcomes can ensue as when a dependent wife learns that she can work and support a family in a time of crisis. If the husband needed her dependency to stabilize his own psychic economy, his problems of adjustment, and therefore *theirs*, will face other complications.

A companionship marriage could be less adversely affected, unless economic strains prove unbearable. Such relationships are most common among advanced-age marriages; often, the specter of future disablement already has been acknowledged and some psychological preparation made. Nonetheless, no elderly couple is really prepared for the nightmares that accompany the serious disablement of one of them, especially those who want to stay in their own homes. A single, disabled, elderly person is apt to be placed in a caregiving facility; and while the pain of such change may be great, a measure of security is gained. When a spouse is present, however, the couple may fight to stay in familiar surroundings despite poverty, extreme hardship, and almost total inability to procure even the few supportive services that are available. All over the country, frail, elderly husbands and wives, who themselves are eligible for attendant care, are struggling to provide it to even more disabled spouses. In cases such as these, it is not the love relationship that is in jeopardy, it is survival itself.

A specific aspect of the relationship to consider is the nature of the experienced, expressed love between the two partners. Holistic health spokespeople remind us that we are tripartite in nature: we are body/mind/ spirit. So, too, can love be conceptualized, and each love relationship may stress one or two of these aspects over the other(s). This pattern will affect a couple's postdisability adjustment, but not in uniformly predictable ways. It simply must be contemplated in putting the pieces back together, in understanding what actually has been lost due to disability, what has not, and what will require attention in rebuilding.

Whether or not sexuality was a central or peripheral part of a relationship prior to disablement, it almost certainly will become an important adjustment area afterward if significant changes are entailed. Sexual arousal is highly vulnerable to stress (such as changed physical or emotional circumstance), and sexual behavior patterns that have yielded satisfaction in the past are very reluctantly relinquished. Since sexuality is a major topic of the following chapter, this aspect of the marital family's adjustment to disability is only mentioned here.

Equally important is whether love is experienced as either possessive or enabling; that is, whether the partners are motivated to ensnare each other and maintain the psychological and "political" (powerbase) status quo, or to facilitate each others' growth through mutual support, caring, and sharing. Obviously, the prognosis for possessive love relationships is poor under any kind of stress, while that for enabling love relationships is favorable.

In addition to the couple's relationship with one another, the impact of disability—in one or both of them—on parenting practices and success in child rearing creates still another important set of issues that must be examined.

An essential characteristic of any marriage that survives the onset of a severe disability and continues to be rewarding to both partners is that of balance. Both partners must be able to make valuable contributions to the other, and both must be able to receive. A situation in which one person becomes responsible for caring and the other is the recipient of care is doomed to failure (or abject unhappiness, at best). The rehabilitation team needs to be sensitive to this potential pitfall and help both partners to recognize and maintain their unique contributions to the relationship.

Child Rearing

Many questions are asked on this topic, but little research has been done and few answers are given (Kirshbaum, 1996; Olkin, 1999). According to Buck (1993), the literature is impoverished in this area, and what little exists is preponderantly speculative exposition, purporting to answer such questions as: should disabled individuals attempt to raise children? how can discipline be maintained? can a disabled parent serve as an appropriate role model? what if a father can't play ball with his son? The fact that such questions are asked may be part of the problem. Buck and Hohmann's (1983) own research on parenting found no support for the foreboding speculations found in the prior literature on these and related issues. The questions seem to reflect proclivities for stereotyping disabled people and their lifestyles.

Much of the writing about "parentification" blatantly reveals such prejudicial assumptions. This concept maintains that children of parents with disabilities are at risk for taking on physical or emotional caretaking roles at inappropriately young ages. The concept was originally applied to parents who abused alcohol and other substances, and then it was applied without evidence to parents with other kinds of disabilities. Throughout the society, expectations and practices differ with regard to tasks that children are given to carry out. Olkin (1999) points out that although anecdotal reports indicate that inappropriate responsibilities may be put upon a minority of children, the problem is likely to stem from the lack of adequate support services for the family rather than pathology attributable to the parent's disability.

Apart from fears of parentification, it usually is expected that children who are part of a family when parental disablement occurs will manage to grow up relatively unscathed. Nonetheless, disabled individuals confront strong social pressures against having children if they have not done so yet; occasionally, they are urged to relinquish children they already have. The questions listed previously, and many others, are posed as challenges. No negative answers can be supplied, but the absence of positive data is treated as if that should be sufficient deterrent. Much more research is needed to explode the myths related to parenting with a disability, and some of this work is underway at Through the Looking Glass, a service and research program located in California. This research, educational, and service center was established in 1982 in Berkeley with the following mission: "To create, demonstrate and encourage nonpathological and empowering resources and model early intervention services for families with disability issues in parent or child which integrate expertise derived from personal disability experience and disability culture" (Design, 2002). They have conducted a number of studies, including one slated for completion in 2002 on parents with disabilities and their teens.

Buck and Hohmann's discussion (1983) suggests that while emotional disabilities may pose serious problems for effective childrearing, physical disabilities do not necessarily do so. It is the parents' general emotional health and attitudes about their disabilities—not the disabilities per se—that can create problems. For example, if a man believes his inability to play ball with his son is a problem, or if his wife does, then the child-parent relationship may suffer. Another man with an identical disability, who believes the verbal guidance he offers compensates for any physical incapacities, can be a better than average father regardless of the severity of his disability.

A substantial body of literature exists on parenting youngsters who have developmental intellectual disabilities, but only a few studies have focused on parents with mental retardation. There appears to be a presumption in society that mentally retarded people cannot possibly serve as adequate parents; however, one occasionally observes or hears of an "exception" to this "rule." Ehlers Flint's (2001) qualitative study revealed that mothers with cognitive disabilities have common positive feelings about parenting and their abilities to nurture their children, although those who had a personal history of trauma were less confident. Another study (Llewellyn & McConnell, 2002) indicated that family members were extremely important in the lives of women with learning disabilities and those who lacked family involvement often were quite socially isolated. These findings underscore the danger of simplistically attributing isolated findings about parental functioning to disability when so many other social and environmental correlates may be contributing to observed relationships.

A rehabilitation psychologist interviewed by the first author quoted the famous eight-word maxim on correct parenting—"Have 'em, love 'em, and leave 'em alone!"—and added, "There's no reason a disabled parent can't do that as well as anyone else." Additional interview material from rehabilitation psychologists tended to agree with Buck and Hohmann's findings (1983) that the children of reasonably well-adjusted disabled parents differ from children of nondisabled parents mainly in that they are more affectionate and appreciative toward their parents and more responsible or mature than the typical child of the same age. This probably results from being assigned household and other responsibilities out of necessity, and is reminiscent of earlier times when children were a needed, valued part of the family work-force. (The loss of a role of economic importance to the family is suggested frequently as a causal factor in today's serious behavioral/emotional problems among children and adolescents.) The child of a blind father was described as follows:

> At 3 years old, Christin could guide her father anywhere and she loved it. Whenever she was along, that was her job and she guarded it jealously. Once, she inadvertently walked under a barrier that laid her father out cold. She was mortified but was finally consoled that it was an understandable error and she still had her job.

In some cases, children of disabled parents are thought to be old beyond their years, but this is attributed more to the emotional health of the parents than to the existence of a bodily disability.

When a disabled individual can produce children, and especially when a coparent is present, the opinions of others as to suitability for parenthood are of little practical consequence. Criticizing the childrearing practices of others is a very popular indoor sport, hardly limited to people with disabilities. However, there are several circumstances in which an individual's right to be a parent arises as an issue: when nonvoluntary sterilization is considered (for retarded women usually); when a social agency or estranged spouse attempts to remove a child from a disabled parent's custody, on the grounds that disability renders him or her unfit for parenting; and when a disabled individual is unable to produce children and seeks—often fruitlessly—to adopt. These and other issues relating to parental rights will be treated in Chapter 9.

5

Pairing

Sexuality and Intimacy

The urge for pairing is almost ubiquitous, and, despite long-lasting rumors to the contrary, it does not disappear when disability intervenes. In fact, as will be seen, it sometimes grows stronger. Part of the urge is biological; we seem to be preprogrammed with a drive to continue our own particular gene pool. Too, the process of procreating feels good and we have strong proclivities to act on the principle, "If it feels good, do it."

Throughout recorded human history, social pressures have been exerted toward sanctioned patterns of pairing, and our immediate forebears endorsed one as permanent as the ravages of childbearing would allow. That is, in earlier times, males could be expected to wear out a wife or two, then avail themselves of another, creating a pattern of serial monogamy. As medical advances made childbearing less lethal, however, single, lifetime pairings became the social ideal in what is referred to as "the civilized world."

With monogamous pairings the accepted standard, sanctions against other patterns developed. Individuals electing not to conform were regarded as suspect, and those unable to procure mates were treated with contempt (tough) or pity (tender). For both biological and social reasons, individuals with functional defects were not prized as mating candidates and could expect to be rejected. The social order saw no earthly purpose in perpetuating what might have been defective gene pools, and survival requirements placed negative value on mates who could not pull their own weight. Happily, as survival has become less contingent on physical abilities to secure food and shelter, the rejection of disabled mates has lessened.

Next enters ego. With developing self-awareness, the urge for pairing became not only a matter of biological and social survival, but survival of the ego as well. To be mateless became a public humiliation, a clear message that one was regarded as inferior stuff. On the other hand, to have a mate of your own offered proof of your being worthwhile to someone and, therefore, salvation from ignominy.

Last, but assuredly not least, and true to the topic of this chapter, pairing offers a convenient, effective means for gratifying the human needs to give and receive love. Love seems to evolve in such a way that much of its power to gratify takes time to develop, and this can occur only in an extended relationship. Moreover, considerable attention to one's object of love is required.

Thus, many forces converge to reinforce the urge toward pairing, and with some degree of exclusivity. None of them are neutralized by the advent of disability, and some are enhanced. If you are disabled, your peers may prefer that you not reproduce, but you are likely to have the same desire as everyone else to do exactly that. When the sensual pleasures associated with sexual contact occupy a high proportion of public media space and time as well as private conversation, the chances are that you'll want to get in on that, too.

When it comes to social and ego survival, a disabled person may have stronger than ordinary motivation to pair off on a long-term basis. Having someone who has promised to be there, for better or worse, can allay many anxieties about being able to fend for yourself. You may know that a quasiwelfare state will not let you starve, but it will not provide a very desirable lifestyle. As for your ego, it already has taken a beating and it doesn't want any more. For once, the ability to attract lovers becomes an excessively important proof of continuing worth in the face of self-rejection due to disablement. Although disability can be one of many factors that contribute indirectly to impaired ability to love, in the main, it does not neutralize this desire either; and it virtually never extinguishes the need to be on the receiving end of love.

Not all nondisabled people are interested in pairing, and this obviously holds true for disabled people as well. Some people can't stand children; others can't stand sex; and still others may have enjoyed either or both in the past, yet moved beyond them. Countless other reasons for the avoidance/ neglect of pairing exist, and they apply equally well to the disabled and nondisabled. But, given that for most the urge is strong, the process of pairing is problematical enough under ordinary circumstances to have generated billions of dollars worth of business enterprise to aid or exploit it. The cosmetic and fashion industries; the entertainment industry, especially records and films; the preponderance of self-help publications; the popularity of liposuction, breast enlargement, and other forms of plastic surgery; and body-building gymnasiums and spas are among the most obvious of such applications.

In addition, an overwhelming proportion of people who seek counseling, psychotherapy, or human potential development offerings do so because their love lives aren't satisfactory. When a disability is present, "normal" problems are apt to be exaggerated and new ones almost surely will emerge. Unfortunately, those with special needs are not only deprived of the extra attention they require, they are altogether ignored by mainstream "pairing industries." The first area in which help may be needed is that of developing readiness to attempt pairing behavior, because of the vulnerability such a commitment creates.

Readiness: Self-Confidence Plus Know-How

Many grown men can recall the courage it took to ask for their first date. "What if she laughs?" Or worse yet, "What if she tries to be nice but can't hide the fact that she'd rather be dead than be seen with a creep like me?" Similarly, many adult women can recapture the agony of wishing he would call—anyone would call—when a dates-only party was but a week away. The vulnerability of being (exposed as) unselected in the game of pairing is a fearsome one for both sexes. Adjectives fail when individuals have disabilities that the objects of their desires may reject. In a society that venerates beautiful people, serious flaws seem intolerable.

Harnessing the confidence to confront a challenge for which one feels ill equipped is no easy matter. The necessary preparation can be divided into (1) making the most of what you have, and (2) developing a philosophy of life that places more value on the achievable and less on the unachievable. The "up front" resource in pairing is physical attractiveness, and frequently this is impaired by disability. The clutter of wheelchairs, braces, and crutches; the appearance of disuse atrophy, joint and bone deformities, absent appendages, sunken eyes, scarring, and the bodily irregularities that may accompany mental retardation are harder to camouflage than a flat chest, a receding hairline, or thick ankles. In addition to these tangible accoutrements of disability, the onset of disability may bring distressing changes in self-concept. A group of women with spinal cord injuries rated their bodies as being only half as attractive as they had been before the injury (Kettl, Zarefoss, Jacoby, Garman, et al., 1991) and reported that their perceived change in attractiveness was one of the most difficult effects to accept.

Maximizing Physical Attractiveness

Sometimes, physically disabled people feel embarrassed about making the effort. They are so convinced that the end result will fall short of even modest success that they prefer not to advertise that they've tried and failed. Imagined success usually involves idealized images of what they might have been had disability not intervened—or of other unattainable standards of comparison. People with mild to moderate mental retardation are aware of the degree to which their bodies fall short of cultural ideals. A study of 17 women found that, like most women without disabilities, they were hard-pressed to identify anything positive about their bodies, and a majority were particularly dissatisfied with their weight (McCarthy, 1998).

Years ago Robert Shushan (1974) conducted an exciting doctoral dissertation on appearance and disability. The project was initiated by his preschool-aged daughter. Riding in their car one day, she observed a child in a passing car and asked, "Daddy, is that little girl retarded?" Shushan responded that she appeared to be, and then he began to question this event. "No wonder mentally retarded people are put at a distance by others, if their differentness can be 'diagnosed' by a 4-year-old in a passing car. If concerted efforts were made to help them look more 'normal,' would they be accepted more?"

In the project that ensued, he took "before" pictures and then spent approximately twenty minutes with each subject, applying corrective grooming and coaching them to adopt facial expressions that maximized their good features and minimized their flaws. (For example, if they had good teeth, they were encouraged to show them when they smiled. If the teeth were bad, they were encouraged to do the opposite.) Wigs, cosmetic eyeglass frames, and everyday makeup were the only props he used. Then, "after" pictures were taken, and the resulting album is a dramatic presentation of the difference twenty minutes can make. On the left, one sees pitifully unattractive mentally retarded individuals; on the right is a collection of average to outstandingly appealing people. The panel of judges was unable to correctly identify the "after" pictures as those of retarded people when they were interspersed with pictures of nonretarded individuals. Shushan (personal communication) indicates that seeing themselves looking attractive had some lasting effects on the subjects, shown in efforts to maintain themselves in the more attractive mode; however, these would deteriorate over time without "booster shots" to keep the improved images fresh in their minds.

Obviously, the subjects of this study can't go on forever keeping a lock of hair over a sunken jaw, not smiling, or doing whatever was required to get a "normal looking" snapshot. However, if looking better has a positive impact on how they are regarded by themselves and others, the appropriate dental work or plastic surgery to make the improvements permanent would seem to be worthy investments. At least as much should be done as would be done if the person weren't intellectually disabled.

The appearance of mentally retarded people has been neglected for a number of reasons, some not altogether a tribute to those who care for them.

At the most benign level, the neglect reflects an attitude that, if they aren't aware of their own appearance, there is no reason to create a source of concern for them. In addition, however, the neglect is sometimes an intentional effort to discourage pairing behavior. Operators of residential facilities find that management of their charges becomes more difficult when romantic or sexual alliances are formed, and they hope that utility haircuts and nonattention to dental and grooming needs will be deterrents to such unwelcome complications. Moreover, the prospect of sexual activity among people with mental retardation is disturbing to some individuals, similar to the discomfort experienced by adults over the sexual drives and experimentation of children.

Although data are not available on the subject, it seems likely that issues of appearance also are overlooked in other kinds of rehabilitation programs, though perhaps for different reasons. Sensitized to the problems of negative public attitudes, counselors and others in the field are trained to view appearance as a shallow concern and to deny it credence. Reports of more recent studies like Olushan's have not been located in the psychological literature, and even demonstration articles are rare. One exception is a chapter by Kammerer-Quayle (2002), who has created a hospital-based "Center for Image Enhancement" which provides consultation regarding corrective cosmetics, flattering clothing, and positive self-esteem to individuals with visible disabilities. The center grew from Kammerer-Quayle's personal experience with facial disfigurement and her desire to be recognized as a worthwhile human being rather than shunned because of appearance.

It may be slightly ironic that while rehabilitation professionals assiduously look beneath the surface and avoid responding to appearance, people with disabilities generally are more attuned to the importance of maximizing their attractiveness today than was true only a few years ago. For example, some male college students have found that participation in sports and physical activity can improve their appearance as well as strength (Taub, Blinde, & Greer, 1999). The heightened consciousness issuing from the disability rights movement has affected nearly every realm of being. As a result, many people are trying consciously and conscientiously to make the best of what they've got, not only with respect to looks, but also by exploiting in positive ways the unusual aspects of their experience. Once pairing efforts are made, they find that having successfully combatted adversity has given them qualities of character that are valued by potential lovers and mates; and that, although what they have to offer is different from what the ordinary person regards as requisite, it is no less worthy of appreciation.

Attention is paid to both the inner and outer determinants of beauty. Such encompassing "figure flaws" as total-body disuse atrophy accompanied by full-time use of a motorized wheelchair are dealt with as matter of factly and effectively as possible. What can't be changed can be compensated for, and the human-potential/holistic-health movement of the 1970s contributed materially to helping everyone understand that beauty has more to do with what comes from within than the perfection of physical attributes. Part of what comes from within is the message that "I care about this body enough to make it as aesthetically pleasing as possible (without pouring excessive time and energy into it)." That message of self-respect helps to generate respect flowing from others, and an expectancy that "This person likes who he or she is, so maybe I would, too."

Although such a level of self-acceptance is reached by a sizable proportion of disabled people today, it does not come quickly or automatically. Each individual seems to follow the entire phylogeny, which begins with self-loathing that becomes neutralized and, hopefully, finally transforms into a positive view of self. Dana, for example, says she burst into tears when she first saw her thin, lower legs after six months in bed. She wore ankle-length dresses during the fifties counter to fashion to hide their awful truth from view. Fifteen years later, she joyfully showed as much of them as possible during the miniskirt era because:

> Miniskirts were so easy to cope with in a wheelchair, and by that time, skinny legs didn't seem so bad. No guy ever rated my legs as one of my better features, but at least I got "ho hums" instead of the "yecchs" I had expected. I figure if your ego can't take a few "ho hums," you're in deep trouble!

Personality Resources

Maximizing physical attractiveness seems to be one of the few areas of "resource development" that can be accomplished through direct striving. The others, which fall under the general rubric of "personality," are more likely to develop as by-products of less specifically goal-directed efforts to mature and grow as a human being. For example, a self-conscious effort to become a good listener is apt to end in a manipulative facade where inattentiveness to what is being said is masked while the "listener" busily checks out whether the performance is having its desired effect of entrancing the speaker. The genuinely good listener, on the other hand, is such because of sincere caring about the other person, not because of skillful use of a technique. The speaker almost surely will sense the difference and will find the latter more attractive, whether or not he or she can articulate why.

There is little doubt that people with disabilities face special challenges in the dating game (Gill, 1996; Rintala, Howland, Nosek, Bennet, & Young, 1997). What is important for disabled people (or others who are/feel handicapped in the pairing process) is to be aware of the personality resources they do possess and place appropriate value on them; to know that "This is what I have to offer and that's not bad!" Even more important is to recognize that this is precisely what everyone needs, too, in order to approach pairing with confidence. Having a disability does not, in this way, create a unique or peculiar situation.

Courtship

Bach and Deutsch (1970) introduced the term "pairing" as an alternative to the term "courtship" in an effort to distinguish the traditional "put your best foot forward" approach (courtship) from a more honest and open style of "being yourself" (pairing). They point out that traditional courtship rituals often lead to rude surprises because flaws, foibles, and inconsistencies are hidden until after a commitment is made. "All's fair in love and war" is the slogan of such old-fashioned trickery. Because romantic duplicity has been idealized throughout a long span of history, both parties willingly collude in the deception. Unfortunately, both parties also pay.

People with disabilities have the usually unwelcome advantage of being less able than most to play courtship games. In this context the well-worn phrase, "What you see is what you get," has a poignant ring. To illustrate, it's hard to feign fascination with the art galleries your intended adores if you're blind. Or, if you're deaf, how do you display a rewarding response to sweet nothings whispered in your ear? Also, it's definitely not easy to stage a sexy entrance in a wheelchair. More basic than this, if you have a disability, a sizable proportion of the field of potential lovers will classify you peremptorily as ineligible for courtship consideration because of the functional and/or aesthetic liabilities you present. Being confronted with this form of dehumanization while you're trying to maintain confidence and hope can stimulate insight and growth in the strong, but it can virtually destroy those whose egos are weak.

As pointed out, a normal degree of boldness must be tempered lest advances by a disabled person be viewed with alarm. It takes time and experience for one to develop the inner surety to accept, philosophically, a rejection so automatic that it is barely recognized as such by the rejecter without, at the same time, accepting the rejecter's opinion of oneself. Once such assuredness is gained, however, automatic rejections can be dismissed in the knowledge that others exist who will look beyond the disability to decide whether they like whatever else is there.

Mikhail was an energetic, fun-loving fifteen-year old who was just beginning to explore his sexuality and relationships with girls when he sustained a spinal cord injury. Afterwards, he avoided flirtation or dating, and just worked at being a good buddy to his classmates. His first dating experience came during college when he met an attractive student and struck up a friendship. Several weeks later he got up the courage to ask her out to a movie—his first real date. She accepted, and for the next few weeks they enjoyed the delightful experience of new attraction. Then, on their fourth date, his worst fear came true—an involuntary bowel accident while they were driving to a party. Sure that this would be the end, Mikhail said that he wanted to "crawl into a hole and die." Jeanne, on the other hand, just suggested that he open the window and go home to change clothes before continuing to the party. Their relationship grew and led to marriage during their junior year. They have now been married for more than ten years, and they have a young son and daughter.

More authentic sharing may take place when one or both courters has a disability, but this is not always so. It may be necessary to tell a prospective lover that you use a leg bag, yet cover up completely how wretched you feel about that fact. However, if anything is going to destroy the relationship later on, it will not be the leg bag, it will be the wearer's failure to integrate it into a positive self-image. As usual, it is lesions in self-acceptance that disrupt long-term love relationships.

Some of the problems arising are less philosophical than practical, such as fitting two wheelchairs into a car, or one into a sports car. In addition, a frequent complaint of people who find themselves attracted to individuals using wheelchairs is that the chairs make it impossible to "accidentally" get physically close. Also, so much of the courtship process centers about looking, talking, and doing together that impairments in any of these functions can damage spontaneity and require adjustments to be made. The dimly lit restaurant, so important in traditional courtship rituals, can be devastating to someone who needs good light to lip-read, barely discern the writing on a menu, or avoid bumping into other diners' chairs.

Assuming the necessary adjustments are made and an alliance survives the tragicomic buffeting it has in store, the disabled lover may be in for a new set of tests and surprises. As Dana put it:

> If you think Tracy and Hepburn looked astonished when their white middle-class daughter brought Sidney Poitier home to dinner, wait until Mr. America brings

home a crip! One guy said his mother went into a diatribe about how girls like me should be locked up in institutions where they can't get out to try to marry people's perfectly normal sons. Hell, I hadn't even planned to ask him to go steady!

It's not easy to be objective when a guy wants you to reassure him that he's not somehow abnormal for having fallen for you—and variations of that happened several times—but it's even harder to stay cool when he asks for advice on how to deal with parents who have dismissed you from the human race.

Courtship isn't solely a time for convincing someone you'd be a good partner for fun, sex, or maybe even marriage; it is also a time for screening out those willing candidates who might not be good for you. As illustrated by Dana's experiences, disabled people may have a particularly difficult task in this regard. People who are attracted to persons who are dependent on others for basic life functions may need to be needed in ways and for reasons they themselves don't fully understand. Sensing an unwholesome flavor to a lover's solicitousness, and rejecting it when it is found, are two equally difficult challenges, especially when the field of choices is limited. Developing the inner strength and emotional independence to say, "I'd rather be alone than used, controlled, or exploited," is likely to evolve from a sequence of valuable mistakes.

In addition, people who think poorly of themselves also may tend to seek out visible underdogs with whom to form romantic alliances. In relationships with physically disabled individuals, they may feel more worthy simply because they are physically intact. People with such tenuous self-respect may prove difficult to be close to, and this can be particularly troublesome to a partner who is not fully self-reliant. From the other's point of view, to choose a mate or lover who seems like a pussycat because of a disability and then find oneself linked to an emotionally stronger, more independent tiger can feel like a disaster. A similarly misguided view of women with disabilities has reportedly led some pornographers to portray them as passive and hence the ultimately compliant sex objects (Elman, 2001).

Dana claims that if you are disabled, the ideal is to search for someone who wants you in spite of your disability, not because of it. She points out, however, that this requires you to have the emotional stamina to withstand a period of indecision and torment on your lover's part while he or she decides whether you're worth the various sacrifices that must be made. Others disagree. Max counters that he and his wife got married because:

We felt sorry for each other. I was a quad and she was tall, gangly, and no one else even looked at her. It has all worked out, though. We gave each other the love and support we needed and we've built a good life. As a matter of fact, Joy's become quite attractive as she's matured. I'm still a quad, but I *have* gotten rich, so I'm not such a bad catch either!

The Sexual Encounter

When the relationship either evolves or catapults into sexual activity, still another set of tests and surprises awaits. There are the usual concerns that generate a continuous market for the publishers of sex manuals and less didactically oriented erotica. Since most people seem to have at least a few "hangups" with respect to sexual functioning, there is no reason to believe that people with disabilities would have been free of them had disablement not intervened. In fact, there is evidence indicating that people with early-onset disabilities are significantly disadvantaged compared with their peers in terms of basic sexual knowledge (Erikson & Erikson, 1992; Swartz, 1993; Szollos & McCabe, 1995). Still, one generally can assume the presence of doubts, fears, and confusions that bear no particular relationship to disability. In addition to this base of "normal" perplexity, disabilities frequently create further complications of attitude and action in the sexual role.

Body Image

Attitudinally, a central issue is body image. If a disability has altered one's appearance and/or mobility away from an accepted norm, antipathy toward the body may assume interfering proportions. Fears that a prospective lover may find it grotesque or uninviting are heaped upon the normative baseline of anxieties about a pending sexual encounter. Disability-related body aberrations that can be masked somewhat by carefully selected clothing will be revealed when the couple retires to the bedchamber. Moreover, limited mobility may threaten to render one the unpardonable in these days of sexual liberation and preoccupation: a lousy lay. If urinary or fecal collection devices are added to the equation, positive regard for the body requiring them may plunge precipitously. At the root, if you hate the way your body looks and behaves, it will not be easy to offer it joyfully to a lover.

Learning to love your body, no matter how far it falls short of the cinema-induced ideal (or even a more reasonable standard) takes time and is part of a larger process of self-acceptance. As this process advances, ideals can be relinquished for the apparitions they are and reality, of whatever sort, can become beautiful simply because it is. All over the world, disabled people and the rehabilitation workers who serve them are paying attention to such matters, and many have come forward to testify that they know such attitudinal transitions are possible because they have made them. They have found their bodies are loved because they are loved, spasms, deformities, collection devices, and all. A surprising number of both men and women who have severe disabilities report being told by nondisabled lovers that they "look better with their clothes off." This may be partly a function of eliminating fear of the unknown and partly due to the simple fact that some figures just don't wear clothes as well as others. Newly disabled people aren't likely to believe such hopeful messages right away, but, given time, most can learn. This is a relatively new awareness, and it has grown out of conscious, concerted efforts to retrain attitudinal tendencies and to make room for a wider range of differences that are not only accepted but appreciated and loved.

Interestingly, some disabled people have come to be in the vanguard of the sexual revolution, opening doors to self-exploration for people in general. Sexuality is seen as a right that has been denied to people with disabilities; as a result, the problems are being discussed openly and exhaustively today, not only in rehabilitation settings, but even on television. Perhaps because the surface problems are related to politically important attitudinal barriers and practical issues that are somewhat distinct from the more usual psychodynamic factors that frighten people into silence, they are somehow easier to approach and examine than the typical problems of sexual dysfunction. Rehabilitation workers and others thus observe increasing numbers of disabled people modeling what seems to be an extraordinary degree of openness about their sexuality and related concerns. This gives them permission and encouragement to be more open and less fearful about their own.

Many of the problems discussed relate to sexual action as well as attitudes: the practical problems that arise when one or both lovers are paralyzed, deaf, or otherwise impaired. The sexual performance and enjoyment problems of people with motor disabilities receive most of the attention, but people who are blind or deaf have their share of problems, too. Harris, for example, points out that as a result of losing his hearing he still has occasional trouble "diagnosing" whether some of his wife's physical movements during intercourse are the sequelae of her passion or efforts to let him know that he is hurting her.

The list of practical problems that can ensue when one or both lovers has a physical disability is virtually endless. Paralysis creates one set of problems, pain another, amputations yet another, and neurological impairments affecting erotic sensation and bowel and bladder control produce still more. The literature contains information about sexual issues that are common in specific disabilities, including spinal cord injury (Donohue & Gebhard, 1995; Sipski, 1993), multiple sclerosis (Dupont, 1996; Stenager, Stenager, & Jensen, 1994), brain injury (Medlar, 1993; Zasler, 1993), chronic pain (Monga, Tan, Oster-mann, Monga, & Grabois, 1998), amputation (Bodenheimer, Kerrigan, Garber, & Monga, 2000), and cerebral palsy (Shuttlesworth, 2000). When an individual is very severely disabled, even masturbation may be impossible without assistance; or, if both lovers are severely disabled, an attendant's help may be necessary to make sexual contact possible. Fortunately, this era of sexual liberation has brought with it at least a few good-quality guidebooks that disabled people can profit from reading, both for technical advice on solving specific problems and for their overall message that, as far as the need for and right to sexual expression and enjoyment are concerned, however you are all right. The internet offers a cornucopia of information on sexuality and disability, some good and some questionable. As always, the key is relying on reliable sources, such as the National Institutes of Health or the Sexuality Information and Education Council of the United States (see, for example http://www.siecus.org/pubs/biblio/bibs0009.html) (Meade, 2002). One Web site, designed to educate women with disabilities about reproductive health care was shown to be effective in meeting its goals (Pendergrass, Nosek, & Holcomb, 2001), confirming the generally held belief about the great potential of the internet for conveying knowledge. Accessing enlightened perspectives can provide people with disabilities freedom and courage to meet their own needs. A couple may be unaware that hundreds of other severely disabled couples are asking their assistants with varying degrees of comfort to help position them for lovemaking. This couple, then, must make a far bolder move to broach the possibility with their own assistant(s) than an informed couple.

The long silence on the conjoint subject of sex and disability was, in part, an outgrowth of devaluative attitudes. (As for the other part, everyone in the "civilized world" has been sexually oppressed for a long time.) Overvaunted values placed on physical attractiveness led inexorably to the multilevel conclusions that disabled people are distorted and/or ugly; therefore, no one will want or permit sexual contact with them; therefore, the kindest thing to do is help them keep their minds on other things. Moreover, the thought of disabled people wanting sexual involvement carries an implied threat that "If they want it at all, they might want it with *me*—and what would I say? I wouldn't want to hurt such a person's feelings." Disabled people held similar values and attitudes, and a conspiracy of silence ensued. But today is an era of massive attention to the acceptance, even celebration, of differences whether related to race, nationality, gender, age, disability, or individual temperament. Although the silence currently is broken more by lip service than genuine clamor to embrace the unknown, such is a first step, and more palpable gains may follow.

Unfortunately, embracing differences sometimes takes unwholesome turns. The attraction of some men to women with amputations has long been considered as a form of sexual varietism that stems from emotional disturbance. As disabled people began to talk among themselves and go public with their experiences, it came to light that individuals of both sexes may be sexually drawn to a wide range of disabilities more than to the people who have them. Several disabled people who unknowingly formed alliances with such individuals describe as nightmares their dawning recognition of the source of their partner's titillation. Realizing that she had been sought out as a "freak" led Peggy to contemplate suicide. On the other hand, Naomi, after a period of time, was able to place the pathology where it belonged: not with herself, but with her former partner.

> He thought having sex with me would be kinky. When he first blurted that out, I was destroyed. Now I just think he was a little bit crazy, but I'm not going to get crazy, too. If I were "normal," I wouldn't blame myself for accidentally getting hooked up with a foot fetishist as long as I got out when I realized he was a kinko, that is.

Another side of human acceptance is illustrated by a story told by Marya. A bilateral, above-knee amputee, she had been married to Emory for over three years when he confessed to her one night that he had, since early adolescence, entertained fantasies of having relations with women such as herself; and that her disability had been the prepotent source of his attraction to her initially. By then they had established a solid marital relationship and were viewed as an ideal couple by many of their friends. Marya recalled:

> I wanted to die. I wanted to vomit. Actually, I wanted to kill him. But somehow, the next morning, when he begged me not to leave him, because he had grown to love me for many other reasons, I weakened. He had trusted me enough to tell me something that still bothered—no, terrified him. He had given me love and support and now he was asking me to accept *his* disability—a psychological problem that he was repulsed by and didn't understand. I agreed to stay if he would go to a psychiatrist. That was ten years ago. I don't know that he has completely resolved all of his hangups, but our marriage is a good one . . . and whatever crazy thing he has for my stumps, he is a lovely guy I'm glad I hung onto.

Personal anecdotes come down on both sides of the question regarding the motives and wholesomeness of devotees. The scientific literature is similarly unclear about whether this attraction empowers or exploits people with disabilities (Aguilera, 2000). Perhaps, as with other relationships, there is no single answer but it depends upon the individuals involved.

Sexual Abuse

As the subjects of sexuality and disability were opened to public discussion, it became known that people with disabilities have been victims of sexual abuse, probably with even greater frequency than have nondisabled individuals (Nosek, 1996). Cole (1991) and others have described the once-hidden problem and cited reasons for its prevalence. Persons with severe disabilities are more likely to live in institutional settings where they can fall prey to unscrupulous aides and other staff (Sobsey & Mansell, 1994). Sexual abuse may also be perpetrated by other residents in congregate settings. In a five-year study that identified 72 substantiated cases of abuse by disabled people, Furey and Niesen (1994) found that although most of the perpetrators were men, both men and women were vulnerable to assault. Individuals who are unable to speak or who are viewed as being unreliable reporters have been particularly vulnerable because they are unable to effectively defend themselves. Children with disabilities often are subjected to repeated examination, handling, and undressing by medical personnel, and they may become confused about what kinds of touch are appropriate, again adding to their vulnerability. Further, people of any age who are physically dependent upon others for care, may be reluctant to complain and possibly alienate people whose help they require to live. Although further study of this issue is needed, recognition of the problem is a first and important step to reducing its impact on the lives of people with disabilities.

The Mythology of Sexual Perfection

Several states have legislation requiring specified health practitioners to acquire continuing education credits in human sexuality. These training sessions rather consistently attend to the matter of exploding myths surrounding sexual experience. Included among these is "the myth of the orgasm." It is yesterday's news that the fictional ideal of simultaneous orgasm seldom exists in reality. Somewhat more current are the considerations that the orgasm may not be essential to sexual fulfillment at all. As people have become free to tell the truth about their sexual experiences, it turns out that many couples—disabled and nondisabled alike—place a high value on sex lives that seldom if ever culminate in, or otherwise include, the phantasmagoric orgasm.

Again, people with disabilities have been in the forefront of myth exploding. Individuals with neurological impairments to genital sensation report both satisfying sensual/sexual expression that does not include orgasm and orgasmic experiences produced by fantasy and/or localized in nongenital areas. Hearing it said by people with sensory impairments has made it possible for numbers of nondisabled people to acknowledge that a similar pattern is familiar to them, too. It has become common practice in sex therapy clinics to de-emphasize striving for orgasm among women and men who find that it does not flow naturally from them. Instead of focusing massive efforts upon bringing it about, as in earlier days, clients are encouraged to savor the other pleasurable sensations associated with sexual activity and avoid creating a climate of weary, frustrated negativity because a particular sensation is not readily forthcoming. Not surprisingly, a number of them find that when they cease their desperate striving, the orgasm occurs. Those who do not have this experience are likely to find that nonorgasmic pleasurable sensations are sufficient reward in themselves. For all, the sensual pleasures and spiritual fulfillments of physical intimacy with a lover are stressed.

The 1970s and 1980s were a time of sexual freedom and exploration for many Americans, including those with disabilities. As the bans on formerly censored speech and activities were been lifted, the new message became, "Whatever with whomever is okay." This message became less acceptable a few years later, however, with the spreading of sexually transmitted diseases, particularly HIV/AIDS. The unbridled enthusiasm for sexual education and counseling within rehabilitation centers has abated, but the total silence of earlier eras has not returned.

As wholesome as the increased attention to sexuality was for both disabled and nondisabled people who were viewed or viewed themselves as desirous of activities and fulfillments that were somehow taboo, it concomitantly produced a new mythology of sexual perfection. This, in turn, created further barriers to self-esteem when the quantitative and qualitative ideals described in the sex manuals are not achieved or achievable. Moreover, once sexuality was legitimized, it was no longer so legitimate to regard it as an inconsequential or a sometime thing. As a result, people with low levels of sex drive (and, like other human traits, sex drive is assumed to be distributed along the normal curve) are forcing themselves to become the sensuous man or woman regardless of their natural proclivities. Disabled people have been caught up in this just as much as nondisabled people and, in some cases, perhaps even more.

Certain people whose disabilities so severely inhibit mobility and/or sensual gratification that they would just as soon leave sex alone feel that they are not permitted to do so now. The message coming from every direction is that in order to be psychologically "whole" they must be, in the words of Ernie, "hornier than thou." Although this is most likely to be heard from people with phobic feelings about sexuality that are unrelated to their disabilities, such is not always the case. Ernie also provides a good example of a related problem that arises. He bitterly denounced the efforts of a psychologist at his rehabilitation hospital to help spinal-cord injured patients adjust sexually.

> She came in there wearing her miniskirts and strutting around and using four letter words and I wouldn't have trusted her any farther than a quad like me could have thrown her. She was working out her own thing, not helping anyone else . . . and she didn't pay any attention to the women, just the men.

Ernie's wife indicates that their sexual adjustment was relatively uncomplicated; in fact, he became a better lover for her because much of his pleasure centered about satisfying her. Her view of the "help" he was offered was this:

> I think [the psychologist] glommed onto the big furor about sex and disability as a way of dealing with her own problems. She was some kind of zealot and that really turned Ernie off because sex was the one area he kind of had together. I wish someone had been that interested in helping him see that he could still do some kind of work. It's been seven years now and our sex life is fine, but he's still not doing much of anything else. That's what's beginning to turn me off.

And thus the pendulum swings. An era in which the sexual needs of disabled people are ignored may be followed by an era in which at least a few must face having the sexual problems of others imposed upon them in ways insensitive to their values and needs. In the main, however, the attention paid to sexuality among disabled people has been a positive influence, enhancing recognition of the breadth and depth of sexual expression possible. In this respect, the field of rehabilitation already has contributed significantly to filling the gap left by the mainstream "pairing industries," as the latter are only beginning to acknowledge and respond to their disabled markets.

Recent literature on sexuality and disability has included some attention to gay and lesbian issues. Some articles have addressed the special needs of these populations, including rectifying myths, coping with the negative attitudes of health care workers, and countering isolation (Corker, 2001; McAllan & Ditillo, 1994; O'Toole, 2000; O'Toole & Bregante, 1992). Sexual preference statistics that have been touted in the public media indicate that as much as 10% of the population may choose same-sex individuals as lovers—a significant minority that is still misunderstood. The need for counsel is great; disabled gays express more fears than nondisabled gays about "coming out of the closet" because of their dual devaluated status. Believing rejection by the straight majority could threaten their very survival, many stay silent and their problems of establishing love relationships remain unresolved. The issue of AIDS is also a serious one for disabled gay men (Saad, 1997), especially given the inadequate sexual education that is typically provided to people with disabilities.

Why is it that sex is such a powerful subject? Probably in part because it is potentially a vehicle for manifesting nearly every facet of human consciousness and of meeting the demands of almost every level in the human hierarchy of needs. This is true not only for the most basic levels of consciousness reflected in the needs for security, sensation, and power, but also for the "higher" levels of consciousness reflected in the needs for self-esteem, love, self-actualization, and spiritual enlightenment. This aspect of sexuality is only mentioned here, but these concepts will be developed fully in Chapter 8 ("Transcending").

The fact is, the development of a truly intimate relationship may be far more difficult for many to achieve than an imitation of sexual perfection. It has become almost a cliché in sex therapy circles that failures of intimacy are the primary causes of sexual dysfunction. Perhaps, contrary to expectation, this does not change with the advent of disability. There may be organic bases for certain aspects of sexual dysfunction, but these do not explain an unsatisfactory sex life or love life. When genuine intimacy exists, couples whose sex lives consist of lying quietly together may report more satisfying erotic experiences than sex-manual gymnasts who reach orgasm but feel strangely empty and displeased nonetheless.

Intimacy

Intimacy seldom, if ever, happens suddenly. A special rapport is sometimes almost instantaneous, but true intimacy takes time to develop. It may or may not include the sense of being "in love," but it involves loving. Caring about the other person's needs and ways of being, and freely sharing one's own, are the hallmarks of intimacy. Several years ago, one of the popular psychology magazines carried an article that asserted that the sense of being "in love" had only two basic requisites: (1) the loved individual keeps one in a state of arousal, and (2) that state of arousal is labeled "love." This was thought to explain such phenomena as possessive love and the renowned hairline difference between love and hate. If the state of arousal generated by another is confounded by possessiveness or unresolved resentments (hate), there is very little chance that a truly intimate relationship will evolve from it, however powerful the chemistry appears to be. All of this holds true regardless of whether disablement is a factor in the relationship. When it is, however, it is poignantly relevant because of the heightened likelihood of the emergence of both possessive and resentful feelings.

As they relate to disability, feelings of possessiveness are most apt to be experienced by disabled lovers who feel insecure about their ability to "hang on" to a lover or spouse. Whether or not it is true, they are likely to attribute their insecurity in this regard to their disabilities. Possessiveness is also an important issue with nondisabled people who choose disabled lovers/spouses partly in the belief that they will be less subject to being wooed away by someone else. Resentments can emerge for a thousand reasons. The disabled partner may resent over- or under-solicitude, or may simply be jealous of the other's freedom from disability-related constraints. Gratitude for caregiving is notoriously mixed with resentment over its necessity, and those feelings tend to be directed toward the caregiver. A nondisabled partner may resent what feels like a burden, yet be afraid of alienating or hurting the other and thus say nothing but continue to seethe.

If the couple finds that such feelings can be shared and thereby de-energized, a step toward greater intimacy has been taken. If not, it becomes more remote, and ultimate dissolution of the relationship looms likely. Because the building (or rebuilding) of an intimate relationship is so central to marriage and other unions involving formalized commitments, these concepts will be pursued further in the following sections dealing with marriage and alternative lifestyles.

Building a New Marriage

If a marriage takes place after disablement is a fait accompli, statistics show the chances for success are greater than for marriages established previously. There are two fairly obvious reasons for this: (1) the marriage will not have to endure the emotional weathering associated with the acute stage of illness or injury, and (2) both partners make their commitments in the face of known disability-related conditions. Each makes a positive choice that acknowledges the reality of disability; it is not a seemingly unfair, fateful event that is thrust upon them. There will, nonetheless, be the usual needs for adjustments, some of which will center on the disability. The problem areas will be little different from those of couples whose marriages predated disability. A signal example is the temptation to view every conflict as a "disability issue." Naturally, an early order of business is learning to sort what is from what is not an issue related to disability.

A disabled partner may have projected fuller acknowledgment of disability during courtship than was true at a deeper level. He or she may even have expected that having someone to "love and honor 'til death do us part" would magically make the pain of disablement go away. In one way, this is little different from the usual images of bliss that surround romantic alliances, and it must be brought into line with reality as the marriage matures. However, when failure to accept part of oneself that is frequently in the forefront of consciousness is at issue, efforts to "force" the partner to make everything better may redouble. Frequently, people who feel they have had much taken away from them look to their closest family members—parents, children, spouse—for compensation. It is a hard but important lesson to learn that others cannot make up for one's losses.

Linked to this are the problems of jealousy and fears of spousal abandonment whenever a nondisabled or less disabled spouse becomes interested in activities that can't be shared. A woman executive with one paralyzed leg resulting from polio described the panic she felt when her husband first took an interest in skiing:

> I was miffed that he wanted to do something I couldn't do. I thought, "How insensitive can he be?" I was very threatened by the fact that even though I could succeed in business, I still couldn't join my husband in what he wanted to do. For awhile, I really got paranoid; I refused to go along and then tortured myself with fantasies of him falling in love with some winter Olympian who looked like Sophia Loren. I damaged our relationship by trying to make him feel too guilty to go.
>
> Finally, one of our friends told me what a jerk I was being. He really laid it on. After the sting went away, I knew he was right. Why should I force Jed to be cripple just because I'm one? That's real dog-in-the-manger stuff. Anyway, now I go and have a good time sitting around the lodge, visiting, knitting, enjoying the beauty of the setting, and watching Jed ski. It took him awhile to trust that I wasn't pulling some kind of martyr act or spying on him, but now even that's behind us. The good part was when he admitted it was nice to find out I had a scared side, because the supercompetent businesswoman had kind of scared him!

This couple did not have to clear the issues that arise when a spouse is called on to provide all or part of such needed services as attendant care, interpreting, reading, and driving. When this is true, delicate problems can arise.

The caregiving spouse may come to feel "used," like a "servant"; and the recipient may feel dissatisfied and angry over untimely or inattentive care. Moreover, the effects of caregiving responsibilities on sexual attraction to the disabled spouse create highly fabled concerns for numerous couples. Nondisabled individuals contemplating marriage to disabled men or women regularly are counseled, by friends, family, and professionals, to reconsider: "You may think you are in love now, but you'll get turned off fast after you've had to take care of him/her like a baby for awhile." The disabled parties, especially those who have not yet integrated their dependency into a positive self-image, inwardly and fearfully agree with such pronouncements. When marriage takes place anyway, chronic dread that proof is imminent may follow.

If frank discussion of all such issues is inhibited by fears and resentments, alienation can only increase. Both parties must struggle to be fair and realistic, while at the same time protecting their own rights and needs. Sound marriages are generally the product of equivalent giving and taking, and understanding equivalencies (not equalities) of contribution requires very balanced perception when disability creates highly visible areas wherein one gives and the other receives.

Two examples illustrate compensatory patterns that can reduce the extent to which a couple feels an imbalance in giving and taking. Harris has found that work colleagues are so used to his bringing paid interpreters to meetings that on social occasions they may treat his wife as if that were her only role. At her request, he now points out beforehand that she will interpret for him, but will be present, first and foremost, for her own social pleasure. Carol, whose husband provides her morning and nightly attendant care, says she tries to "repay" him by pampering him with breakfast in bed on weekends, and dinner in bed during football season, where he likes to lounge while watching the games.

Roy, the nondisabled husband of a very severely paralyzed woman, lamented,

> I wish Toni could just realize that I married her because she made me happy . . . she was so tender and understanding when we were going together and that's all I wanted from her. Hell, I knew she was disabled! But now, all she does is brood about what she can't do . . . says she's afraid she's going to lose me because she can't cook and keep house and raise kids. If that was what I wanted, I would have married someone else. If she loses me, it will be because I can't take her constant gloom anymore.

Learning that the best you can offer to someone else is to be the best you can be for yourself—and the happiest—is a sophisticated human lesson to learn. People with severe disabilities have the seldom-envied advantage of a great incentive to learn it well, regardless of whether they adopt lifestyles of traditional marriage. The urge toward pairing also can be satisfied in other ways, including quasitraditional marriage, living singly and dating, and forming committed unions with more than one other individual.

Alternative Lifestyles

The first to be considered is more an alternative to poverty than to marriage. Many couples, wherein one or both are recipients of Supplemental Security Income and/or Medicaid benefits, may wish to marry but find it would entail a devastating loss of income. Administering agencies are reluctant to pay spouses for providing attendant care, so many couples remain unmarried, living ostensibly as "recipient" and "provider" when, in fact, their lifestyle is one of common-law marriage. Other couples, both of whom are "recipients," meet similar disincentives to legal marriage. On the positive side, "living together" is no longer regarded with the social disdain it once was. People do still marry, however, so the ritual, the contract, and the commitment of marriage continue to have deep and widespread meaning. Many disabled people/couples want to sanctify their love relationships in this way and enjoy the sense of security a marriage commitment connotes, but, because of the economic disincentives built into the income system on which they rely, they feel unable to do so. Couples such as these and others who adopt nonlegalized marital lifestyles for other reasons (for example, previous marital ties undissolved, preference for avoiding long-term or legal commitments, or gay marriages) experience essentially the same issues and problems as the married couples described in the previous section.

A truer alternative to marriage exists in communal living arrangements that both serve familial functions of mutual support and offer opportunities for love relationships. Some disabled people join established communes, others select from the extant range of independent living arrangements (ILAs) referred to in Chapter 3, and still others create communal or independent living situations for themselves. Group marriages, though generally rare, occasionally include one or more disabled partners. ILAs are likely choices for severely disabled individuals, who need their practical features as much as their opportunities for love relationships. However, some residents are married couples who enjoy the sense of a large extended family in addition to the special facilities and services available. Cohousing is a current and expanding phenomenon throughout the country that is attracting people of all ages and abilities. Individuals and families own homes or condominiums that are grouped around green space and a shared great house, where some meals and activities are held. The goal is to create the kind of interactive and interdependent community that seemed to be more typical of rural society in past centuries.

Finally, the alternative of living singly (with whatever assistant or other help might be needed) has become "respectable" in society at large. It now carries less connotation of having been unchosen, since many people, including increasing numbers of women with ample opportunities to marry, are making singledom their choice. Here, the women's movement has had a beneficial side effect for single disabled people, by reducing the sense of stigma associated with unmarried life. Nonetheless, Karen, the disabled feminist cited earlier (see Chapter 2), expresses the opinion that:

> Being single and disabled is still a little bizarre, especially for women. It's true that the stigma is reduced, but it's still a problem. If you're single and disabled, other people assume it's because you have no choice, even if that's not true. And if you haven't gotten past being concerned about your image, or being pitied, that bothers you. Also, realistically, dates aren't all that easy to get for most of us, and it's easy to get caught up in the "one night stand" syndrome, just for the momentary proofs that someone wants you. Many people don't want the obligations of marriage, but few people want to be alone—and marriage or living together or even having a steady are ways to combat that. Also, when you're disabled and have trouble finding jobs, having a lifetime partner is very reassuring. Economic security is still one of the main reasons people team up in marriage . . . and disabled people want that even more than most.

As cited in several earlier contexts, a couple's or family's economic situation can have significant impact on their interrelationships. Severe financial hardships are notorious for eroding love, whether or not disablement is a factor. Obviously, the major cause of fiscal difficulty among disabled people is the problem Karen alluded to: under- or unemployment. Job barriers abound for the disabled population, and they begin being erected at least as early as elementary school. The following chapter will examine the education and employment processes as they relate to disabled people's work lives.

6

Working

Getting Educated and Employed

People disabled in infancy or childhood may begin very early, and without knowing it, to experience what one day will prove to be serious hindrances in getting and keeping jobs and in advancing their careers. This is because all aspects of one's education—not just the formal, didactic schooling, but the experiential parts as well—have the power to shape or misshape people for their eventual work lives. The well-known studies of creative artists and scientists consistently show that enriched early life experience—from world travel to simply being read to a great deal—is a commonly found factor among those who are most successful. Compare this with the homogeneity and stultification potentially present in the life of a child who is sheltered and relatively isolated from peers for long periods of time due to a disability. If this happens, problems that will beset getting vocationally established in the practical world begin even earlier than the first day of school. They are apt to increase markedly when that day arrives, however.

Special Education, Mainstreaming, and Inclusion

Many people alive today have seen public education for disabled youngsters progress from no education at all, to "special" education in segregated settings, to a concerted effort to integrate disabled students into mainstream schools. The accompanying change of attitude from "Tough luck, Charlie" through "separate but equal" to the recognition that separate is as inherently unequal here as elsewhere reflects growth in a positive direction. This trend, like others cited earlier, is a product of civil rights concern and legislation at national and local levels.

The special education era—which has by no means ended despite massive efforts to desegregate disabled students—itself came into being as a result of dire societal need. In its time, it reflected important social progress. As other conditions changed, however, and the artifact of segregation was observed to create its own set of problems, further change was seen to be required. This has culminated in the passage of legislation requiring all young people with disabilities to be educated in the "least restrictive environment" appropriate to their condition. The Education for All Handicapped Children Act (EHC), passed in 1975 and renamed the Individuals with Disabilities Education Act (IDEA) in 1990, called for maximal integration into mainstream schooling, with a minimum of segregated programs. To accomplish this, a multidisciplinary team of education/health professionals is required to evaluate each child. Parents and team members then jointly develop an individualized educational plan (IEP) to guide decisions about the provision of educational services. An appropriate education is guaranteed to be free from approximately 3 years of age until 21 or graduation from high school, whichever comes first. (Earlier intervention, from birth to 3 years, is allowed but not mandated.) The school district is required to provide the services needed to implement the IEP (e.g., transportation, special equipment, and supportive or corrective therapies) without regard to the financial resources of the parents. IDEA also provided for due process rights for students with disabilities and their families who disagree with the IEP.

Most recently, merely bringing students with disabilities into regular school buildings has also been viewed as insufficient, and advocates are insisting upon full inclusion in education. This means bringing students into regular classrooms and involving them the same lessons and activities as much as possible. By the 1998–99 school year, approximately half of students with disabilities who were receiving special services spent at least 40% of their school time in classes with nondisabled students and the remainder in "resource rooms" (U.S. Department of Education, 2001). More than a quarter spent most of their day in resource rooms, and about 24% attended separate schools or other facilities.

The wisdom of the move toward mainstreaming is controversial. While its proponents have been dissatisfied when the mandated changes have been implemented slowly, incompletely, or reluctantly, dissent comes from several different quarters. One group points out that the cost of providing an equal education to certain extremely disabled youngsters exceeds the value of the objective. That is a heavy message for disabled people to receive. School districts complain that the requirements were mandated by federal and state laws, but that no special resources were provided to offset costs. Others believe that the quality of education for all suffers. Depending on their interests, they may lament a regular classroom teacher's time being overly directed toward a few disabled students, or they may stress the teacher's inability to do an effective job with disabled students. Many of the displeased are teachers. Some complain because they dread having disabled students in their classrooms; others protest because they envision their special-education expertise being wasted. All reactions reflect a mixture of fact and unreality laced with fears of the unknown. Many disabled youngsters who are aware of the controversy are hurt or angered by it, as are disabled adults who can assess the implications for their social status more fully.

For the purposes at hand, disabled students might be viewed as comprising three distinguishable groups: (1) those whose learning ability is impaired, (2) those whose communication ability is impaired, and (3) those whose disabilities affect neither learning nor communication abilities. The reasons differ for segregating the education of each of these groups from the mainstream.

Students whose ability to learn is impaired by intellectual limitation, emotional/behavioral disorder, or other neurological dysfunctions may be segregated so that their slower learning pace does not retard the progress of more capable students, and to allow the extra time and attention needed for them to absorb material. Accommodating both the faster and slower learners may require some segregation by classroom, but it no longer is clear why it once seemed necessary for them to attend school in altogether separate facilities. Desire on the part of the nondisabled populace to avoid contact with people thus limited is the most logical explanation for society's having taken this extra step.

Historically, students whose communication abilities are affected by vision, hearing, or speech disorders have been segregated into settings that specialize in presenting educational material in modes they can "receive" adequately, and that provide the extra time and equipment needed for them to "transmit." By segregating their education, regular classroom teachers were freed from concern over students with unusual communication needs, and school systems found it cost effective to provide special services and equipment in a single location, rather than at each mainstream school. These arguments for expediency have given way to other values, however. Most schools for the deaf or blind have been closed, and students are being educated in regular schools.

Students with physical disabilities affecting neither their learning nor their communication abilities frequently used to be segregated simply to avoid the architectural barriers characterizing mainstream schools. Also, when severe disabilities require personal assistant services during the school day, having it available at one rather than all schools seemed to be cost effective.

The problem is that separating disabled from nondisabled people early in their lives created other social costs to be paid for later, such as expensive programs designed to break down the attitude and job barriers early segregation fostered. It is no wonder that employers, most of whom are relatively nondisabled, found it difficult to imagine that disabled job applicants could function in their work settings when, as children, they were led to believe that disabled people couldn't even function in the same elementary schools. It also is not surprising that disabled and nondisabled people had trouble simply relating to one another when they had no opportunities for contact from their earliest years. After schooling is over, they hardly could be expected to come together at last with ready-made mutual understanding.

The artifact of segregation is not the only problem cited with respect to special education. Maria, and many other disabled people who attended "special" schools, express the belief that they did not get an education equal to what they would have obtained in a mainstream school. They say both academic and socialization standards were relaxed far beyond the levels needed for many of the students, and that orientation toward college preparation was virtually absent. Mindy, a rehabilitation counselor whose disability is leg weakness secondary to polio, states:

> There was no reason for me to be sent to a school for the handicapped except that my parents didn't know how to say "No." My disability in no way affected my scholarship, and I could even climb stairs. At the school, everything was geared to the slow learners, who were in the majority, and those of us needing challenge were out of luck. No one talked to me about college, so I never considered it until I found my way to the "voc rehab" bureau. This was four years after I finished high school . . . for four years I hung around home with no idea of what to do with myself. I'll never forget how amazed I was when my rehab counselor said she thought I'd be good at her kind of job. That compliment clinched my career choice . . . I never considered anything else. It's a good thing it was a good choice because I would have accepted anything she suggested. Ignorance makes you very, very vulnerable.

Occupational Choice

This brings us to the matter of vocational decision-making. The matter of transitioning from school to the next phase of life is an important issue for all students. They face the challenge of choosing a college, a job, military service, or even taking a little time off to see the world. The ultimate goal of the transition process typically is finding a suitable career. In this society, most people grow up expecting—and wanting—to work. A few people, born into families that have been recipients of welfare programs for several generations, may not share this expectation, but even they are being pushed into the labor market by changes in welfare laws. Most others have primary role models (parents, usually) who work, and they intend to follow suit. Thus, occupational choice is not generally a matter of deciding whether to work; it is deciding what kind of work to do. Depending on the prepotency of geographic and familial occupational tradition, this may entail a simple or complex process of decision making. For example, if you live in a "textile town" and your parents, grandparents, and great-grandparents all worked at the mill, your occupational choice may appear automatic, a simple conformity to custom. At the other extreme, if you live in a megalopolis and your father's family are professionals and your mother's are in business, you may confront a dizzying array of options to choose from.

When significant disablement enters into the equation, the transition may become exceedingly complex, or it may be overlooked altogether. In the past, schools have often assumed that their responsibilities extended to the point of graduation, and little thought was given to planning beyond that point. The disability may have been so severe that no one could envision any suitable job, so it was assumed that the individual would rely on public or family support rather than earn a living. Without any outside evidence to the contrary, the student may be led to a similar conclusion.

Along with the move toward inclusion in regular classrooms, however, another development has helped to change this perspective. Transition planning is now required for all students with disabilities, beginning at age 14. By age 16, a full plan must be developed by the student, family, and educational team. A representative of the vocational rehabilitation system typically participates as well, ensuring that work or higher education is part of the plan.

Why Work? Incentives and Disincentives

For most people with severe disabilities, whether early or adult onset, welfare, Social Security, and Medicaid benefits make it possible to survive without employment. Nonetheless, the incentives for working are strong. Although one can survive on a welfare income, the lifestyle it affords is marginal and stigmatized. Moreover, work is a vehicle for acquiring such socially revered external rewards as money, prestige, and power, as well as the inner rewards associated with self-esteem, belongingness, and self-actualization. Unemployment generates sociopolitical and economic powerlessness, and powerlessness is the basis of learned helplessness—a form of depression. A vicious cycle can develop in which these, in turn, lead to a reduction in one's actual power to influence the course of events in one's life.

The demise of the work ethic has been predicted for several decades now. Automation was expected to usher it in, as were more recent spiritually oriented shifts in human values. So far, however, the reports of its death have been highly exaggerated; in fact, many young professionals claim to be working longer hours at a more hectic pace than ever before. Consequently, people with disabilities are still under pressure, from within and without, to establish themselves vocationally, to have an occupational identity, to reap the materialistic rewards that accrue to wage earning, and to luxuriate in the good feelings that accompany being "a productive, contributing member of society." These are powerful incentives.

Disincentives rooted in the welfare system have been a tremendous barrier to employment, however. Fortunately, after long and emotional years of testimony, Congress recognized the double bind facing many citizens with severe disabilities and passed the Ticket to Work and Work Incentives Improvement Act in 1999. The Supplemental Security Income (SSI) program provides more realistic cash allowances to disabled recipients than general relief programs do for the nondisabled unemployed. Moreover, it is complemented by Medicaid coverage of sometimes extremely costly health-related needs, including a regular, monthly outlay for personal assistance services when required. Frequently, severely disabled recipients are unable to earn anything approximating these forms of income, and certainly not from an entry-level job.

When individuals drawing (and needing) large total benefit amounts moved into employment (thereby relinquishing eligibility for SSI and Medicaid), they placed themselves in serious financial jeopardy. Work sometimes offered no additional income and sometimes even entailed a reduction. This is especially true when personal assistant salaries were paid, as group medical policies available through work will not cover this expense. Even more demotivating, the threat of failure or delay in reestablishing eligibility for benefits following an abortive job attempt generated fears of catastrophic life disruption or even institutionalization. Under such circumstances, the decision not to work and to opt instead for a life on welfare hardly can be viewed as social irresponsibility. It was simply a very rational decision.

The problem stemmed partly from a carryover of earlier thinking regarding the employment capabilities of severely disabled individuals. Predecessor programs were labeled "aid to the totally disabled," on the presumption that severe disablement rendered one totally nonfunctional in the labor market. We now know that even extremely severe disability may not entail being vocationally handicapped at all, as blind, deaf, and completely paralyzed persons secure increasing numbers of high-level positions.

With the passage of the Work Incentives Improvement Act, disincentives have not been eliminated, but they have been greatly reduced. The goal of advocates who have lobbied for the new legislation is to allow people with severe disabilities more freedom in choosing whether to pursue a career. Those who decide that they want to try, like anyone in the throes of making an occupational commitment, immediately face three major questions. What are the options? How does one learn about them? How does one decide which option to choose? When a significant disability must be incorporated into the decision making, a difficult process becomes even more convoluted.

The Perception of Vocational Choices

Clearly, disabilities do not limit vocational options to the extent people have been led to believe. Nonetheless, the functional limitations associated with disabling conditions do eliminate certain jobs from consideration and surround others with impaired probability of success. This still leaves a vast assortment of options available for most disabled people, who then must try to sort the good-chance options from the risky, and the risky from the foolish.

When no role models can be found who demonstrate concretely that a blind, deaf, paralyzed, or learning-disabled person can land a given job and perform in it well, it is easy to conclude that the job in question must be among the impossible. However, because of prejudicial hiring practices in the past, this is not necessarily the case. Therefore, many disabled people entering fields uncharted with respect to track records of disabled workers must make subjectively high-risk decisions in choosing what, objectively, may be sure things vis-à-vis the interaction of functional limitations with job demands. Happily, with the advent of protective legislation regarding employment opportunities for disabled workers, role models are becoming easier to find.

Some disabled people go through many iterations of choosing vocational goals, only to be told, time after time, that their choices are unrealistic and they should choose something more in line with their capabilities. Sometimes this is accurate. Tim, a totally paralyzed youngster who insisted he wanted to be a carpenter like his father, provides an unarguable example. In other cases, such advice reveals the limited imagination of the advisor. This was true for Carol, a triplegic psychologist whose undergraduate advisor said she should not pursue psychology because she could not operate a stopwatch and record IQ test responses simultaneously with only one functional arm and hand. Later, her rehabilitation counselor suggested that clerical work would be a more realistic level of aspiration. Tim went through a painfully disappointing series of confrontations before acceding to external opinion.

Carol suffered needless anxiety before gaining enough experience to discredit faulty advice and pursue her chosen career.

Others may be unable to formulate even one vocational objective; everything seems beyond the range of feasibility. When a firm commitment has been made to a given job or field—through prior work involvement, highly developed interest or talent, or both—relinquishment may seem unbearable. Narrowing of vistas and refusal/inability to shift focus may obliterate the perception of other options, some of which might yield equivalent satisfaction if given the chance.

Any of these situations may call for professional assistance, in the form of testing and other evaluative procedures, and counseling and guidance to improve the person's chances for getting appropriate training. ("Appropriate" here means that the job objective and therefore the type of training are in accord with both the person's and the labor market's realities and that the quality of training, given the objective, is good.) Some disabled people claim the professional help they got was heaven sent. Others describe it as an additional handicap they had to overcome.

Professional Assistance

Vocational counseling is a service most people would find beneficial, but few get it. Oddly enough, disabled individuals have a better chance than most to get more than cursory guidance, because of the barriers to employment they face. Far more extensive services have been made available to them through federal legislation than are available to the general public through the state-federal employment service plus private sector programs. Most people consider this a dubious advantage, but it is a potentially valuable opportunity nonetheless. Interestingly, the Workforce Investment Act of 1998 moved toward the integration of core employment services for the general public and individuals with disabilities, establishing a system of "one-stop centers." The state-federal rehabilitation system will participate in these one-stop centers, and they will also maintain separate programs for specialized services.

Some are able to utilize vocational services with little ado. They understand, or are helped to understand, the reasons for esoteric-seeming evaluation procedures; they know how to participate or are coached to participate actively in drawing conclusions from the findings to formulate a vocational goal and a plan leading to it. From there, they know how to proceed on their own or are given the help they need when they need it. They have moral/emotional support from their own family and friends or find it available from the counselor and other professional helpers.

Many others, however, have found the vocational rehabilitation system to be an extremely complex and confusing, multilevel stress test that was one more trial to adjust to. They were forced to go to doctors and psychologists whose inputs seemed unrelated to their desires to learn a trade. They were forced to take tests that seem embarrassingly silly, or embarrassingly difficult. The counselor didn't seem to have time to see them or seemed dictatorial about what they should do. Nobody ever told them how they did on all those tests, so they assumed the worst. The counselor finally agreed with what they wanted to do, but then the supervisor said, "No." Or the counselor went along with the plan, the supervisor agreed, and after two years of training the job market dried up.

Happily, the state-federal program has evolved in philosophy and practice away from a system that viewed the counselor as the expert who had final say on the use of resources and approval of vocational plans. Now individuals with disabilities are recognized as the central figures in the development of rehabilitation plans, and counselors are primarily consultants and facilitators. They may encounter an occasional old-time counselor who resists the changes, but they should not be afraid to make their desires known. Even programs that work with individuals who have severe developmental disabilities are required to use "person centered planning" which recognizes the right of any individual to be supported in making personal decisions.

Accommodation in Education

In most vocational rehabilitation plans, some form of training or education will be called for. This ushers in a new phase of adjustment to new settings, people, and demands. For example, the availability of distance learning programs has grown exponentially, to the point where the University of Phoenix, a virtual university, is now one of the largest institutions of higher education in the country. How far this trend will go remains to be seen, but some people believe that on-line programs work best for continuing education of people who are already employed in their chosen professions. Real campuses, where students can interact face-to-face with each other and with professors may continue to be the first choice for those who have the opportunity to attend a traditional program. Traditional programs pose special challenges for people with disabilities, however. Whether for reasons relating to the nature and/or severity of disability, financial inability to obtain a car, the lack or inaccessibility of public transportation, or all three, many people in all categories of disability will find their first problem to be, "How do I get there?"

Severely physically disabled students also may need to resolve personal assistance problems in order to get to class on time. Assistants who are accustomed to getting their employers out of bed, dressed, and ready to function in their own good time may resent and resist having to meet an earlier deadline. Vision- and hearing-impaired students will still, all too often, be confronted with serious barriers to learning once they arrive on campus because lecture (for deaf) and written (for blind) materials will be inaccessible to them without extraordinary measures of accommodation. Physically disabled students also will confront barriers in the long distances between classrooms and in architectural design.

Like access to other parts of American society, access to higher education has been a long, arduous struggle that is not yet finished. Still, the doors were opened with the passage of the 1973 Rehabilitation Act and were swung wide with the arrival of the ADA. Institutions are required to make their programs accessible to students with disabilities. That doesn't mean that every historic building must be retrofitted with elevators, but it does mean, for example, that a class needed by a student with a mobility impairment must be moved to an accessible building.

Some of the needed accommodations are being made on the campuses, and the state-federal vocational rehabilitation program is footing the bill to meet additional needs. For example, on-campus "resource" programs for disabled students dispense information, advice, advocacy, and other valuable services. School libraries stock recorded and Braille materials for vision-impaired students and occasionally distribute amplification devices that allow hearing-impaired students better access to lecture presentations. Schools provide reader services for blind students and interpreter services for deaf students. The state-federal vocational rehabilitation program provides many additional types of adaptive equipment and personal services to students with all types of disabilities. In addition, consumer-run independent living programs offer help to students needing to tighten their off-campus support systems to allow reliable school—and, some day, work—attendance.

Once the major problems have been resolved and the student is matriculated safely and regular in attendance, other problems arise. These relate to "other people." The law clearly requires that reasonable accommodations be made to allow students with disabilities to participate in classes and campus activities, but any given instructor may encounter special needs rarely and have to be educated about appropriate responses. Some instructors are reluctant to flex their teaching styles to accommodate disabled students. If they don't use ample handouts ordinarily, they are unwilling to adopt the practice for the sake of current and future deaf students. If they do use ample handouts, it is the responsibility of blind students, with the assistance of the disability resource center on campus, to get them read. Although it may be illegal, some teachers still refuse to allow students unable to take notes to record their lectures. Students physically unable to participate in laboratory activities may find instructors hesitant to allow them to play a modified role in meeting laboratory requirements. When these situations occur, students need to remember that the law is on their side and perseverance will prevail if the requested accommodations are reasonable. These problems, obviously, are felt most acutely by disabled students lacking in social presence and assertiveness. As a veteran rehabilitation counselor with a college student caseload once remarked, "I've never seen a client who was gracious and poised get hassled by teachers who didn't want to make allowances." Thus, attractiveness and assertiveness again arise as critical resource variables in the adjustment process. Both on-campus resource programs and off-campus independent living programs are directing some attention to helping people who do not have these traits naturally to develop them to a level that will contribute positively to their school (and life) success.

School is a legitimate part of one's career. It is, in a sense, a full-time job, a time- and energy-absorbing endeavor that also becomes one's center for social relationships and recreation, as well as a place in which to prepare for future economic stability. Just as life can't be all work and no play, it can't be all scholarship and no socializing. Making friends and getting dates are avowed goals of many students, but they may be harder to accomplish when one has a disability. Deaf students may find others' desire to include them in social discourse waning as the effort required becomes evident; blind students may be as unseen as they are unseeing. Physically disabled students may fare better in the long run, but only if they are able to reduce others' anxiety over someone who looks markedly different.

A tendency exists for disabled students—like ethnic minority students—to group together, focusing on their visible core of shared experience. Special service programs may inadvertently or intentionally reinforce this by establishing social functions that prove to be of interest only to disabled students. This is especially true in schools that have set aside special housing for disabled students needing personal assistance services. A tight in-group camaraderie may develop, but social intercourse outside of the group may be inhibited. Although facilitation of relationships with other disabled students is a positive contribution, the lack of impetus toward building social contact with the nondisabled majority seems to detract from the overall social gains that could be made in school.

Thus, segregation of disabled from nondisabled students sometimes develops even in an integrated setting. Other disabled individuals do all or part of their vocational training in explicitly segregated settings established for the purpose of preparing disabled workers for jobs. These settings are referred to generically as "work preparation programs," and they exist primarily in rehabilitation centers and in work-oriented rehabilitation facilities.

Entering Work

Just as segregated special education programs have given way to inclusion, so specialized work preparation programs have changed quite dramatically during the past two decades. Once sheltered workshops were a major part of the rehabilitation establishment, providing both training and long-term employment for people with severe disabilities. The logical assumption that people need to be trained before they can be expected to function in a work setting was turned on its head with the advent of the supported employment (SE) paradigm. SE advocates placing people on the job and then providing necessary supports in situ to help them become able to function with increasing independence. It encourages people to work in the community, integrated with coworkers who do not have disabilities. The advantages of SE are many. First, greater diversity of both types and levels of work can be secured. Second, it eliminates some of the guesswork in predicting how clients will fare in mainstream jobs after being tested and trained in settings that are, at best, simulations of the ordinary world of work. Third, just as well-publicized findings have shown that standardized tests predict job performance poorly for ethnic minority job applicants, experience suggests this is also the case for disabled employment seekers. Consequently, actual job performance sampling has been cited as the best predictor for both groups, and the SE approach is becoming an important means for obtaining it. Fourth, it aids placement efforts because employers get to know disabled workers through the relatively nonthreatening, noncommitted evaluation and training processes, thereby becoming less resistant to hiring them. This trend yields an additional boon for disabled people: the opportunity to enter into mainstream occupational life at a much earlier point in time. Months or even years of segregated rehabilitation and work preparation may be eliminated, and social relationships with nondisabled coworkers can begin.

The SE model has, itself, evolved over time. At first, professional helpers known as job coaches were typically used for extended periods of time to help a client learn a job and continue to function up to an acceptable level. Later, more attention was given to finding natural supports existing within the work environment and using them to facilitate an individual's functioning. A job coach is often used for a short period of time to help a person learn a job and to find ways to perform it most efficiently, and then the coach fades from the scene, encouraging coworkers and supervisors to provide the day-to-day social support and guidance.

Despite the increasing shift of rehabilitation services into the community, some specialized facilities continue to provide evaluation, training, and employment. This genre of training does far more than impart the skills and knowledge necessary for performing jobs. Work evaluation, work adjustment, and job placement are as integral to these programs as skill training per se, and oftentimes moreso. They are oriented to disabled people with serious and multiple barriers to employment that stem not only from the nature and severity of their disabilities, but from other factors as well. Some of these include histories of being overprotected or neglected, lack of prior work experience, educational deprivation, and behavioral aberrations that could make it difficult for them to succeed on a mainstream trade-school or college campus, or in the world of work. Some of these programs do excellent jobs of preparing their multiply handicapped clients for work. Individuals who have failed in mainstream work settings or to qualify as feasible for service by the state-federal vocational rehabilitation program have obtained the remedial help they needed to take the next step from private sector workshops. Such facilities are used extensively by counselors in the state programs when work evaluation, work adjustment, and specialized job placement measures are needed.

At the same time, the very nature of these settings creates certain problems for both the clients who use them and referring counselors as well. The work available may be intrinsically repetitive and boring, and pay may be very low. Further, the organization may be pulled in opposite directions by its rehabilitation mission and its need to keep functioning as a business. On the one hand, it has a responsibility to help clients develop and transition into competitive jobs in the community, and at the same time it needs to meet production standards on the contracts that keep the facility in business. While keeping the best workers would promote the latter goal, it would violate the former, so staff is continually challenged to face ethical choices.

Further challenges emerge from the fact that workshops are serving increasingly diverse populations. Some facilities that initially served only individuals with disabilities have broadened to include other groups with barriers to employment such as refugees and nondisabled Americans referred by the court system. Workers on the same production line may speak different languages and come from contrasting cultural backgrounds. Besides bringing differing histories and expectations about work, they may also bring problematic attitudes about working with those who have disabilities. Even clients with milder disabilities sometimes are frightened or angered at being placed alongside extremely limited workers. They wonder if they are seen as like individuals by the professionals who referred both to the same setting, and they want to escape quickly from such an unwelcome confrontation. Providing effective services in such rich and complex settings demands flexibility, a willingness to understand and meet individual needs, and a real commitment to a shared mission.

Getting a Job

The world of work in America changed to an astounding degree during the last two decades of the twentieth century. Young people entering the workforce are told they can expect to have not one career but a series of careers during their lifetimes. Technology has provided new tools that are indispensable to most jobs in the economy: computers, cell phones, faxes, and silicon chips that drive machinery of all types, from the robots on the factory floors to the appliances in our homes. Bridges (1994) forecasts that jobs themselves will disappear as the primary means of earning a living, turning us into a population of entrepreneurs and consultants, working, but not as employees.

These changes, and others, have implications for the work future of people with disabilities. Historically, people with severe disabilities have had an abysmally low rate of employment (less than 30%). Among the developments that should result in greatly improved opportunities include the following:

- The passage of the Americans with Disabilities Act (see Chapter 9), which prohibits discrimination in hiring, retention, and promotion against qualified persons with disabilities.
- ADA provisions that require employers to provide reasonable accommodations to allow people with disabilities to perform jobs.
- The explosion of technological innovation that has reduced the physical labor involved in many jobs and provided alternative ways of carrying out many tasks.
- The passage of the Ticket to Work and Work Disincentives Improvement Act, which will allow individuals who leave the Social Security rolls for work to maintain Medicaid or Medicare coverage. Under

certain conditions, the act also allows them to obtain reinstatement of benefits without a new application and disability evaluation if they are unable to continue working because of the disability.

- The development of new vocational rehabilitation services and philosophies that emphasize community integration and consumer choice.
- The creation of a system of independent living centers that provide peer counseling and assistance with aspects of housing, transportation, and personal assistance that are prerequisites to employment. In addition, some independent living centers are becoming directly involved in employment services.
- Increased attention to the transition from school to work for individuals with developmental disabilities, reducing the tendency for people to spend years inactively after leaving the educational system.

With all of these positive developments, it would seem that the employment problems faced by people with disabilities have been solved. Unfortunately, reality is lagging behind the promise. In fairness, some of the developments, such as Ticket to Work, are so new that they have not yet had time to bear fruit, but the statistics are still disappointing. The rate of employment among people with chronic health conditions or impairments remained constant at about 52% during the period from 1990 to 1994 (Kaye, 1998). Less than one-third of people with severe functional limitations were employed during that same period.

Yet, summary statistics may not tell the whole story. Duncan Wyeth (personal communication, June 29, 2000), an activist who has been involved with disability issues for many years, believes that the employment rate among younger people with disabilities has increased significantly during recent years, but this is masked by the increasing numbers of older individuals who develop disabilities and take early retirement. Given the aging of the population and the higher incidence of disability with increasing age, this seems to be a reasonable conclusion.

Where does all this leave the individual with a disability who is trying to make decisions about his or her place in the world of work? The first question is whether it makes economic sense to work. Individuals who require full-time personal assistance services or who have high medical expenses know that they cannot afford to be without comprehensive health insurance. These expenses simply cannot be paid out of pocket by anyone earning an ordinary salary. Since the group insurance available from employers rarely covers personal assistance or medical supplies, maintaining access to Medicare or Medicaid coverage is essential. Until recently, there was no way, over the long run, to be self-supporting and retain that lifeline. As noted above, this dilemma has been addressed with new legislation, and a solution may now be available. Individuals who receive SSI or SSDI and who are considering the possibility of going to work should obtain the most current information available from the Social Security Administration or from a reliable source on the Web (e.g., www.ssa.gov/disability/) (Social Security Administration, 2002). They should also make sure that any adviser is fully informed about the new regulations, both federal and state. Some family members, caseworkers, and others may be so concerned about avoiding risk that they warn against doing anything to jeopardize the status quo. If a person really wants to work, however, a genuine opportunity may now be available.

Job Search

The availability of information and advice regarding effective methods of job seeking is now ubiquitous. Software programs can help a person develop a resume in dozens of different styles, and the neighborhood copy center can print them on parchment or in any style requested. You can prepare for job interviews by using an inexpensive diskette to review hundreds of frequently asked questions. Of course, books are available on these same topics. An internet search of "careers" will turn up hundreds of sources of information about job openings and requirements. You can even post your resume and wait for the headhunters to begin calling.

People with less technological sophistication may not feel comfortable accessing these resources without a coach or mentor, however, and these general sources may leave many questions unanswered for the seeker with a disability. Fortunately, many individuals with disabilities have one or more professional experts coaching them and encouraging them to follow through. These supports are necessary because of the uphill battle they face in convincing employers to take a chance on them.

The quality of support offered by job-placement programs varies. Counselors in state vocational rehabilitation agencies are renowned for their dislike of doing job placement. Accordingly, many offer impoverished services, enjoining their clients to conduct their own job searches and rationalizing that such is the correct way to foster client independence. Others may contract out the job-placement process to specialty programs offering it as part of a package deal including work evaluation, adjustment, and training. Bringing in new players who do not really know the client may be inefficient or disheartening. In all, this key element of the job search often has been shortchanged in the rehabilitation process, possibly helping to explain why the unemployment rate of people with disabilities remains so high despite decades of services.

The Selection Process

Some of the most egregious barriers to applying for a job have been corrected by the ADA. The application process must be accessible to potentially qualified persons. A blind person cannot be discounted simply because he or she cannot read and fill out a printed application form. Tests cannot be used that would have the effect of screening out applicants with disabilities regardless of their qualifications. For example, people with upper extremity impairment may be predestined to fail a vocabulary test, not because they don't know the answers, but because they are unable to fill in the little boxes on the scoring sheet quickly enough. This is no longer defensible. Any screening tests must be valid predictors of essential functions of the job in question. If extensive vocabulary is, in fact, a bona fide requirement for a position, then the test must be given in a format that does not inadvertently disadvantage certain groups, or alternative formats must be available.

Before the ADA, employers were allowed to ask general questions about whether an applicant had various medical conditions. The applicant then faced the choice of acknowledging the condition (and probably not being hired) or of denying it and running the risk of being fired if the condition were to be discovered later. People with invisible disabilities such as epilepsy or bipolar illness were particularly threatened by this eventuality, and they have been particular beneficiaries of ADA's prohibition of such questions. Of course, this aspect of the law can do little to protect individuals with visible disabilities such as cerebral palsy. In fact, the applicant may have an increased burden to raise the issue of disability and proactively demonstrate the way in which he or she will be able to meet the job requirements. Otherwise, since interviewers are not free to raise many questions, they may base their hiring decisions upon unwarranted assumptions to the ultimate disadvantage of disabled applicants. This is not fair, and it may be illegal, but it is reality.

Doing a Job, Keeping It, and Advancing

From a psychological point of view, one of the most important aspects of doing a job is where you do it. What kind of work setting is it? Such issues as the industry (its size, location, personnel policies, and work conditions), its organizational climate, and other factors too numerous to mention all play roles in determining whether the quality of work life for employees will be good or bad. In addition to these usual variables, two others become critical when the workers in question have disabilities: (1) the extent to which the work setting is integrated into the mainstream world of work, and (2) the extent to which disabled workers are sheltered, as opposed to accommodated.

"Shelter" is the word traditionally used to denote ways in which job situations are allowed to conform to the needs of workers with disabilities. However, contemporary employers have become increasingly open to employee requests for a four-day work week, flex-time, job sharing, and on-site child care facilities. These are ways in which job situations can be altered to conform to worker needs not necessarily related to disability. Often, they relate to parental obligations. In such cases, we don't speak of shelter, we generally use the term "accommodation." This is an era in which many aspects of jobs are being modified to meet the needs of workers, rather than forcing them to make all of the necessary adjustments. Providing accommodations for disabled workers is only one facet of this. The ADA requires employers to make "reasonable accommodations" to enable qualified workers with disabilities to do a job effectively. The term "shelter," then, is reserved for cases in which some degree of reduced production quantity or quality, or inappropriate work behavior, is tolerated. Thus, accommodation is something an employer offers selected employees to enable them to produce up to standard, whereas shelter is something the employer provides for selected employees who are unable to meet the standards.

Supported employment now represents a middle ground between competitive employment (with or without special accommodations) and sheltered work. An individual with a severe disability may begin a job with substantial assistance from a coach and develop work skills and appropriate behavior over time, eventually reaching the point of satisfactory productivity without assistance. Enclaves represent another approach that is often used for individuals who either need to develop employable skills and behaviors, or for those with disabilities that intermittently affect work capacities (e.g., those with recurrent mental illness). Competitive work is carried out in regular workplaces by a team of workers with disabilities and one or more coaches or supervisors who ensure that standards are consistently met. Since these workers function in teams, any one person can be replaced temporarily by others in order to get the job done.

At one time, competitive work was done in integrated workplaces, and sheltered work was done in special facilities. Now, the correlation between setting and productivity is no longer clear. Supported work, by definition, is done in community settings. Home-based work, once considered the ultimate in shelter, is being done by increasing numbers of professional and technical workers as well as by individuals whose conditions make it difficult for them to leave home. Many people, with or without disabilities, prefer to work in mainstream settings, but others find they are happier and more productive without the demands of commuting, restrictive work schedules, and the distractions of office politics. With computers and instantaneous communication, a wider range of well-paying jobs can now be done out of the home. Employers are becoming more accepting of the practice, finding that it is still possible to monitor productivity from a distance and that they may actually save money that would have gone to support office space and equipment.

Job Performance Problems—Technological Solutions

Disabled people now are entering occupational fields heretofore undreamed of because technology has generated solutions to job-performance problems created by their disabilities. Just as the widespread use of motorized wheelchairs inaugurated an era of increased independence and expectation for one group of disabled people (see Chapter 3), other applications of technology have vastly improved the functional capabilities and quality of life for people with nearly every type of bodily disability. Many serious problems, encountered in activities of daily living, communication, transportation, homemaking, recreation, and, of course, meeting job demands, are melting under the torch of twentieth-century technology. We now have calculators that speak answers to blind users, machines that use air currents to separate materials for people with poor coordination, miniaturized teletypewriters for deaf individuals, and a seemingly endless array of more and less exotic devices. Disabled people are reaping spinoff gains from the space and defense industries; in fact, they are becoming, in the opinion of some, their primary beneficiaries.

In reality, though, all workers are relying upon technology to an unprecedented degree. Voice recognition software, for example, was once available only to people, such as those with tetraplegia, who had funding to cover the $12,000 price tag. Now anyone with $200 can walk into their local software store and carry home an equally sophisticated program. It may be just a matter of time before a majority of executives trade in their keyboards for microphones. Amusingly, some employers used to argue against the use of assistive devices by workers with disabilities on the grounds that "if we get this for him, everybody will want one!" Of course they did, with the result that technology has produced unparalleled growth in the American economy during recent years.

Sensory aids for vision- and hearing-impaired workers and mobility aids for motor-impaired workers are proliferating under the relatively generous federal funding of rehabilitation engineering centers. Information about their accomplishments is disseminated systematically to consumers and professionals, especially through such resources as the Job Accommodation Network (JAN) on the worldwide web. As a result, the psychological well-being of multitudes of disabled people is being enhanced, not by psychological methods, but by sophisticated modifications of their physical world and capabilities. In effect, technological substitutions for absent sensory and motor capacities are restoring occupational options previously considered lost to those with given disabilities. This allows them access to higher-level and more interesting kinds of work.

Quality of Work Life

Until fairly recently, disabled people were considered lucky to get any job at all. Intrinsically interesting work offering opportunities for career advancement was beyond expectation. Rather than focusing on resolving this dilemma, the more frequent course taken was to cite work-life research findings that the same is true for many nondisabled workers as well. With the impetus of the civil rights movement for people with disabilities, attention finally is being paid to work as a source of life satisfaction for disabled people, as well as a means for reducing the size of the welfare rolls.

Welfare recipients of any kind seldom find agency workers highly motivated to help them locate gratifying work. Agency workers appear to reflect taxpayers' attitudes that recipients are obliged to accept any available job and have little right to be choosy. In some agencies, the workers themselves have not found satisfying work and cannot envision it for their clients. In others, it may be an outgrowth of pressures to accumulate high numbers of job placements with little official concern for their quality. Whatever the reasons, it has required social pressure from consumers and other advocates to initiate changes in entrenched operating philosophy. The technological developments described previously also have contributed significantly by making more intrinsically rewarding fields feasible.

Increasing numbers of special projects are being funded to encourage disabled people to enter the fields of technology and science. A few even encourage disabled artists to pursue their painting, acting, writing, or other creative expression, but artists are not as generously supported in this country as scientists are. The emergence of consumer-run independent living programs and affirmative hiring of disabled people in rehabilitation organizations is opening up professional and management options. Service agencies are developing better methods for helping clients with entrepreneurial interests and talent to establish independent businesses. Since time immemorial, the secondary labor market has been the primary work resource for disabled people. This market consists of undesirable jobs that no one but the desperate want. They disappear in times of economic crisis and when they exist they offer minimal salary, no fringe benefits, no security, poor working conditions, no inherent rewards, and no opportunities for advancement. Now, at last, its mindless use is going out of style.

Since work occupies fully half of our waking lives, it seems only reasonable to expect it to be an important avenue through which we learn to be, do, and get what we want from life. Most of us have these three types of goals. We want to get specific materialistic rewards, such as homes, cars, adult play toys, and so forth. We also want to engage in identified activities, either for the pleasure of the process, the outcome, or both. And we want to appear a certain way, viewed by ourselves or others as good or honest or tough or whatever characteristics are deemed desirable. Disabled workers have little chance of reaching these goals through their work, or at all, if they are relegated to traditional or conveniently available jobs. They may eat, pay the rent, buy a few clothes, and successfully avoid returning to the welfare office, but a quality work life entails much, much more.

As the Strong Vocational Interest Inventory reveals, a crucial part of job satisfaction is working with and around compatible people. More than this, work provides the major avenue for many people to form friendships. Thus, people working in areas suited to their temperaments are more likely to find coworkers with whom they will want off-the-job social and recreational contacts. Friendship and recreation are the subjects of the following chapter, but before turning to them, there is a last, brief point about employment opportunities for disabled people to be made.

The Last Discrimination

As reported earlier (Vash, 1980), the fact that disabled people are unabashedly discriminated against with respect to participating in the federally funded military services has long been an irritant to this author. Consumer groups are not clamoring for their rights to be inducted for both obvious and not-so-obvious reasons. Some disabled people, specifically young men during wartime, figure being 4-F is one of the few benefits of disability. Most, however, don't realize the magnitude of benefits they are giving up by maintaining this protected status.

I recall an abortive attempt to discuss this issue with a recruiting officer during a television program on which we both were guests. The officer nearly exploded and the moderator quickly changed the subject, since I obviously had lost my senses by suggesting that severely disabled people may have not only a responsibility but an inalienable right to serve their country. Recalling this, I asked Dean Phillips, then president of Goodwill Industries of America, what he thought about the issue. For a moment he was silent. Then he cocked his head to one side and spoke:

> Well, you kind of got me there. I just hadn't thought of it. Why of course disabled people should have the opportunities military service provides! The Marine Corps is the only branch that requires everyone to be combat-ready at all times, so disabled people ought to be inductible into every other branch. The opportunities for trade training and the many benefits of veteran status should certainly be available to disabled citizens. The Peace Corps and VISTA are alternatives, but they don't offer anything comparable to the fringe benefits of military service . . . complete health care for self and family, lodging, meals for self, cheap/convenient supplies for self and family, experience, and salary, plus the whole host of benefits that accrue to the veteran, whether from peace or wartime. (Vash, 1980, p. 116)

Most military occupational specialties have civilian counterparts, and most civilian jobs can be done by people with disabilities. If a person with paraplegia, say, can do a clerical job in the civilian sector, there is no reason why he or she cannot do it in the military; therefore, he or she should have the opportunity to reap the benefits like anyone else. So far, the efforts of Phillips and others to initiate discussion on this issue have proved fruitless.

7

Playing

Friendship and Recreation

Play has many different functions for human beings. For children, many kinds of play (e.g., playing house) serve as rehearsal for adult roles. Sports and games help them learn to function within a team, to follow rules, and to discipline themselves through training. And the importance of play does not end with maturity. John Nesbitt (1979) delineates the "four R's" that he believes play fulfills in the lives of both children and adults: recovery from the rigors of working and learning; relaxation; reward for work (school) performance; and renewal for returning to such responsibilities. He points out that the reward function also may be seen as the satisfaction and fulfillment that issue directly from one's chosen play activities. Very simply, play may be what you choose to do because it feels good rather than what you have to do to survive. At the same time, Nesbitt and others observe that it also can make survival-related activities less arduous and more effective.

This dual nature of play—as a source of primary gratification and an enhancer of success in survival-related activities—means that it serves different functions for different individuals. People devoted to their work, domestic, or scholastic pursuits may use it primarily for recovery, relaxation, and/or renewal; whereas those who are bored with their jobs may use it as their primary source of reward in life. Either way, because of social and economic changes that are occurring, play—or leisure time—is becoming more sharply focused in the thinking of today's society than has been true in the past. For some people, work days have become shorter and labor saving devices have lightened chores at home. "Early retirement" has become popular, and the baby boomers are approaching that stage in life in great numbers. Travel has become more available to the middle class, and new forms of entertainment (such as virtual reality games) appear weekly to tantalize us on television, the Web, and in print media.

As usual, the disabled population has been largely left out of the social planning for use of leisure time, at least until recently. Museums, parks, and other recreation areas were built for years without regard to their usability by people with disabilities. Now, because of disability-related civil rights laws and improved social consciousness about disability, efforts are being made to correct the errors in physical facility and program design. Recreation therapy has been included among the rehabilitation disciplines; and both the primary and spinoff values of avocational pursuits are receiving rapidly escalating attention. Some of the developments, as well as remaining gaps, in recreational opportunities for people with disabilities will be described in this chapter. First, however, let us look at a topic concerning play that is still receiving little attention.

Friendship

Friendship ties receive very little emphasis in this culture, compared with others. To cite an extreme example, certain African tribes have ceremonies as elaborate as marriage rituals to solemnize primary friendship bonds. In Mexico, the ties to one's chosen compadre or comadre are enduring and strong. History tells us that Native Americans have long ritualized "brotherhood" bonding by an exchange of blood; it is a deeply felt friendship commitment made with solemn reserve. Today, the formal celebration of friendship ties in the dominant culture grows ever less frequent. Antique jewelry stores display the "friendship links" of a bygone era; friendship rings are exchanged still, but primarily during fads of decreasing frequency and duration. It is not just the ritualization that is passing; with increasing geographic mobility, friendships become as disposable as consumer products. At the same time, the honorifics "brother" or "sister" are bestowed casually on strangers with little or no place in the speakers' lives. Many people enjoy remarkable friendships, but the trend described is nonetheless real. Acquaintanceships proliferate with increased social and physical mobility, but committed friendships may not survive socioeconomic or geographic separation.

This trend is particularly disadvantageous to disabled people for several reasons. First, friendship bonds are often more important to unmarried people than those with spouses and children to fulfill their needs for companionship, love, and interpersonal interaction; and a large segment of disabled people spend a significant part of their adult lives unmarried. Second, people who are not socially or physically mobile miss opportunities to form acquaintanceships that meet some interpersonal needs; and disabled people often lack mobility. Third, friendship ties are particularly important to people who might be termed "social underdogs" because of the extraordinary practical and moral support needs their devalued status generates; and disabled people are unquestionably social underdogs.

Children with disabilities are similarly disadvantaged in making and keeping friends. One dissertation (Gold, 1996) described attempts of adults to establish "circles of friends" around children and teens with disabilities. In four of the six attempts, friendships failed to materialize over time, perhaps because there was a tension for the other participants between being a helper and being a friend. Ironically, mainstreaming children into regular schools may be contributing to the social isolation that many children with disabilities feel. Despite the undeniable advantages of integration, the only deaf child in a classroom may find it more difficult to make friends than did such children who lived at a school composed entirely of deaf youngsters.

The foregoing illustrates several different functions that friendships fulfill. Friends are more than partners in play; they also figure importantly in meeting one's needs to love and be loved and to have practical and emotional support. Thus, friendships, like marriages, can be characterized or "typed" according to the needs being met and the interactive styles used to meet them. Let us next look at some of the effects of disablement on friendship patterns and satisfactions.

Old Friendships, New Disability

Here we will consider the interaction between disablement and friendships established prior to its occurrence. Naturally, the viability of such relationships will depend largely on their nature and solidity before being subjected to such a test. This is important because friends can be crucial to the adjustment process, lending—or failing to lend—practical and emotional support during the acute, postacute, and rehabilitation phases.

It is difficult to assess the importance of popularity. An individual's ability to develop a wide circle of friends and admirers may prove to be invaluable in some instances; whereas only one or two devoted friends may be equally helpful in others. Clearly, however, an attractive, magnetic personality will elicit more concern and desire to help. An individual's involvement in a large friendship group (usually tied to organizational affiliation, such as a church, school, or club) may have especially positive implications for group-motivated support efforts.

Despite the reported trend away from the centrality of friendship in many people's lives, instances are known wherein friends have given heroic aid to recently disabled individuals. One such case was described by a rehabilitation nurse as follows:

Ed had just passed the bar exam when he became a c4 quadriplegic in a car accident. He and his wife had many friends, but one couple was particularly close. They left their jobs, moved to the town where the rehabilitation hospital is located and rented a house nearby so Ed's wife could stay with them and Ed would have a place to go home to on weekends.

Far less extreme measures of friendship than this can also be vitally important. It is amazing how many disabled people would not part with their collections of get-well cards, years or even decades after their illnesses or injuries. Families need help and support from their friends, too. Kevin pointed out that his mother particularly needed a friend who could confront her with the pitfalls of "self-sacrifice." Others simply need help with the shopping, a small loan, or a shoulder to cry on.

Many people who sustain disabilities as adolescents or adults report a flurry of attention from their friends shortly after onset. As the weeks of recovery stretch into months and years, however, many of the old friends visit less frequently and eventually drift away. Whether this happens to a particular individual depends largely on the nature of the relationships and their potential for adapting to changed circumstance.

"Being" Versus "Doing" Relationships

As is true for marriages, friendships can be characterized as based on intimacy or parallel play. An intimate friendship is a form of "being" relationship; a parallel-play friendship is a form of "doing" relationship. The terms are almost self-explanatory, but some elaboration may be useful. People involved in "doing" relationships simply enjoy doing the same activities together. Not all "doing" relationships are parallel play; there may be central and considerable interaction between the friends. People involved in "being" relationships enjoy being together, communing or communicating, sharing feelings and ideas, or simply feeling good because of the presence of the other. The degree of intimacy may vary. "Being" and "doing" relationships are in no way mutually exclusive; in fact, most relationships combine both aspects but have one that is predominant.

A friendship that is predominantly a "being" relationship is apt to be little affected by the functional losses resulting from disability. Poor tolerance, on the part of either friend, of emotions stimulated by the disability may strain or disrupt it, but seldom will the disability itself. A friendship that is predominantly a "doing" relationship may be in serious jeopardy no matter how well disability-related emotions are handled, if the shared activities cannot be resumed or replaced by new or modified ones. Sometimes a friendship that entails a great deal of conjoint playing actually has a strong basis for intimacy and sharing on a feeling or ideational level that was masked or overridden by activity. Such relationships have good potential for enduring and deepening after their active play aspect is interrupted. Just as work can be play for people who enjoy the process as much as the outcome, so can feeling and idea sharing be relaxing, renewing, and rewarding. Naturally, many "doing" relationships endure simply because the modality impaired has little relevance to the shared activities. For example, concertgoers can continue to enjoy each other after one becomes blind; chess players can go on with their games whether or not one begins to use a wheelchair.

Friendships help people avoid loneliness, whether by connecting with another at an intimate level or by filling time and consciousness with activities and absorptions. The styles differ, but the goals may be much the same. For anyone, the dread of being alone may stem partly from a failure to distinguish solitude—which can be richly rewarding—from that state of deprivation labeled "loneliness." But whatever the genesis, people with disabilities, like people who have grown old, frequently express dismay over the extent to which they find themselves alone.

Either kind of friendship can alleviate the immediate need for human interaction, but certain types of "being" relationships can help people learn to enjoy their solitude as well. Friends such as these may be thought of as teachers, guides, counselors, or gurus, or their beneficent influence may go consciously unnoticed. At other times, both friends see these qualities in each other. Such friendships may be "made in heaven" and are as rare as the individuals who reach high levels of personal development. Nonetheless, numerous disabled people report life-changing experiences facilitated by friendships with highly evolved personalities. Carol, for example, declares of her friend Kate:

> She helped me see that it's okay to just be; I didn't have to do, accomplish, act, achieve all the time. At first, when she talked about how she treasures her alone time, I didn't even know what the devil she was talking about. But somehow I learned from her all about just being, enjoying solitude, and enjoying the time I do spend with others even more . . . they are all interrelated. My block was fearing to be alone because of my physical dependency, yet longing for it and not recognizing that fact. She saw it all right away. Actually, the best thing she did for me was like me. I thought she was so fantastic that if she picked me for a friend, I had to be okay . . . any friend of hers is a friend of mine . . . even me!

This last remark may encapsulate the core meaning of friendship, but the description also shows that friendships can assume the quality of a counseling relationship that supercedes commonplace supportive listening, validation of ideas and feelings, and advice giving. A friendship that stresses mutual counseling support is one form of symbiotic relationship.

Symbiotic Relationships

Such friendships (or marriages) are sometimes considered alternatives to intimacy—which may be accurate—but symbiosis also can coexist with intimacy. All that is required is for the relationship to serve certain practical purposes as well as provide pleasurable human exchange. When friends serve as each others' confidants, sounding boards, advisors, or counselors, this can reasonably be viewed as a form of symbiosis. Without such informal "services," either or both might find it necessary to seek, and pay for, professional help.

Along with growing awareness of the value of "peer counseling" for people with disabilities, the counseling role of friendships is becoming more salient among disabled people. Informal friendships may begin as a result of formal peer counseling contacts, and established relationships may take on counseling aspects as their benefits come to be more widely advertised, legitimized, and personally experienced. It is important to keep in mind that symbiosis implies roughly equivalent give and take on both sides, but not necessarily identical. It is just as likely that one friend will offer counseling in exchange for a different kind of support that is needed.

Programs designed to train paraprofessionals to work with disabled (or other service-needing) populations sometimes refer to their work as training students to form helping friendships. Perhaps when the public grows weary of sex manuals, the next interpersonal how-to-do-it fashion could focus on how to become a truly helpful friend who fosters growth and avoids reinforcing maladaptive tendencies. People with disabilities who have been associated with independent living programs might be in the vanguard of such a movement. Because of the peer counseling emphasis in these programs, they now have head starts in a direction that could benefit everyone, whether or not they have disabilities.

The "using" aspects of relationships are often overtly disdained, but nonetheless constitute a benefit of many friendships. Friends may have contacts useful for anything from quick, cheap appliance repair to landing prestigious jobs. People with disabilities find it particularly desirable to develop friendships with their neighbors, people who will be close by in times of crisis. There is nothing inherently selfish about using friendships in such ways, assuming the friendly caring is authentic and the giving and taking are more or less balanced. When they are not, the friend with the deficit is likely to end the relationship.

Because it is not always obvious to the external observer who is getting what out of a relationship, it may be the apparent "taker" who ends up feeling drained. For example, nondisabled people with strong needs to be needed not infrequently attach themselves to people who are, at first, grateful for their help. After awhile, however, the latter may find themselves emotionally exhausted by the subtle exaction of a price for all services—in such forms as patronization, solicitation of gratitude, and reminders of dependency. As was discussed relative to pairing (see Chapter 5), disabled people sometimes must be wary of friendship candidates who would help too much.

New Friendships, Old Disability

After one has grown used to having a disability, an eventual consideration is making new friends. "Will people still want to be friends with me now that I can't do many things or 'keep up' with them?" "Will they be uncomfortable around me?" Even apart from such deliberations, it is easy for people with disabilities—especially severe ones—to narrow their experiential worlds to the close and familiar. This is a fairly natural reaction to "stimulus overload," which is the prevailing condition when much of life is seen as new, unusual, demanding, or depressing. Such narrowing may include limiting one's associations and seeking to meet all interpersonal needs through parents, spouse, or children who will be part of one's world anyway. This avoids the addition of more sources of unwelcome stimulation. When disability is so severe as to inhibit mobility away from home, associations may be limited still further. The result is friendless individuals who place enormous demands on the family members they live with to meet all of their needs for companionship, needs that usually are distributed among a larger constellation of relatives and friends. A spouse, parent, or child may become virtually the person's only friend—a heavy burden for those who feel trapped by responsibility already.

Some disabled people resolve to associate only with other disabled individuals "who will understand." As indicated earlier (see Chapter 2), this may issue from self-derogation, a belief that one will not prove worthy to nondisabled friends. The act of making a resolution suggests a self-defensive maneuver, and this is most likely to be the case when it happens early in the adjustment process. Others, who have found themselves fully able to attract friends regardless of disability, simply may find that their firmest ties are to those who have shared the disability experience. This is more likely to be the result of need evolvement through learning, and reflects a positive choice, not a defense.

The kinds of people sought as friends always depend on where they are found, whether through school or work, at church, in clubs, or around the neighborhood. For the high proportion of disabled adults who are unemployed, a major source of friendship contacts is eliminated, even for those who have no desire to limit their associations. The Internet, however, has opened up amazing new possibilities for establishing friendships, even for individuals who have little opportunity to leave home. A quick search under the keywords "disabilities" and "friendship" turns up dozens of listings for chat rooms, pen pals, and guides for making friendships around the globe. Of course, there is no need to specify disability in the search: people of all kinds are using the Web to make friends, and there are chat rooms for people with all kinds of interests. Still, these resources can be especially useful for those with visible disabilities who need to overcome attitudinal barriers in many face-to-face encounters. On the Web, everyone starts off on equal footing, and they can share whatever they wish as the friendship develops. Some may wonder whether an electronic relationship can ever become a true friendship, but others can attest to deep personal bonds that may develop over time.

In addition to traditional and electronic routes to friendship, the disability rights movement has opened up alternative opportunities in recent years, through independent living centers and organizations "by and for the disabled." Although most of these have service and political action missions, they are proving to be a better resource for friendships than the "social clubs for the disabled" of an earlier era.

Now that rehabilitation and independent living programs are beginning to train disabled people in how to select and supervise their personal employees (assistants, interpreters, readers, and drivers), an issue that frequently arises is whether the relationship should remain strictly that of employer and employee, or if it also should be one of friendship. There is no simplistic answer. In every kind of work setting, people can be found who prefer to keep their work and social lives separate, as can others whose friends are almost solely work colleagues. Many employers socialize with peers, but believe it unwise to spend time with subordinates outside of work. Others forcefully disagree. In all cases, individual predilection is the key.

Some people can learn to play the dual roles of "boss" and "friend" effectively; others can't. Some fear the practice will lead to exploitation by the subordinate; others simply say they would be careful not to choose an exploitative person as a friend (or employee, if they have that choice). With respect to personal employees, the issue is most salient with live-in assistants. Because the employment relationship is so much more intimate than with the typical live-in domestic worker, social distancing is less feasible. It seems the most satisfactory and enduring relationships do not lose the primacy of the employee-employer responsibilities, but are leavened with mutual caring and concern for the other's needs that could only be termed "friendship." Moreover, compatibility was usually given conscious consideration at the time of hiring.

There is an old saying: "From friendship to love, maybe; but from love to friendship, never!" Although modernized thinking is changing the accuracy of both clauses of this adage, people with disabilities especially find that the likelihood of "friendship to love" is more than a hesitant "maybe. "Many report that most of their romances begin as friendships, contrary to their predisability patterns. The explanation appears simple. Visibly disabled individuals, no matter how physically attractive, are unlikely targets for the random dating efforts that go on in the singles community. They may, in fact, be seen by the nondisabled majority as sexless and therefore perhaps less threatening. While this might not be flattering to the disabled person thus regarded, it does facilitate cross-sex friendships. Once the individuals get to know each other, and the strangeness of the disability wears off, the "sexless" image is recognized as inaccurate and the spark of romance may ignite.

Regardless of the way in which a friendship develops, friends are widely thought of as people to do things with and who can share one's recreational interests. Let us next explore the topic of recreation—refreshment of body or mind through some form of play, whether pursued with friends, strangers, or alone—as it relates to people with disabilities.

Recreation

Almost every conceivable activity or pursuit can be construed as play or recreation by someone, however dull or terrifying or otherwise unpleasant it might seem to someone else. Nowhere is the cliché "one man's meat is another man's poison" more pertinent. The person who relaxes, renews, and gains rewards from engraving The Lord's Prayer on the heads of pins is unlikely to enjoy a deep rapport with the one who prefers driving in demolition derbies. This is an important reason why friendship is such an integral aspect of the topic "playing."

To understand why certain recreational activities are attractive or unattractive to given individuals, it may be helpful to look at them in terms of the processes involved and their outcomes. With respect to process, such polarities as active-passive, physical-mental, delicate-expansive, formalized-spontaneous, and creative-fixed can be used to characterize them. The first two are self-explanatory. The engraver and derby driver just cited reflect the delicate-expansive polarity. Bridge is formalized; so is football. Fifty-two pick-up and catch are spontaneous. (Irrepressibly spontaneous players in formalized games are apt to be unappreciated by serious devotees to the rules in question.) Dancing ranges from the precision of ballet and the tango to the spontaneity of a street dance.

Outcomes can be described in terms of such qualities as their relative benefit to the individual or society, their potential for becoming vocations as well as avocations, and their "therapeutic" value. Perhaps, if the use of leisure time becomes a more critical societal concern, such process and outcome variables will be used for an "avocational interest inventory" to help people discern, with less trial and error, the types of recreations that will meet their needs best. This, of course, would overlook the possibility that the trial-and-error process is itself recreational.

Few conclusions can be drawn, prima facie, about the kinds of recreations appropriate for disabled people. True, many people with high-level quadriplegia may be uninterested in "active, physical, expansive" activities, but others can and do pursue vigorous and potentially dangerous pastimes. Peggy was one such person; several years after her injury she finally fulfilled her dream to fly an ultralight plane. It is not unusual for those whose diversions seem incredible to the general public to appear in the news as inspirational examples to others. Ironically, this can have the opposite effect on disabled people whose motivation levels are more nearly normal but who nonetheless would like to identify hobbies or other leisure activities within grasp. At the other extreme, severely disabled people are apt to be encouraged to try to enjoy such "passive, mental, individual" recreations as art, music appreciation, or reading, despite protestations that they meet none of the person's felt needs.

Failing to find other sources of recreational gratification, some choose pastimes held in social disdain, such as the recreational use of alcohol and drugs, or television viewing taken to extreme. Both are renowned favorites among people with disabilities and are viewed as escape rather than renewal activity. They involve little effort, and they offer little opportunity for growth. This is an important reason for efforts to discover and educate people with disabilities about both traditional and new recreational possibilities.

Recreational Advocacy

In recreation, as in education and employment, mainstreaming has become an important issue. Activist groups all over the country are turning some of their attention to the wide range of indoor and outdoor recreational accommodations: museums, galleries, parks, amusement centers, beaches, forests, sports arenas, hiking trails, theaters, skating pavilions, boat harbors—the list is endless. With the backing of the ADA, they are requiring that all public recreational accommodations be designed or modified so that artificial barriers to their use by disabled citizens will not eliminate recreational outlets that otherwise could be enjoyed.

The base-level demands are for (1) buildings and grounds that are accessible and safe for all disabled users, and (2) user information available in forms accessible to people with sensory differences. Stairs, and lack of guidebooks on tape, for example, are artificial barriers to the use of available programs. The next level of advocacy is for programmatic change toward inclusion of more recreational activities feasible for disabled people. If none of the planned activities can be done by a person who can't see or hear or walk or think quickly, accessible/safe facilities will be of little import. The third level of advocacy involves the reduction of natural barriers for designated populations. Tactile replica exhibits for blind people wishing to experience ancient artifacts that cannot be touched provides a prime example.

Early efforts to make mainstream recreational facilities accessible often resulted in intramural segregation, with disabled viewers being seated together, apart from their companions. Such disappointing experiences led to refinements, often coming from advisory panels of individuals with disabilities. More appropriate, scattered accommodations are now common, and individuals who use wheelchairs are seldom turned away at the entrance (as sometimes happened in the past). When an amusement area has historical significance, however, disabled citizens are apt to find themselves in political combat with the local historical society, which oftentimes values authenticity of style more than the rights of disabled people.

Not all recreational advocacy is aimed toward mainstreaming. Interestingly, just as the concept of "special education" was losing favor, the parallel term "special recreation" was coming into vogue. The best-known examples of special recreation are the Paralympics, for physically disabled athletes, and the Special Olympics, for athletes with mental retardation. The Paralympics grew out of the British Stoke-Mandeville games, and the first Paralympic Summer Games were held in Rome in 1960. The Paralympics attract world-class athletes who compete in an array of sports similar in scope to those of the Olympic Games. More than 4,000 athletes from 120 countries participated in the most recent summer games (U.S. Paralympics, 2002). The International Paralympic Committee is formally recognized and funded in part by the International Olympic Committee. Despite the protestations of some who believe both should be integrated into the Olympics, most see these programs as offering invaluable experiences to disabled people with outstanding athletic prowess. The Special Olympics have a different purpose and format (Special Olympics, 2002). Rather than focusing on elite athletes, it provides opportunities for participation and competition to individuals 8 years of age and older who have mental retardation or cognitive delays. All participants are considered winners.

Special recreation and fitness centers in some areas offer facility design and programming specifically tailored to accommodate disabled participants. Crosstrainers Fitness Forum in Clinton Township, Michigan is a new facility that goes beyond being "wheelchair accessible" to being "wheelchair friendly" (Boyd, 2001). Christopher Grobbel, himself paralyzed from the chest down as the result of a 1994 motor vehicle accident, created a facility that serves both people with disabilities and those without, side by side. Educational programs and special events complement such offerings as strength training, wheelchair aerobics and yoga, and diet consultation. Among the machines is a new multivector strength-training machine that accommodates anyone's range of motion, however limited. For example, it is being used to help one young man to develop enough strength to use a joystick for driving a van (Grobbel, personal communication). Grobbel hopes eventually to take the concept to national markets through expansion or franchises.

The Vinland Center, which was founded with a bicentennial gift to the United States from the government of Norway, provides an example of a different kind of structure and mission. It is located on a lake about 35 miles west of Minneapolis and offers both day and residential programs for persons with physical, cognitive, and substance abuse disabilities. The grounds and facilities are fully accessible, and the programs combine recreational, educational, and rehabilitative elements.

Adventure therapy programs, sometimes aimed specifically at persons with disabilities and occasionally integrated with other participants, have also attracted attention during the past two decades. These programs put participants in unfamiliar and highly challenging situations such as traversing suspended rope bridges, canoeing in icy waters, and climbing rock faces. By pushing themselves beyond their ordinary capabilities, participants may learn that they need not accept the limitations they previously assumed were inevitable. One study (Herbert, 1998) found that participants gained self-esteem and professed a greater internal locus of control compared with a control group, although these gains did not persist during a one-year follow-up. The author indicated a need for more research and varied programs to provide further information about the potential of this approach for changing life perspectives.

Perhaps, with time and experience, special recreation can go the way of segregated education, i.e., be limited to an ever narrowing band of the population. It might even be that the Paralympics one day will be integrated—or at least more closely combined—with the Olympics. Further advocacy will be required for any of this to occur. In addition, preparation for recreation is needed by many disabled people at various stages in the rehabilitation process.

Recreational Preparation

Because sports and recreation are so strongly associated in the American consciousness, nonathletically inclined individuals may ignore programs labeled "recreation," expecting them to be composed of wheelchair basketball, bowling, archery, and little else. At one time, this was true of the first author, who related to a recreation therapy symposium:

> Until I recognized the prevocational potential of recreation, I was never very interested in the field because I identified it with sports. When it comes to athletic prowess, disability helped me avoid a distressing source of embarrassment. In school, when team captains chose up sides, they fought over who was going to get stuck with me. The loser would tell me to go to the backfield and under no circumstances to touch the ball. I wouldn't have anyway. My unvarying reaction to having a ball thrown at me was to cringe and duck. I consider this a sensible reaction to this very day. Looking over the program for this symposium, however, one sees how much more than sports is entailed. There's music, dance, arts and crafts, drama, gourmet cooking, water play, puppetry—literally something for everyone. [Vash, 1978b]

During the years when the onset of severe disability was often followed by long periods of inpatient rehabilitation, recreation programs were an important part of the recovery process. With changes in health care funding, hospital stays have been drastically shortened, and many of the ancillary services have been pared away. In some areas, independent living centers have added recreational components to their programs. For example, the Capital Area Center for Independent Living in Lansing, Michigan, has a lively collection of "circles" that offer informal opportunities for participants to engage in crafts, writing, and many other activities. Such examples aside, recreation is seldom a top priority for CILs. Issues more central to community survival (for example, financial advocacy, assistant recruitment, and transportation) tend to usurp the funds available. When a volunteer instructor is available, good recreational programs may take place. When the volunteer disappears, however, so does the program.

As noted earlier, recreational participation can serve as a powerful prevocational tool, especially for individuals whose work experience and skills seem limited. Sometimes competencies can be discovered and developed in the less challenging milieu of a recreation program from which there is no threat of "mustering out" that later can be translated into a vocational plan. Sometimes what is needed is not so much preparation as instigation. This can be illustrated best by an additional passage from the author's previously cited address to a recreation therapy symposium:

> Dance was an important part of my life before I became disabled. My sister was a dancer and tutored me from preschool days. My unheroic career as an athlete became less painful in high school when modern dance was offered as a physical education option. When no one was throwing balls or hockey pucks at me, I did okay. Since then, with two significant exceptions, which I will share with you, the only "dancing" I've done is with men who are strong enough to carry me while leaping about a dance floor.
>
> The first exception was at a party a dozen years ago where a woman instructed me, at inebriated length, on how to "dance" in a wheelchair by shaking my shoulders and torso to the music. I was having so much fun I almost missed seeing her march over to my date and beg to be carried, "like you do her!" Then her date asked me to dance. I made the usual gesture of someone expecting to be lifted, but instead he looped his belt through the arm rest of my chair and sent me spinning. Everyone got off the dance floor, including our respective dates. Mine almost dropped his. He had an uncanny knack for making a wheelchair with a ninety-pound load go where he wanted it to. This was purely passive on my part, but it was a lot of fun. The shoulder/torso dancing was active but, somehow, the disinhibition I needed for such a routine—and got from an instigator—hasn't happened again.
>
> The second exception reinforced the important role of an instigator. While serving as a VR administrator, I visited an independent living center. A movement and dance group was going on and the director made clear that there would be no observers-only participants, including bureaucrats. The others had gait problems, poor coordination, or weakness, but I was the only wheelchair user present. Since it was motorized, I was the most mobile person there. I had a ball . . . creating routines that took advantage of both the chair's movement characteristics and my own. My lack of inhibition amazed even me, but, again, I had instigators: one said, "You must" and a dozen showed that they were game. [Vash, 1978b]

The motorized wheelchair is not the only rehabilitation engineering aid available for recreational purposes. The Assistive Technology Sourcebook (Enders & Hall, 1990) presents case examples illustrating the use of a broad range of recreation-related assistive devices and aids. Expositions of equipment for people with disabilities are hugely popular, both as stand-alone events and as adjuncts to rehabilitation-related conferences. The current Abledata Web site, for example, lists 21 national and international conferences scheduled for the coming year. Some involve specialized topics such as augmentative communication, and others appear to cover a broad sweep (e.g., First Annual

World Congress & Exposition on Disabilities). In recreation, as in other aspects of life, technological advancement offers expanding means to enhance the quality of life, yielding more and more to discover.

Recreational Discovery

Most discovery of feasible and rewarding recreations comes about adventitiously. One hears about hobbies, sports, and games from associates and, occasionally, one of them "clicks." Recreational fads are common in the general population, and the same is true for specific disability groups, especially when popular pursuits prove feasible for people with given functional limitations. For example, ham radio operation was a perennial favorite among people severely disabled by polio when that portended being homebound, as was frequently the case. Later, trap/skeet shooting and radio controlled model airplanes enjoyed prolonged vogues among wheelchair users with good arm function.

In recreation, as in so many other spheres of life, the Internet is now available to supplement accidental discovery as a prime means of generating fresh ideas for enjoyable activity. Accessible resorts, tours, and adventures, adaptive sports and recreational equipment, and information about travel by plane, train, bus, automobile, RV and even motorcycle are at your fingertips in moments (Lubin, 2002). Whether your destination is the Everglades National Park, Ireland, Tokyo, or the Puerto Rican rain forest, you can instantaneously call up information about accessible transit, accommodations, and attractions. Examples of other kinds of recreation abound. The National Center on Physical Activity and Disability (Accessibility, 2002) offers papers reflecting the variety of possibilities, including, for example, *Therapeutic Horseback Riding, Instructional Tips for Golfers with Disabilities, Big Game Hunting with Long Arms,* and *A Day at the Zoo.*

Abledata (2002) offers a treasure trove of information about assistive technology in 20 categories, including recreation. The links include information about specific items and suppliers as well as some detailed publications on aquatic sports, winter sports, and recreation equipment. Among the aquatic devices are flotation platforms, harnesses, balls, pool lifts, adaptive swimwear, amphibious wheelchairs, and several models of water skis. For winter sports, skis with outriggers or stabilizers, sit-skis, mono-skis, and sleds are just some of the products available to eliminate barriers to participation in outdoor recreation.

Not all recreations look like play on the surface. Volunteerism, for example, looks like work; however, if the individual is not being paid (and is not using volunteer work to expiate sins), the chances are that the intent is pleasure. It is very convenient for people with well-developed social consciences to be able to play and contribute to the social good at the same time. In addition to church, civic, political, and other traditional types of volunteer work, disabled people now have independent living programs and organizations "by and for the disabled" eager to receive their help. Some examples include Adapt and Not Dead Yet. Adapt is an activist organization that has staged many episodes of civil disobedience to prod cities to develop accessible and integrated transit systems. Most recently, they have worked to change the incentives in social systems so that people with disabilities are not unnecessarily confined to nursing homes. Not Dead Yet is opposing initiatives that would legalize assisted suicide, reflecting concern that people with disabilities might be led to end their lives for reasons stemming from negative attitudes or inadequate resources and services.

Membership in a group, and the opportunities for human contact and belonging it provides, is often the prime motivator for doing volunteer work. Perhaps equally often, it offers a way to secure a sense of doing something worthwhile when one is not employed, or such satisfaction is not forthcoming from one's work. Because the unemployment rate for disabled adults continues to be exceedingly high, this is an especially important motivator for disabled volunteers. Disability-related advocacy also offers the promise of personal benefit.

Professional efforts to guide recreational discovery do not always happen within the confines of planned programs. A retired recreation therapist related to the author that his most rewarding venture in this respect occurred spontaneously, after a planned outing for severely disabled child patients of a rehabilitation hospital. Passing a grassy slope on the return trip from an amusement park, one child murmured, "Wouldn't it be fun to roll down that hill?" On cue, the therapist stopped the bus and spent the next two hours wrapping disabled children in heavy sheets kept aboard the bus, rolling them down the hill, and returning them to the bus. A few weeks later, none of them had much to say about the official outing, but he reports that they never stopped talking about the hill rolling. He believes the rare opportunity for severely paralyzed youngsters to experience the kinesthetic pleasures of gross and rapid body movement was as therapeutic as it was enjoyable, and that such spontaneous adventures should be encouraged.

Sadly, he also reports that he "caught hell" from his supervisor for doing anything so risky, although not one child was hurt in any way. This brings to mind the well-known poster of a child wearing leg braces who is perched on the limb of a tree. The caption reads, "There is dignity in taking risks." This is an important reminder in general and is particularly applicable to recreation.

Guided discovery also is taking place within an exciting cluster of relative newcomers to the field of recreation: therapies based on the transcendental arts and a host of techniques imported from the Far East. Sometimes viewed as psychotherapy (or psychogogy, see Chapter 11) and at other times considered recreation, these approaches can be both, simultaneously. The transcendental arts therapies include such modalities as art therapy, music therapy, dance therapy, psychodrama, and poetry therapy. Their use is greatest with people who have emotional disabilities, but their potential for people with bodily disabilities is becoming appreciated. Dana illustrated the potential value of poetry therapy to her (see Chapter 1) and made the further observation that:

> Certain insights seem to fall out of your brain when you write poetry . . . as if the rhythm pulls them out, in a way that doesn't happen in reverie, conversation, or writing prose, however hard you are searching.

Yoga and the martial arts are being incorporated gradually into therapeutic recreation programs, too. Their practitioners cite their value as play, as well as their physical and mental health benefits. Martial arts training for disabled people has the added value of reducing feelings of vulnerability. More will be said in Chapter 11 about this entire constellation of new techniques based on ancient arts, and their roles in psychological strengthening.

A number of disabled people who, by and large, did their own recreational discovery without professional guidance, are serving now as guides to others. Louise Sauvage, who was born with spina bifida, has earned Olympic, Paralympic, and World Championship gold medals in track (e-bility, 2002a). This elite athlete partnered with the Northern Eagles NRL Club in 2000 to establish the Aspire To Be a Champion Foundation, which provides financial help to young athletes with disabilities. Robert Ott, who is blind, holds the rank of 5th degree black belt by the Korean Hapkido Association. As President and Chief Master of the World Kidokwan Federation, he gives motivational presentations for schools and other organizations (Ott, 2002). Judith Geppert, an adventurer with cerebral palsy (e-bility, 2002b), searched for several years before finding a skydiving instructor who would make a jump with her strapped to his back. These and other disabled people have found ways to have fun, as well as survive, and are sharing their methods with people newer to the process. They have, in a sense, transcended their disabilities—and this is the topic of the following chapter.

8

Transcending
Disability as Growth Experience

Acceptance of disability, for most people, evolves gradually over a span of years filled with instructive experience. It comes seldom, if ever, as a *coup de foudre* followed by getting on with life. Instead, the process of living teaches, little by little, that disablement needn't be viewed as an insurmountable tragedy. It may be only a complication or an irritant—and whose life is without those? As the struggles to survive, work, love, and play show evidence of some success, individuals find awareness of disablement slipping longer and oftener into the background of consciousness. Eventually, for some, it may come to be seen as a positive contributor to life in its totality—a catalyst to psychological growth. Since these changes take time, trial, error, and correction to unfold, forward movement does not always look like progress.

The initial chapters of this volume described the effects of devaluation on acceptance of disability and on reactions to disablement, especially in the early stages of adjustment. This chapter will augment those descriptions with a finer analysis of the lifelong process of acknowledging disability, physically, intellectually, emotionally, and spiritually. It also will pursue the process further than usually is done, beyond the range of "normalization" to higher levels of self-actualization that are fostered by the disability experience.

Acknowledgment of Disability

The late Nancy Kerr, a psychologist who was paraplegic as a result of polio, describes five major stages in the process of adjusting to permanent disability: shock, expectancy of recovery, mourning, defense, and, finally, adjustment (Kerr, 1977). She hastens to point out that the stages are points on a continuum, not discrete categories, and that they describe common, but not inevitable, behavioral phases. During the shock stage, the individual has not really comprehended the fact that he or she is ill or disabled, so little anxiety is present. The realization that something is truly wrong is often accompanied by expectancy of recovery, including preoccupation with improvement of the disabling condition. There is no motivation for learning to live with the disability, however, since it is expected to vanish. When this does not transpire, mourning may follow. Acute distress, readiness to "give up," and thoughts of suicide are common. Reprimands for self-pity may engender hostility, and some resign themselves to their fates and remain at this stage indefinitely. Most others progress to the defense stage, characterized by coping efforts and interest in learning to be as normal as possible. Barriers are acknowledged and either conquered or circumvented. This is considered healthy defense. The defense stage is considered neurotic if the person employs defense mechanisms to deny that barriers exist. Kerr believes that reinforcement from others to "look on the bright side" and reprimands for sadness are conducive to the use of defensive denial. People who reach the adjustment stage no longer consider their disabilities as barriers to be fought, have found ways to satisfy their needs, and feel that they are adequate persons.

The Value of Denial

Different variants of denial are evident in the shock, expectancy of recovery, and defense stages. Traditionally, denial is viewed as maladaptive, but Kerr draws no such inferences respecting the shock and expectancy of recovery stages. Only when it appears later, in the defense stage, does she describe it as neurotic. Arnold Beisser, a psychiatrist who was quadriplegic as a result of polio, has discussed the adaptive value of denial in surviving myocardial infarction and other life-threatening conditions (Beisser, 1979). He indicates that the view of denial as a psychopathological sign of poor ego strength is fading as research supports its survival value, and he exhorts physicians to judiciously consider whether, when, and how to interrupt it. Most of his examples reflect the shock and expectancy of recovery stages; however, in all cases, the physician is enjoined to consider foremost the patient's psychic economy and at what expense to self he or she must adhere to a particular view.

The following account of personal experiences with denial (Vash, 1977) illustrates its multiform nature as it evolves over time.

> I became paralyzed over a matter of three or four hours. Until I finally collapsed, I simply refused to believe it was happening. I felt weak but not ill, and kept struggling out of bed to walk around and prove to myself that what seemed to be happening could not possibly be happening until I fell flat on my face—at which

point I was more or less convinced, at least temporarily. That is plain, old fashioned, *primitive denial*. The facts are there and you deny them admission to consciousness.

When the doctor told me I'd had a slight case of polio, I breathed a sigh of relief. I'd read an article about how awful polio used to be until the Sister Kenny treatments, but now the main requirement was determination to do your exercises. As an erstwhile gymnast and dancer I wasn't afraid of exercises, so I figured in a few weeks I'd be fit as a fiddle again. That form of denial is called *selective attention*. You admit some of the data to consciousness, but not all of it—not the part that would be upsetting.

About three months later, when I'd gotten back some use of my left arm and hand but not much more, I hesitantly asked my physical therapist, "Hey! I don't mean to get worrisome about this but is there any chance that I might not get all better?" Her answer was classic: "Well, you hardly ever hear of a case that doesn't anymore." She belonged to the school that professed, "Give them an ambiguous answer that permits them to hear what they're ready to hear." I was ready to hear that recovery might take a few more months, and that I might have to settle for choreography instead of performing dance, to the extent that I continued dance as either vocation or avocation. I had heard a rule of thumb which stated, "If you don't get it back within a year, you won't get it back." I turned that around to mean, "Don't worry for a year." So I didn't. This goes beyond selective attention; I was working very hard to keep the facts out of consciousness.

The year went by. I was about to adopt an alternate rule of thumb. By then I had heard of cases taking up to two years for full return of function. It was beginning to look like I was one of those. The issue was forced by the school psychologist during a vocational counseling session. In the seventh grade I had decided that I was either going to major in psychology and minor in dance, when I went to college, or vice versa; but in the ensuing five years, I had never decided which. I told the psychologist it was looking like a forced choice but I wasn't ready to give up yet. He suggested it was time to ask my doctor, since college was only a few months away. I did. He said, "Better prepare for a sedentary life." I said. "What's sedentary?" Now, I was known in school as a walking dictionary, but all of the sudden I didn't know what "sedentary" meant. Isn't denial fascinating?

He explained and I said, "Oh shit." Mother frowned but didn't chide. I cried on the way home, straightened up my act, called my two best friends, told them, swore them to secrecy because I feared the other kids couldn't handle it and might start avoiding me, and two weeks later I ran off and got married. Everyone knows what that one is called. It's called *acting out*. It's one of the niftier denial mechanisms; it drives other people crazy. They can't believe you are just ignoring the whole thing.

I wasn't ignoring it. I was relieved. It took much less energy than that damned two-year plan. And I was depressed. No Gloomy Gus on the outside, I smiled and smiled and smiled—another form of denial. But on the inside, such self-loathing, such world weariness, such cosmic depression as few are privileged to experience. I'd wake up and look across the room at my wheelchair and the hydraulic lift used to put me in it and say, "No. No human being was ever meant to be like this—a useless blob of protoplasm that has to be moved from one place to another with a crane."

I had moved through one level of acknowledgment—facing the facts—only to find myself immediately embroiled in a struggle with a second level—acceptance of the implications.

Reasons for Denial

Aside from practical reasons for wishing disability were not so, there are additional reasons, issuing from devalued status in society. The social implications are either known or sensed by newly disabled people, and experience tends to confirm the worst expectations. Disability leads to devaluation, which in turn leads to segregation and its ubiquitous companion, oppression. Until the passage of ADA and other civil rights legislation, the person was seen as outside the law, too aberrant to be included under constitutional or statutory protection. Even now, residual discrimination often leads to impoverished education and socialization, with resultant noncompetitive status. Poverty and powerlessness ensue, reinforcing both self-devaluation and devaluation by others. When the vicious cycle set in motion by disablement is examined thus, it is readily apparent why individuals would wish to deny being caught up in it. Conversely, as disabled people are able to escape this cycle, they become able to relinquish the "protection" that denial affords. They then can move into Kerr's (1977) adjustment stage and from there onward to higher levels of psychological development.

Models of Psychological Development

If we're lucky, we all experience the processes of birth, infancy, childhood, adolescence, young adulthood, mature adulthood, old age, and death. The early stages reflect changes in the direction of growth; the latter, decay. Theorists from many disciplines, ancient and modern, have been redividing and renaming the developmental stages with astounding regularity over the years. They also have debated the inevitability of psychological decay; whether psychological (spiritual) development ceases or progresses with death. To illustrate: Freud named his developmental stages after the psychosexual stages he believed we all go through: oral, anal, phallic, and genital (Hall, Lindzey, & Campbell, 1998). Like many Western theorists, he used these same labels for his personality typology; that is, he claimed that we do not all get to be "genital" characters just by virtue of growing older. Some of us, because of certain experiences, get fixated at certain levels and become or remain "oral," "anal," or "phallic" personalities. In this case, psychological growth lags behind physical development.

A very different approach comes from Hindu philosophy. In one system, life is divided into four twenty-year segments. The first twenty years are the time for learning. The second twenty years are the time for getting established in the practical world. The third twenty years are the time to search for oneself and God. The fourth twenty years are the time to renounce the material world and wander about teaching others what one has learned. (Isn't it odd? That is exactly when we in the United States encourage retirement from our schools and universities!) According to the Hindus, psychological or spiritual growth continues and perhaps intensifies long after physical development has sloped downward toward decay.

Kerr's (1977) stages of adjustment to disability are a model of psychological development focused on a particular segment of the population in a limited aspect of their lives. It purports only to describe the developmental process of regaining or establishing a normative adjustment under nonnormative conditions. Following is another such model, one that offers a different emphasis.

Levels of Acknowledgment

The model put forward by the first author (Vash, 1978b) condenses the five stages described by Kerr (1977) into two levels of acknowledgment of disability, and then adds a third level that goes beyond the resumption of normalcy to what might be construed as development into higher consciousness—catalyzed, in part, by experience with disability.

Level I: Recognition of the Facts. Here the person understands the nature and the extent of the limitations, the probability of permanence, and the realities of social stigmatization, but detests every bit of it. Disability is seen as a tragedy and has negative valence.

Level II: Acceptance of the Implications. Here the person acknowledges the realities of his or her condition without a sense of loss and shows acceptance of what "is" without recrimination. The facts and implications of the disability are integrated into a chosen lifestyle. Disability is seen as an inconvenience that can be mastered and has neutral valence.

Level III: Embracing the Experience. Here the person recognizes that without the disability he or she would be different from what he or she is, and there is no desire to be different. There is appreciation of the fact that disability has been, is, and will continue to be a growth catalyst if allowed to be so. Disability, like all other life experiences, is seen as an opportunity or gift, and therefore has positive valence.

Naturally, there is a period of time before reaching Level I when the person fails to acknowledge even the facts; and acknowledgment and denial alternate in and below consciousness throughout life for most disabled people. With varying degrees of difficulty, most people advance into the second level of acknowledgment. Individual differences in the degree to which most "old hands" have acknowledged their disabilities usually could be described in terms of how far *within* that level they have progressed. Few get stymied at the first level any more. This has not always been true, and the consciousness raising going on of late regarding disability is largely responsible for this positive change. How far one has progressed within Level II could be defined in terms of the extent to which one accepts without rancor the conditions life presents, versus tendencies to lapse into moments or days of disappointment, rage, despondency, self-hatred, or other erosive emotions related to the facts and implications of disability.

At the same time, relatively few people even conceive of the third level— embracing the disability experience as a positively valued opportunity—and fewer still actually progress into that level. In part, this simply reflects the reduced numbers of people who progress into higher levels of consciousness generally, regardless of experience with disability. At Level III, one embraces disability as an opportunity for psychological growth and spiritual development which has few parallels in life; an opportunity that can be wasted or exploited, a gift in disguise. The individual arrives at faith in the maxim, "You don't always get what you *want*, but you always get what you *need*" (for progressing toward spiritual goals). To the extent that we learn through pain, disability is an excellent chance for learning. It's a little like getting hit by the proverbial two-by-four. If you're not strong enough, it may kill you. But if you survive and it gets your attention, it can be the beginning and the way of a great adventure.

One reason so few people aspire to this level of development is that it is not ingrained in Western culture. The biblical story of Job is as close as we get to it in our widely-read writings. It is integral, however, to Eastern psychology and philosophy, which are now being read eagerly in the West. The concept would strike most newly disabled people as a cruel hoax or sardonic joke, and may strike others as an example of "sweet lemon" rationalization. Easier to accept is a related concept, reflected in the claims of numerous disabled people, that severe disability has made them strong. While there is little doubt about that, there also appears to be a level beyond strength,

where such individualistic qualities are surmounted. People who have survived, accepted, and transcended painful loss—and disablement is but one
example—may be uniquely enabled to grow beyond the limits Western
thought has allowed for. They can move into a realm we are only beginning
to appreciate and aspire to as the spiritual East and the technological West
discover that each has ignored a vast part of life for centuries, and if the
human race is going to survive, they must begin to learn from each other.

Moving Forward

Rehabilitation: A Lifelong Process

A television interviewer once asked the first author if she felt she were fully
rehabilitated at that point in her life. She responded that she doubted she
ever would be, and asked if he felt *he* were, although he had no discernible
disability. He understood quickly what was meant and agreed that the term
"rehabilitation" tends to be substituted for phrases connoting "human development" whenever a person has had such catastrophic life experiences as disablement or incarceration.

People working with disabled children assert that the concept of rehabilitation doesn't apply well to people who had not established themselves physically, socially, and vocationally at the time of disability onset. They self-
consciously speak of *habilitation*, to stress the illogic of trying to restore a
person to a previous level of functioning when applied to individuals disabled
since childhood.

It may not make very good sense when applied to other disabled people,
either. "Going back" to a previous state is not the natural direction of growth
at any age, and language suggesting it as a goal may not be a wholesome
influence. It has the weakness of any regressive effort: it is a growth retardant.
It says, "The past was better, the present (and maybe the future) is (are) not
so good; I was something then, I'm not much now." Worse, the concept of
restoration to a previous state denies the validity and value of the disability
experience as a potentially powerful stimulant to psychological growth. The
following quote elaborates on this point of view:

> I have been disabled since I was sixteen, yet hardly a week goes by nearly thirty
> years later, that I don't make some discovery or improvement that in one way or
> another makes my disability less handicapping. Since I hope that happy process
> never stops, I have to say that I hope I am never fully "rehabilitated." My physical

abilities are still increasing. When, with age, they begin to decrease. I fully expect to continue or accelerate in the psychological and spiritual discoveries that make my disability not only less handicapping, but a matter of trivia compared with the nonphysical realms of discovery and improvement I am experiencing. Each in its own age, but all part of my own human growth . . . or psychological development . . . or rehabilitation . . . or whatever you prefer to call it. Sometimes I'm not sure what my disability is. Is it being paralyzed, or does that add a laughably small increment to the primordial handicap of being mortal human? The core of psychological development is realistic acceptance of one's limitations—be they physical, intellectual, spiritual, or of some other realm. We are not perfect; we are never what we would wish to be—however beautiful, good, gifted, serene, or strong we appear. These imperfections must be accepted without rancor before we can get on with the real and simple business of psychological development—doing the best we can with whatever we've got. (Vash, 1976, pp. 2–3)

Thus, the continuity of the "rehabilitation" of disabled people with the "human development" of people in general is stressed. The developmental tasks are the same; the unique aspects and different situations created by disablement are of secondary importance. In the context of this chapter, growth relates to such tasks as achieving self-actualization, maximizing human potential, and developing total mind-body-spirit health.

Devaluation: Both Block and Catalyst to Growth

A sense of being devalued is not unique to disabled people or even to minority-group members in general. At an individual level, it is probably the primal human "hang up." Feelings of worthlessness are central to nonorganically caused mental disorders, and self-esteem is a cornerstone of mental health. The issue has simply become highly salient to the psychology of disability because of the extreme self-devaluation that stems from inability to perform ordinary functions that others take for granted. Having to be led, fed, taken to the toilet, or helped in other ways associated with infancy highlights helplessness, which is conceptually linked with incompetence, and the individual feels (and often is) devalued. The spiraling ramifications outlined previously can block growth severely for a period of time. However, those with the resources to break free from the spiral often find that the process has freed them from human hindrances to growth in a more encompassing way. Being forced to "put away childish things," such as needs for approbation and material comfort, and to do so successfully, constitutes a giant step toward the higher levels of psychological maturity and spiritual development.

Thus, current social and technological advances are making it possible for disability to catalyze rather than block growth for an increasing proportion of disabled people. When disability took away too much, it seemed to stultify growth for all but a few. But the *zeitgeist* is right for change, and the civil/human rights movement, plus rehabilitation engineering technology, are rescuing seriously disabled people from being too overwhelmed to look upward. When they do, some find they have advanced beyond their peers and their own expectations, to a level of existence where more than disability is transcended.

Transcending Disability

Before disability can be transcended, it must first be acknowledged at the three designated levels: recognition of the facts, acceptance of the implications, and embracing the experience. Here, keeping the distinction clear between "disability" and "handicap" is particularly important. If one is to function effectively in the world and enjoy life at the same time, it is necessary to accept without rancor the fact that one is blind, deaf, paralyzed, mentally retarded, or otherwise disabled. However, it is neither necessary nor desirable to accept such handicapping sequelae as no friends, no sex life, no fun, and—most importantly—no job. It is not even reasonable to accept, unquestioningly a secondary-labor-market job, a disappointing love life, and unreliable moments of pleasure that always happen at someone else's caprice. This occurs when external, stereotyped definitions of "handicap" are accepted instead of discovering through personal trial and error what is truly beyond the range of capability.

The first author was once a member of a rehabilitation hospital team that defined a young man's disability (severe cerebral palsy) as an immutable handicap to driving a car. He wisely rejected that definition and independently obtained driver training from a private school. Five years later, he had an unmarred driving record and the author had the privilege of presenting an award to the driving school. From this and countless other similar illustrations that could be given, it is clear that the handicapping effects of a disability must be accepted reluctantly, not only by disabled people themselves, but also by the professionals who work with them. Only when the actual limits for a given individual are determined from sufficient experience should the type and degree of handicapping associated with a person's disability be accepted. The next step, as for disability itself, is transcending the handicap.

"Transcendence" connotes rising above or beyond the limits imposed by certain conditions. With respect to the present topic, those conditions may be the disability itself, societal expectations related to it, or emotional reactions to either or both. Transcending disability requires one, first, to escape from the mind-body trap, the Cartesian duality that eliminated spirit from commonplace consideration. As indicated earlier (see Chapter 2), overlooking or denying a spiritual aspect of human life is particularly subtractive to people whose minds and/or bodies are disabled. Once a spiritual component has been admitted to consciousness, then the components vulnerable to disablement are placed in a less potent, more favorable perspective. It becomes progressively easier to say, and mean, that disability doesn't matter much most of the time. The accompanying perceptual mechanism is illustrated by a passage from Beisser (1979).

> The author of this paper is a postpoliomyelitis quadriplegic with severe respiratory paresis [who is] confined to a wheelchair. He is actively engaged in his profession, and when doing so, is absorbed with the tasks at hand. He is frequently asked questions such as. How do you bear spending your life in a wheelchair? When he is, he is aware that his attention is redirected from what he is doing in an affirmative way to what he is unable to do in accordance with the standards implied by the question. Thus, when what he cannot do becomes foreground, he is aware that he is disabled; while working or carrying out his social or family activities, his disability becomes background and his competence and health are foreground. (pp. 1026–1030)

This reflects the basal level of transcending disability. Its reality is no longer either struggled against or denied. It simply fades, irrelevantly, into the background until rare, extreme circumstance, or someone else, calls it to the forefront of consciousness. Once there, it is experienced with neutrality or, as growth progresses, with positive regard.

Transcending Normalization

"Normalization" is a term used by professionals and some consumer activists to describe the goal they envision for disabled people. It connotes having equal rights and opportunities, taking equal risks, assuming equal responsibilities, and expecting equal heartaches and disappointments. It is an unimpeachable goal for those whose lives might otherwise be deprived and disadvantaged, but for many others, striving for normalization is aiming too low. Carl Jung (1929) captured the essence of this in a passage indicating that to be normal is a splendid ideal for the unsuccessful, for all those who have not yet found an adaptation; but for people who have more ability than the average, for whom it was never hard to accomplish their share of the world's work, for them, restriction to the normal signifies the bed of Procrustes, unbearable boredom, infernal sterility, and hopelessness.

Disabled people are present in the ranks of those gifted with "more ability than the average," and the experience of being nonordinary physically may catalyze acceptance of being nonordinary in other respects as well. We tend to forget that the "normal" curve (Bell Curve) has two tails, both of which are "abnormal." For example, it is not "normal" to be exceedingly beautiful and wise, or to abjure triviality and pettiness. Fred, a postpolio respiratory quadriplegic who heads an $80 million public agency, is abnormal in a number of highly desirable ways: he is brilliant; powerful; earns a large salary; and lives with a talented, beautiful wife. Although he values normalization as a goal of rehabilitation programs for many, it is doubtful that he would want to return to normality himself.

Olivia, a double above-knee amputee, describes incisively the insight experience that led her to discard normality as a goal, having found it maladaptive:

When Tom proposed to me, I said, "Yes, I want to marry you, but there is something I must tell you first. I have decided not to try to use these damnable prostheses any more. I'm tired of falling down, and I've finally caught on that the rehab people only want me to use them because it's important to them that I *look* as normal as possible. They don't seem to tune into the fact that I'm totally unfunctional when I have them on. I look the way I look and if other people don't like it, that's their problem. I'm not making it mine any more. From now on, I plan to scoot around the house on my ass, because that's what *works* best, and I'll use a wheelchair when I go out; but I will never put on those dumb legs again. If you still want to marry me, I want that very much; but I won't change my mind just to meet any needs you might have for me to look more normal."

Olivia, obviously, is unusually confident about her own human worth. Tom proved to be fully in accord with her decision and has since developed some rather stringent opinions:

I think you rehab people are really messing up by pushing so hard for disabled people to be and look "as normal as possible." What's so great about being normal? To me, that means being dull, drab, run-of-the-mill, and who needs it? You *ought* to be out there educating the general public to be more open and acceptant of differences. Then, when something happens to one of them, they won't be so apt to fall apart because they're not normal any more.

The first lines of the credo of the Human Resources Center in Long Island, New York, reflect a goal that surpasses normalization: "I do not choose to be a common man. It is my right to be uncommon, if I can." Disabled people, like others who have been forced by usually unwelcome circumstance to recognize, accept, and then embrace their differentness in one respect, sometimes have a head start on acknowledging other nonordinary aspects of their being. An outstanding exemplification of this is Ken Keyes, Jr., a postpolio quadriplegic who was a spiritual leader in this country for several decades.

Ken Keyes, Jr.—Transcending Lower Consciousness

Keyes (personal communication) relates that despite being almost totally paralyzed, he was a successful real estate broker living on a yacht in the Florida Keys when he was introduced to the writings of Baba Ram Dass, John Lilly, and other significant figures of the still-current spiritual revolution. These stirred him to further studies, which culminated in his major work, the *Handbook to Higher Consciousness* (Keyes, 1975), and the establishment of a training center where students can learn to apply his living love methods to the science of happiness. His analysis of the human condition and methods for improving it (on an individual basis) draw notably from the ancient philosophical writings of India and the conceptions of modern biological, behavioral, and computer sciences—a remarkable melding.

Central to his system is the Indian paradigm of seven levels, or centers, of consciousness (chakras), which he describes in Western idiom. The consciousness of people operating at the first and lowest level is concerned with maintaining survival, safety, and security. It is usually referred to as the "security" level of consciousness. The second, slightly higher, level is called the "sensation" level of consciousness. Here, the individual is not solely preoccupied with matters of survival, but has opened his or her consciousness to sensual pleasures, such as sexual activity, gourmet foods, music, and the arts. Thus, "sensation" consciousness may run the gamut from the carnal to the lofty. The third, still higher, level is considered "power" consciousness. People operating at this level are motivated primarily to gain ascendance over others. Keyes (1975) indicates that most people operate within these three lower levels of consciousness most of the time.

He goes on to describe four higher levels of consciousness, associated with love, fulfillment, enlightenment, and cosmic consciousness. People living at the fourth level of consciousness are attuned to their lovingness toward others and others' lovingness in return. The fifth level Keyes refers to as "the cornucopia center of consciousness," in that one becomes aware that whatever is needed is available, whatever happens is what was needed, and one must

only learn to appreciate these facts. Keyes believes that a significant proportion of the population can learn to live at the fourth and fifth levels of
consciousness most of the time. On the other hand, the sixth and seventh
levels, associated with enlightenment and cosmic consciousness, have been
reached by only a few hundred individuals throughout history, and can be
aspired to realistically by a very small number of totally devoted spiritual
aspirants.

Keyes advocates advancing beyond security-, sensation-, and power-
oriented consciousness into love- and fulfillment-oriented consciousness because the lower three levels have a painful, addictive quality that virtually
guarantees a high proportion of unhappy moments. When survival is at stake,
needs become demands and are associated with intense emotions that are
adaptive for jungle survival but become maladaptive after that stage has been
passed. These emotion-backed demands are tantamount to *addictions* because
you suffer when such demands are not met. Moreover, when they *are* met,
they yield what Keyes calls a "yo-yo" or "roller-coaster" type of enjoyment
that necessarily entails at least as much suffering as pleasure. Table 8.1
summarizes the situation described.

Keyes (1975) believes we are programmed by society and then continue
to program ourselves to approach life addictively, with an attitude of "I must
have/not have" instead of "I prefer to/not to." In a *tour de force* using simple
probabilities, he shows why addictive programming is the mechanism for
unhappiness. If you are addicted to having an event occur (for example,

TABLE 8.1 Lower Levels of Consciousness

Level of Consciousness	Associated Emotions	Why Enjoyment Fluctuates
Security	Fear, worry, anxiety	Constant driving compulsiveness, fear of loss, projections of future worries
Sensation	Disappointment, frustration, boredom	Same as security, plus satiation and boredom
Power	Anger, resentment, irritation, hate, hostility	Same as security and sensation, plus being caught up in defending from counterattack and trying to control

Note: From "Handbook to Higher Consciousness," by Ken Keys, Jr., 1975, p. 59. Adapted with
permission.

martini at five, lover always faithful), you may feel pleasure if it happens, but you will definitely suffer if it doesn't. If you are addicted to having an event *not* happen (for example, charge account billing error, cockroach in the kitchen), you will suffer if it does but will probably not notice if it doesn't. Given equal probabilities for all outcomes, addictive programming yields half suffering and half either pleasure or no effect.

On the other hand, preferential programming virtually eliminates suffering. If you can say, "I would prefer to have such and such happen/not happen, but if it doesn't/does that is all right, too," you have only opportunities for pleasure or no effect and none for suffering. The higher levels of consciousness are associated with preferential programming, and much of the task of developing into these higher levels is reprogramming, that is, converting addictions into preferences. (Only at the highest level of consciousness do even preferences disappear.)

One reason disability is so difficult to adjust to is that it eliminates conditions to which people tend to be addicted. This is also why nondisabled people so often believe that "If it happened to me, I couldn't cope." Moreover, the presumption of similar addictions in others is an important basis for the attribution of mourning (see Chapter 2) to people who have experienced loss. Most presume they have *suffered* loss; however, to people who have transcended the three addictive, lower levels of consciousness, loss may not be accompanied by suffering. It simply may raise awareness that "whatever happened is what was needed" (for spiritual development or elevation of consciousness).

Readers probably can tune into their own pervasive acceptance of addictiveness by examining their reactions to the prospect of being unable to see, hear, or walk: "You'd better believe I'm addicted to seeing, hearing, and walking—who wouldn't be?" One answer is that some people have learned not to be in order to avoid chronic suffering. It is here that disability operates like the blow on the head by a two-by-four that can kill you or get your attention. Some react to it by becoming more tightly bound to security, sensation, and power preoccupations because survival and opportunities for pleasure have been threatened and powerlessness looms imminent. Others, however, in time may transcend not only disability-triggered, excessive preoccupations, but even an average degree of security-, sensation-, and power-oriented consciousness. Somehow, giving up such basic addictions as those to seeing, hearing, and walking can make relinquishment of lesser ones relatively easy, for individuals who have spent some time at the fourth and fifth levels of consciousness. An excerpt from a previous publication (Vash, 1975) illustrates several aspects of the process that takes place:

I wasn't exactly happy and couldn't figure out why. It took a few months to realize that one reason was, I hadn't accepted my disability. When I did, it wasn't at all like [I had] envisioned; settling for second-rate goals and dreams. It wasn't even defusing the disappointment that I would never again hear whistles when I walk, or dance, or ride in a horse show, or walk alone in the rain, or go to the bathroom by myself. It sure as hell wasn't the much touted process of discovering substitute gratifications for the ones I had lost.

It was more like those things not only didn't matter any more, they wouldn't have mattered even if I could still have done them. I didn't need to be able to do them—or to mourn their loss—in order to maintain some image of myself. I felt I understood the relinquishments that come with age. Joys of an earlier era are continuously "put away." Substitutions needn't be sought; new joys simply emerge, appropriate to the new era. I found myself no longer afraid of aging. Acceptance of disability was simply acceptance of myself; and there were parts of me that were harder to accept than my disability by far. I didn't have the language then, but from the personal studies I've done since, acceptance of disability was exactly the process Western interpreters of Eastern mystics speak of as "centering," "ridding oneself of ego," and "casting off attachments [addictions] so they become, at most, preferences." The fact that a few of these attachments were ego images and activities interfered with by disability was just one happenstance of a much larger process. (pp. 152–153)

As a result of the spiritual renascence taking place in current times, more and more people are coming to value and seek the transcendence of lower consciousness, and this includes increasing numbers of disabled people. They are finding that the disability experience has been a powerful contributor to breaking through maladaptive societal programming. Being different and devalued, knowing extreme loss and pain, facing poverty and even death, force one to adopt new perspectives that might otherwise never have been tried; each new vantage point enhances growth and knowledge. Most important, however, is learning to give up addictions—which, without being forced by disability and an alternative of abject misery, one would be far less likely to do.

The disability experience can help one see that preoccupations with security, sensation, and power are "lose-lose" propositions. There *is* no security. No one can work, hoard, or plan enough to guarantee that nothing will ever go wrong. There is also no way to avoid the now-deprived, now-satiated yo-yo world of sensation-oriented consciousness. Finally, you can never achieve total power and until you do, whatever you have is threatened. This brings one to the obvious question: why not give them all up and start living in the higher levels of consciousness? Disability can catalyze this process. First, it instructs: it *can* happen here. Next, one learns: it *did*, and that's okay. This raises a number of growth-inducing questions: Are things perhaps not exactly as they seem? Do some things I thought mattered perhaps not matter? Are there levels of reality I haven't yet comprehended? What is "misfortune" anyway? Once people are in a mode of asking questions instead of imagining or pretending that they have answers, the most important step toward transcendence has been taken.

II
Interventions

9

The Long Arm of the Law

The last chapter of Part I ("Transcending") and the first chapter of Part II ("Legislation"), though contiguous in this text, seem to represent opposite poles. "Transcending" suggested that benefits accrue when individuals can let go of personal power strivings. This chapter emphasizes the psychological and tangible benefits of belonging to a group with a solid, political powerbase. The apparent conflict is resolved only by apprehending the developmental and multifaceted nature of the coping process. Lawmaking is a basic power approach designed to give freedom and equity to groups of people. Transcendence of power approaches, as discussed in the previous chapter, is an individual's step toward liberation of a different kind. It becomes more attainable, it seems, after individuals have experienced the sense of being powerful in ways meaningful to them. Thus, while the previous chapter pointed out that excessive preoccupation with power may interfere with reaching the highest levels of self-actualization, this chapter unabashedly recounts the psychological values of having sufficient political influence to protect one's fundamental, self-evident, inalienable rights.

In earlier days of the civil rights movement, when desegregation of African Americans was the prepotent issue, a conservative United States senator made the pronouncement "You can't legislate morality." This gave a few people pause until it occurred to them that morality is just what we do, legislate—or try to. The Constitution put forth a moral order, and statutory law attempts to maintain it. Ideally, the goals of the law are what's right, fair, and moral to the best of the lawmaker's ability to foresee and implement. Limitations on the ability to foresee have long created socioeconomic problems for disabled people; and these, in turn, generate difficulties in psychological adjustment. (This problem is not limited to issues relating to disabled citizens. It is sufficiently widespread that, in 1974, the House of Representatives passed, by an overwhelming majority, a resolution referred to as the "foresight provision." This stipulates that part of the process of drafting legislation must include an attempt to look ahead at the future implications if proposed legislation were to become law.) Three decades later, the provision seems to have been forgotten by our lawmakers.

As pointed out in the previous chapter, people with disabilities, especially severe ones, were once considered too aberrant to be included under the law, their hopes for pursuing happiness too unrealistic to be considered. The scattered pieces of legislation that emerged from time to time fell far short of constituting a coherent national disability policy. In recent years, however, the confluence of many forces has led to the articulation of a new understanding of disability and the creation of protective legislation. Building upon the energy and vision of the civil rights and women's movements, a disability rights movement began to coalesce and advocate for needed legislation. Once the process of mandating needed changes began in earnest, a snowballing effect occurred. A major role of federal laws is to serve as "enabling legislation," allowing and encouraging similar laws and ordinances to be enacted at state and local levels where enforcement can be accomplished more readily, and many such statutes were passed. At the federal level, concerted and continuous work culminated in the 1990 passage of the Americans with Disabilities Act (ADA) and other critical legislation including the Individuals with Disabilities in Education Act (IDEA).

When efforts to help through legislation have created problems, it usually has been due to limited foresight, but backlash also is an omnipresent reality. For the greater part, however, the long arm of the law, like rehabilitation engineering, has proved to be a nonpsychological tool for vastly improving the psychological status of disabled individuals. The remainder of this chapter will chronicle legislative changes that have come about in recent years, plus advances in regulatory, rulemaking, and procedural design that have been directly or indirectly stimulated by them. The psychological effects of these developments on people with disabilities are often self-evident, but some of the subtler aspects will be pointed out. The discussion will highlight needed changes yet to be accomplished, many of which can be brought about best by the team efforts of disabled individuals and rehabilitation professionals.

The Creation of Benefits and Services

The many laws that have been passed to ensure the rights to life, liberty, and the pursuit of happiness for people with disabilities can be viewed as belonging in two major clusters. The first creates needed benefits and services for the target group, and the second aims to protect them from abridgment of their rights under the Constitution. This section will discuss the first cluster; the second will be discussed in the succeeding section.

The benefits and services created by law can be arranged similarly in clusters designated "basic living needs" and "vocational preparation." Benefits may assume the forms of cash grants, loans, discounts, tax deductions, and goods; services may include virtually any known human service program plus special opportunities to acquire earnings. "Basic living needs" include such elements as food, shelter, transportation, and health; "vocational preparation" includes such elements as education, training, and the establishment of a business.

America's history of benefits legislation rests upon a biomedical model that determines an individual's needs (based upon medically verifiable disabilities that preclude working) and cultural constructs of moral worthiness (based upon innocence for the condition) (Scotch, 1999). It basically involves welfare assistance given to that part of the population that is seen to be the "deserving poor." The earliest pensions were provided to soldiers who had been wounded in the Civil War, and the first vocational rehabilitation services were created for disabled veterans returning from World War I. The country felt a responsibility for aiding individuals who had been wounded in service to their country. Gradually, vocational services were opened to other groups, including all veterans, and eventually to citizens with physical and mental disabilities. The result of this perspective is that benefits and services for people with disabilities have been provided in separate programs with restrictive eligibility criteria. At the present time, advocates, agencies, and legislators are weighing the advantages of continuing to offer programs that provide focused attention to those with disabilities against the drawbacks of segregated services.

In the 1800s, laws provided for the establishment of institutional programs for housing and, later, for treating people with disabilities construed as so severe that they precluded living in the larger society. Mentally retarded, mentally ill, and very severely physically disabled people were the primary occupants of such facilities. Still later, this philosophy was to be reversed and service and benefit programs would be created to allow many who were formerly destined for institutional living to remain in or return to the outside world. Further, in 1999, in the case of *Olmstead vs. L.C. and E.W.*, the Supreme Court interpreted the ADA to mean that individuals have a basic right to services that enable them to live in the most integrated settings. This victory has been threatened by subsequent decisions (e.g., *Rodriguez vs. the City of New York*), which ruled that states are not required to provide additional services to persons with disabilities as "reasonable accommodations." The result was permission "to implement a wholesale cutback in Medicaid home care services" (Griss, 2000), although it is unthinkable that the struggle is finished.

The basic survival programs for individuals with disabilities are contained in the Social Security Act. The Rehabilitation Act has been associated, historically, with vocational preparation, and in the late 1970s provisions for independent-living rehabilitation expanded its coverage into the basic living needs arena. Legislative provisions for veterans cover both areas, and their far greater generosity, compared with available resources for nonveterans, has been a point of contention among the latter.

Workers' compensation laws also contain provisions in both basic living and vocational areas for people who become disabled in the conduct of their work, and "mandatory rehabilitation" provisions in state workers' compensation laws (requiring employers to provide rehabilitation services rather than solely cash compensation to industrially injured workers) became quite common for a time. Each state's system is unique, but rehabilitation has not proven to be a panacea for the problems of injured workers. While the systems can provide resources for living expenses and retraining, they operate under a clear set of priorities that favor return to the same job with the same employer, and failing that, placement in a different job with the same employer, the same job with a different employer, and only as a last resort a different job with a different employer. Retraining is offered only when required to prepare the individual for the different job, and training beyond a year or two would definitely be the exception (Douglas Langham, personal communication).

In the area of personal assistance services, the states have a great deal of latitude in how much they enrich the basic federal programs' allowances. All states that receive Medicaid funds must provide nursing home services, but community services are optional (ADAPT, 2002). In some states, the funding is so limited as to virtually eliminate the opportunity for many individuals with severe disabilities to live outside of institutions. In all states, funding systems are strongly biased in favor of institutional care. The advocacy organization ADAPT (American Disabled for Attendant Programs Today) led in the development and lobbying for passage of a bill that would change the long-term care system and give people a real opportunity to receive needed services in their own homes. MiCASSA (Medicaid Community Attendant Services and Supports Act) was introduced by Senators Harkin and Specter in 2000 and again in 2001, and at the time of this writing the struggle for passage is continuing. As Senator Harkin explained in introducing the bill to Congress, "only about 27 percent of long term care funds expended under Medicaid, and only about 9 percent of all funds expended under the program, pay for services and supports in home and community based settings" (Harkin, 2001). The nursing home lobby is powerful, and is understandably resistant to the diversion of funding to other providers. The Office of Management and Budget (OMB) deemed MiCASSA as "too expensive," even though for the average person community-based services cost about half of those provided in nursing homes. In May 2002, ADAPT blocked traffic to the OMB offices until the agency agreed to a meeting (Gwin, 2002). They also blocked the offices of unions that had opposed the bill. Besides these national efforts, local chapters of ADAPT are working to pass state-level legislation, and they have achieved success in several areas. Few people, given adequate community supports, would choose to live in a nursing home. It seems inevitable that the disability community will win this fight.

In addition to these major entitlement programs, a number of less comprehensive laws have been enacted to create special programs, sometimes for specific disability groups. For example, Part D of the Developmental Disabilities Assistance and Bill of Rights Act of 1996 (P.L. 104-183) provides grants to University Affiliated Programs that conduct research and training to promote the independence and community integration of individuals with developmental disabilities. The Technology-Related Assistance for Individuals with Disabilities Act of 1988 (P.L. 100-407) provides assistance to states in creating consumer-responsive technology programs. The total array of federal, state, and local programs are too numerous to review.

The psychological benefits of such legislative thrusts are enormous. Without them, the concept of "opportunity" is a vacuous hoax; with them, it can be a reality. Possibilities for partaking of the routines, risks, joys, sorrows, excitement, and tedium of ordinary human life begin to exist when such laws are enacted. When they are implemented and emulated, social participation by disabled people becomes increasingly probable. Nonetheless, limited abilities to foresee have plagued nearly all legislatively created means of helping disabled citizenry.

Benefit programs were created without cognizance of the future capabilities recipients would have for entering the labor market; thus, welfare-related work disincentives were to become serious problems for the recipients as well as society. Vocational rehabilitation services were created before independent living services were, guaranteeing painfully demoralizing failures for hundreds of thousands of vocational rehabilitation clients over the years. One reason for such backward planning is anxiety about accountability to the self-interested taxpayer. Services other than those aimed in a straight line toward "removal of the beneficiary from the welfare rolls and into the ranks of the taxpayers" were regarded as frivolous "handholding" that extant taxpayers would spurn. Only when the evidence of greater costs created by failure to attend to such "tangential" issues as independent living and survival systems became massive and incontrovertible did lawmakers and agency heads reverse their orientations and begin to plan for taking first steps first.

As mentioned in Chapter 6, the result of this realization led to the passage in 1999 of Ticket to Work and Work Incentives Improvement Act (TWWIIA). The key purposes of the act are: "to improve work incentive under the Social Security Disability Insurance Program (SSDI) and the SSI program and to expand health care services for persons with disabilities who are working or who want to work but fear losing their health care" (Jensen & Silverstein, 2000).

Recipients of SSDI are subject to continuing disability reviews (CDRs) that serve to determine whether the individual continues to be disabled and eligible for benefits. Since disability is defined as the inability to engage in any substantial gainful activity, these reviews have been triggered when an individual begins to earn income above the specified limit (about $700 per month). Under the new legislation, work alone will no longer serve to trigger CDRs. The new legislation allows for an extended period of time when an individual may remain eligible for Medicaid or Medicare coverage after beginning work, and it allows states to establish programs whereby individuals may continue to "buy in" to coverage on a sliding scale, even if they are earning substantial salaries. Another important provision allows for reinstatement of SSDI benefits without a new application and disability determination for former beneficiaries who attempt to work but are unable to sustain their jobs because of disability. Reinstatement could be requested during an 8-year period following the time when the SSDI payments were terminated because of earnings. Those who lose eligibility for SSI payments would be required to make a new application if the individual passes a 12-month suspension period. For an unlimited time, however, they would be eligible to move back and forth, as their income changes, between eligibility for SSI payments with Medicare eligibility and Medicare eligibility without cash payments.

The Ticket to Work and Work Incentives Improvement Act also includes provisions for outreach programs to provide information and assistance to beneficiaries. It remains to be seen how many people will hear about the changes and decide to risk entering the labor force under the new terms. Frontline service providers (such as social workers in hospital settings or case managers in psychosocial rehabilitation programs) need to be educated regarding the new legislation and encouraged to modify their traditional practice of advising people to work only to the extent that their benefit package remains undisturbed.

Benefits and services also were created before the basic rights of the affected groups were protected. Frustration, anger, and depression are the likely aftermaths when individuals are encouraged to partake of opportunities for education or vocational training only to find, at the end of it, that their rights to secure employment are being blatantly, callously, and systematically abridged. The following sections will address these issues.

The Protection of Rights of People with Disabilities

The problems that faced all of the groups that have come to be protected by civil rights legislation in this society were historically viewed as natural outcomes of the characteristics and limitations of those people. Women were viewed as innately hypersensitive, overly emotional, and therefore unfit to carry out public responsibilities such as voting. Descendents of slaves and others from non-European ethnic backgrounds were presumed to be less intelligent and suitable only for physical labor and other work that demanded minimal levels of education. Even more readily "apparent" to the public was the conclusion that the challenges faced by people with disabilities were the direct consequence of the functional limitations of the disabilities. As a result, the earliest legislation with direct applicability to people with disabilities concerned benefit programs, and laws protecting disabled people's rights to equal opportunity for employment are among the statutory latecomers.

Wage and hour laws designed to protect disabled workers from economic exploitation led the way as early as the 1930s, as did the first state statute advancing the unique right of blind people to be accompanied by guide dogs in areas otherwise restricted to humans. Longmore (1999) recounted the nearly forgotten history of the League of the Physically Handicapped, a group that in 1935 undertook one of the first actions of civil disobedience, protesting discrimination in hiring by the New Deal work programs. Blocked by bias from jobs in the private sector, these New York City individuals also found they were automatically rejected when they applied for municipal work-relief jobs. Six of them went to see the head of the agency responsible for the work program, and they were told that he would not be available until the following week. The group decided to sit-in until they could be heard. Others learned about their strike and joined a picket line in the street outside. The strike lasted for eight days and drew the attention of newspapers. When the protesters were finally allowed to meet with the director he said that he could not promise jobs right away but he hoped that future funds might become available. The activists became formally organized and continued their activities, even making a trip to Washington, D.C. on a flatbed truck. They succeeded in getting some people into jobs, although when the Works Progress Administration began laying off workers in 1937, those with disabilities were the first to go. Despite failing in their efforts to change federal policies that hurt citizens with disabilities, they did manage to open the public sector slightly. Their efforts lasted for about a year, foreshadowing later changes in perspective on disability and disability policy.

Little more was done specific to the protection of rights—as distinct from the creation of benefits and services—until the 1950s. During this decade, concerns over disabled people's rights to use public accommodations began to be reflected in federal and scattered state legislation. Much of the impetus came from a small cadre of disabled people who had managed to become taxpayers and resented supporting facilities they could not use.

The legal statements were generally vague and unenforceable, proclaiming the right of blind or physically disabled people to use public facilities, but issuing no requirements for modifications making it physically possible for them to do so. The major accomplishment of this decade was the heightening of awareness among rehabilitation professionals that their efforts with disabled "patients" or "clients" would come to naught unless the social and physical world were altered to accommodate them. It was rehabilitation providers with political contacts who provided much of the early educating and prodding of legislators to mandate changes they now recognized as necessary. Parents of mentally retarded individuals were equally early advocates for political and legislative change, but disabled individuals themselves were not yet a potent force as their own advocates.

The Right to a Barrier-Free Environment

Near the end of the 1960s, the federal and several state legislatures passed laws requiring that public accommodations funded wholly or in part with federal (or state) monies must be "accessible to and useable by the elderly and handicapped." The laws were strictly proactive; only facilities to be constructed in the future were required to be accessible. Shortly thereafter, a number of states began passing parallel laws requiring privately funded public accommodations to meet similar standards. This reflected responsiveness to local advocates who insisted it was only "right, fair, and moral" to go farther than the federal law had gone. The close of the 1970s saw regulations implementing the "civil rights" provisions of the 1973 Rehabilitation Act (Sections 501 through 504) widely interpreted as either requiring or strongly urging correction of obstructive design in certain public accommodations, regardless of when the facilities were constructed, if any federal funds were involved. Section 502 explicitly established the Architectural and Transportation Barriers Compliance Board for oversight purposes, and sections 501, 503, and 504, which called for affirmative action and nondiscrimination, implied the necessity of barrier reduction.

By this time, disabled activists had taken the lead as their own advocates and were fighting hard to solidify and maintain this hard-line interpretation. Not even in the women's movement, where it began, has the slogan, "You've come a long way, baby," been more aptly descriptive. The advance guard was composed mainly of gifted, disabled individuals who had broken into the establishment without benefit of protective legislation or elevated public consciousness. (As was true for ethnic minorities and women, the early successes were "overqualified.") Their trailblazing, plus the concomitant improvements in benefit and service programs, made it possible for more "average" disabled people to join the battle. Dedicated, driving, volunteer efforts on the parts of unemployed disabled people who joined the barrier-reduction campaign became the first steps out of the proverbial back bedrooms and into the mainstream of social politics for scores, then hundreds, now thousands of people who, not much earlier, might have led more passive, less fulfilling lives.

The Right To Participate in Society

Section 504 of the 1973 Rehabilitation Act rapidly became known as the "bill of rights for the disabled." Many were quick to point out that it was a very limited "civil rights act"; others claimed that the regulations promulgated in 1977 by the (then) Department of Health, Education, and Welfare to implement the law went far beyond what Congress had intended. Both may be correct. Section 504 is a forty-five-word statement that says only this:

> No otherwise qualified handicapped individual in the United states, as defined in section 7(6), shall, solely by reason of his handicap, be excluded from the participation in, be denied the benefits of, or be subjected to discrimination under any program or activity receiving Federal financial assistance.

These forty-five words stimulated nearly twenty-seven pages of regulations with far-reaching implications for expenditures that would have to be made by programs receiving federal funds in order to comply with the law; yet no appropriation was made to cover any part of such expenditures. The attitude of "liberals" on this subject was, "Why should the government appropriate money to pay for affected parties to do what they should have been doing all along?" "Conservatives" on this issue simply awaited the backlash and noncompliance they were sure would come. Nondiscrimination mandates relating to ethnic minorities cost virtually nothing to implement, but those for the disabled minority can engender massive costs simply to render accessible the housing for the targeted programs. Thus, while the law addressed only program accessibility and did not purport to confront physical barrier problems, the regulations incorporated this other, costly issue. In some sectors, concerted compliance efforts began, and in others, massive resistance was mounted, usually because of the projected costs of compliance but sometimes because of disagreement with the principles of integration.

It took nearly four years for the government to produce the regulations that were needed to implement Section 504, and the task was done only at the insistence of disability advocates. Although the section had commanded little attention in Congress (Shapiro, 1993), HEW staff recognized and dreaded the potential fiscal implications of the law, estimating that compliance would cost billions of dollars. In retrospect, the estimates were greatly exaggerated, but the fears nearly prevented implementation of the law.

Despite pockets, and sometimes groundswells, of resistance, Section 504 proved to be a strong card in the hands of disabled people and their advocates as they sought to redress discriminatory practices. Often, educating officials of programs receiving federal money was enough to stimulate voluntary efforts to make it possible for disabled people to participate. However, the card was not strong enough; the first court case elevated to the United States Supreme Court yielded a negative finding (the Davis decision). The Supreme Court decided against a deaf woman who sought to enter nurses' training, indicating, in essence, that they did not view her as "otherwise qualified" and that the law did not require the school to make the extensive curriculum changes needed to make the nursing program accessible to her. They further opined that the DHEW regulations had attempted to create law rather than simply implement it (*Southeastern Community College v. Frances B. Davis*— US, 60 L Ed 2d 980, 99 S Ct 2361 June 11, 1979). For weeks, the activist disabled community was stunned, fearful, and angry over this decision. They were not only angry at the Supreme Court, they were angry at Davis and her attorneys for pursuing what they considered, at best, a "borderline" case, one with slim chances for producing the kind of precedent needed. Soon enough, "all is lost" turned to "the show must go on" and the slow but steady campaign to eliminate discriminatory practices against disabled people proceeded—sometimes with and sometimes without the leverage of Section 504.

Section 504 came under serious threat when Reagan became president and set about to "de-regulate" provisions that businesses found to be burdensome.

These efforts to change Section 504 were defeated when activists resisted with a loud and unified voice. The disability community spent much of the 1980s working to reinstate civil rights protections that had been lost to negative Supreme Court decisions (Mayerson, 1992). In particular, the *Grove City College vs. Bell* decision had severely limited the effectiveness of all statutes that prohibited discrimination on the basis of race, sex, or disability. To counteract this decision, the Civil Rights Restoration Act (CRRA) was introduced to Congress in 1984 and was finally passed four years later. All of the affected groups worked together on this effort, the first time that members of the disability community had teamed as leaders with representatives of minority and women's groups on an important piece of civil rights legislation.

One key to participation in society is accessible transportation, and despite the establishment of the Architectural and Transportation Barriers Compliance Board under the Rehabilitation Act, the public transportation systems in most areas remained useless to people with disabilities. In 1983 American Disabled for Access Public Transit (ADAPT) was founded in Denver by Wade Blank. ADAPT's goal was to get lifts on all city busses, enabling people to get to work, to stores, and anywhere else in the community independently (Shapiro, 1993). The organization grew, and actions of civil disobedience led to hundreds of arrests around the country They used direct, militant protests to instigate change, disrupting every meeting of the American Public Transit System during the following years, and they played a crucial role in achieving passage of the ADA.

The 1988 amendments to the Fair Housing Act marked the first time that discrimination based upon disability was prohibited within a traditional law banning race-based discrimination (Mayerson, 1992). The alliance that was formed with other civil rights groups while working on these pieces of legislation resulted in the active participation of the Leadership Conference on Civil Rights in the later passage of the ADA.

The year 1988 also marked a historic event with the student and alumni takeover of Gallaudet University. The board of trustees had chosen the only hearing person among three candidates to become the new president. Throughout its 124-year history, Gallaudet, the only college in the nation specifically committed to the education of the deaf, had never had a deaf president. Students rallied, blocked the entrances to the campus, and demanded that the decision be rescinded and the chair of the board resign. The board's attempts to explain and mollify the protesters were futile, and many Congressional leaders supported the students' position. A week later I. King Jordan, the former dean of the college of arts and sciences who had been deaf since early adulthood, was named president, and the chair of the board resigned. The students were ecstatic and filled with pride in their deafness and in their achievements.

The third historic event of 1988 was the introduction to Congress of the first version of the Americans with Disability Act. It had been drafted by attorney Robert Burgdorf, Jr. and adopted by the National Council on the Handicapped (now the National Council on Disability). It did not receive much attention at that point, but the disability community began to mobilize support and gather evidence of discrimination that demanded redress. Justin Dart, a man who used a wheelchair as a result of polio, traveled to every state, holding meetings and recording accounts of discriminatory experiences. In September, 1988 a joint hearing was held before the relevant House and Senate committees that afforded people with varied disabilities to testify about the social and environmental barriers they faced on a daily basis. Several key legislators vowed to make a civil rights bill a priority for the next Congress. Both presidential candidates, George Bush and Michael Dukakis, also endorsed the concept.

In May, 1989, a new ADA bill was introduced to the Senate and the House, and a huge coalition of disability organizations, other civil rights groups, and civic and religious organizations geared up to work for passage. For months, lawyers and advocates dealt with complex legal issues that kept arising (Mayerson, 1992). They held tenaciously to the concept of disability as a broad "class" issue, resisting efforts to pare away certain groups such as those with HIV/AIDS or mental illness. The hearings included testimony by people with disabilities from throughout the country and even by Congressmen and Senators whose lives had been affected by attitudinal and physical barriers. The Senate voted overwhelmingly to support the bill (76 to 8) on September 7, 1989, but momentum slowed in the House as four committees held hearings. The disability movement continued to lobby against efforts to weaken the provisions, and the ADA was finally signed into law on July 26, 1990.

The Right to a Free and Appropriate Education

Also in the mid 1970s, the United States Congress and several state legislatures enacted laws requiring that disabled students be educated in the least restrictive environments compatible with their special needs. Both the federal "education for all handicapped act" and parallel state statutes have "mainstreaming" (desegregation) as a prime goal. A great deal of controversy and backlash resulted, from school officials protesting the lack of appropriations to carry out the mandates, teachers fearing disabled students in regular classrooms would drain time and energy from the nondisabled majority, and teachers/parents fearing disabled students would not get the special attention and teaching skills needed (see Chapter 6 for additional discussion). At first efforts toward full compliance were weak. Over the years, however, advocacy groups, especially parents of children with disabilities, have become increasingly knowledgeable and vocal about the rights that have been promised to their children, and now even students with very severe disabilities often are being educated in the same classrooms with their peers. On the other hand, Imparato (2000), head of the American Association of Persons with Disabilities, has cited a study done in January, 2000 by the National Council on Disability that indicates that every State is out of compliance with essential components of IDEA, and "the federal government's efforts to ensure compliance with IDEA over 25 years were found by NCD to be inconsistent, ineffective, and lacking any real teeth." A fundamental problem has been that the federal government has consistently failed to provide the funding that it promised to states to meet the costs of services.

Psychologically, IDEA is among the most important of all legislative accomplishments. Devaluative attitudes, which are at the root of disabled people's adjustment travails, are potently shaped by the separation of disabled from nondisabled in the early, formative years when belief and value systems are being laid down.

The right to participate extends beyond such basic need areas as education. It also includes the pleasures of recreations and cultural activities and the satisfactions associated with making civic contributions. The ADA requires that all programs and facilities available to the public be accessible to people with disabilities.

The Right to Equal Opportunity for Jobs

The most critical area in which disabled people want and need to participate is employment. A few states included disabled people as a protected population under their fair employment practice laws before federal "enabling" legislation was enacted. The 1973 Rehabilitation Act called for affirmative action efforts on the parts of the United States Civil Service Commission (Section 501) and firms receiving as much as $2500 annually in federal contracts (Section 503). Since these federal measures affect only a limited segment of the job market, their primary value was to enunciate the principle to be emulated by local governments. By the end of the 1970s, a survey indicated that at least fifteen states had laws that protect physically and mentally disabled workers, and eleven states had laws protecting physically disabled workers only (Vash, 1980). Since then, most or all states have followed suit. Even after passage of the ADA, these state laws remain important because they are sometimes more stringent (e.g., applying to employers with fewer workers than the 15 specified by the ADA) and because redress may be available by an easier or more effective route than that available through the ADA.

Title I of the ADA addresses employment. Originally applying to employers with 25 or more employees, in 1994 it became applicable to all with 15 or more workers. It requires that employers and labor organizations have application procedures, standards, and selection criteria that do not discriminate against people with disabilities. It also requires that employers provide reasonable accommodations to qualified applicants who request them. Individuals are deemed to be qualified if they can carry out the essential functions of the job, with or without accommodations. The extent of accommodations that an employer is expected to make depends upon such things as the size and resources of the company. The act also forbids employers to ask questions about disability or to require a physical examination prior to making an offer of a job. These provisions eliminate the "fishing expeditions" that used to trap people with hidden disabilities into acknowledging conditions and suffering the effects of discrimination, or else lying, perhaps getting the job and then living in fear of discovery and its consequences. In all likelihood they provide less benefit to those whose disabilities are readily apparent since interviewers would not need to ask prying questions in order for their apprehensions to be triggered. The law prohibits discrimination in terms of promotion, and it also provides some protection against termination for people who develop disabling conditions while employed.

The ADA, as passed, applied not only to private sector employers but also to state and local governments. The 2001 Supreme Court decision in the case of *Garrett vs. the University of Alabama*, however, bowed to a "states rights" argument and denied the constitutional authority of the federal government to impose ADA on the states. This means that individuals cannot sue states for monetary damages because of disability-based discrimination. The further implications of this decision are being examined as this book is going to press. No doubt this decision will serve to highlight the importance of state laws in ensuring the protection of citizens with disabilities.

People who feel that their rights under the ADA have been violated are encouraged to attempt to resolve the problem with their own supervisors or company managers, using the firm's alternate dispute resolution procedures, if available. If those efforts fail, a complaint can be filed with the Equal Employment Opportunity Commission (EEOC), a branch of the U.S. Department of Civil Rights. Procedures for filing are readily available on the Web (http://www.eeoc.gov), but the process of moving a case forward can be difficult and time-consuming. Because of staff shortages, it may take as much as 18 months for a complaint to begin the review process. A large-scale study (Moss, Ullman, Starrett, Burris, & Johnsen, 1999) reported the results of approximately 145,000 employment discrimination cases filed under the ADA and closed by March 31, 1998. The charging parties received some benefit in 15.7% of the cases, although only 1.7% resulted in hiring or reinstatement. The average monetary benefit was $5,646. Individuals with psychiatric disabilities were slightly less likely than those with other kinds of disabilities to benefit (13.6% vs. 16%). These may appear to be rather poor odds for the amount of psychic and tangible investment that goes with a claim. On the other hand, there is no way to measure the amount of good that may have accrued as a result of the law's existence in terms of the effect it may have had on accommodations, hiring, promotion, and retention decisions in cases that never came to litigation.

Case law continues to evolve more quickly than a printed textbook can reflect. Challenges arise to the interpretation and applicability of the law, and the disability community rises to defend its integrity. The Internet and e-mail have proved to be powerful tools informing and mobilizing the disability community on legislative issues. Calls for action can go out across the country—even across the world—with the speed of light, and thousands of letters can reach legislators on a critical issue. Some of the prominent sites include Justice for All (www.jfanow.org); ADAPT (www.ADAPT.org); the Disability Rights Education and Defense Fund, Inc. (www.dredf.org); the World Institute on Disability (www.wid.org); Freedom Clearinghouse (www.freedomclearinghouse.org); and Disability World (www.disability world.org). Many of the government sites also provide relevant and important information about current issues. Some examples include the National Council on Disability (www.ncd.gov); the President's Committee on the Employment of People with Disabilities (www50.pcepd.gov) and disability.gov (www.disability.gov).

Rehabilitation agencies report that their job placement efforts have been aided substantially by the enactment of the various federal and state laws addressing equal employment opportunity for disabled workers. All levels of government are trying to increase hiring of disabled workers through a variety of programs and modernized personnel selection procedures. Private employers are more willing to attend seminars on the subject, to follow through by developing affirmative action programs, and more frequently turn to rehabilitation agencies as sources of workers when they have job vacancies to fill. Legal provisions for offering tax savings to employers who will hire disabled workers and correct mobility barrier conditions in their work settings contribute to the improving trend.

The hard data on employment rates are mixed, however. The Harris Poll, which conducted national surveys of people with disabilities in 1986, 1994, and 1998 found that there has been little or no change in the proportion of people with disabilities who are working (only 32% of those aged 18–64 compared with 81% of the nondisabled population) (Thackeray, 2000). On the other hand, of those who say they are able to work in spite of their disabilities, 56% are employed, and the gap between that figure and the general population statistic of 81% has been steadily closing. Progress has been especially evident among younger individuals with disabilities and among people with less severe disabilities.

In addition to the employment provisions of ADA and other legislation, the transportation and public accommodations components of ADA and the creation of independent living centers have also contributed to the improved employment picture for people with disabilities. Although the Harris Poll showed that people with disabilities are almost three times more likely than others to say that inadequate transportation is a problem for them, accessible mainline buses and dial-a-ride services have become available in many cities during the past decade, making work feasible for their users.

Although civilian employment opportunities for disabled workers appear to be on the increase, as mentioned in Chapter 6, military opportunities are almost nonexistent still. This area needs legislation to enunciate the right of disabled individuals to serve in the military and reap the benefits it affords. The reasons given for excluding disabled people are largely without substantive basis. A sizable proportion of military occupational specialties entail job demands compatible with significant disabilities, and must be performed by someone during armed conflicts or combat training. What is resisted is change—and considerable system change would be required. It seems necessary, however, to eliminate this lingering area of needless discrimination.

The Right to Economic Protection

Related to, yet distinct from, employment opportunity is the matter of protection from economic exploitation. Wage and hour laws that require documented justification for paying disabled workers less than the minimum wage have the longest history. During the 1960s and 1970s, considerable attention was paid to potential and actual exploitation of institutionalized individuals whose work assignments were construed as part of their therapy programs and who, therefore, were paid token wages or nothing at all. Legal foreclosure on such practices benefited some, who truly were being exploited, and created harm for others. The loss of work responsibilities proved to be antitherapeutic for many mentally retarded or emotionally ill residents, and funds formerly devoted to services were diverted to facility maintenance. To a substantial degree, however, these issues have been resolved by the wholesale closing of large, long-term institutions. People who have some capacity for work no longer live for years in situations where they would have to work in the facility or sit idly; their focus is on treatment and early discharge.

Numerous other types of laws can be construed as providing economic protection to disabled people. The federal income tax exemption for legally blind or disabled individuals is one example. Antitrust laws are being used as the basis for efforts to deter manufacturers of durable medical equipment from charging what the traffic will bear in a captive market. All such legislative efforts and accomplishments provide a more stable, higher level, economic foundation for disabled individuals, reducing the emotional wear and tear of wondering how the costs of living can be managed.

The law also provides for workers to organize to improve their working conditions, rates of pay, and employee benefits. This includes workers in sheltered industries, many of whom have been paid less than prevailing rates, ostensibly because of reduced production capacities. This kind of situation has become much less prevalent, however, as sheltered workshops have substantially given way to supported employment as a mechanism for helping individuals with severe disabilities to become employed. A person working in a supported position may be assisted by a job coach (who is paid by a vocational rehabilitation agency) but the individual with a disability is paid at regular competitive rates for the job he or she is doing.

Confidentiality and the Right to Know

Privacy issues are on everyone's radar screen these days. With the unlocking of the human genetic code and the ever-increasing sophistication of data collection and dissemination systems, the prospect exists that prospective employers, insurers, and government could not only obtain intensely personal medical information about us, but also could predict the conditions we are vulnerable to developing in the future. Laws, agency regulations, and professional codes of ethics have long attempted to protect people's privacy by prohibiting improper disclosure of information contained in agency files. "Proper" disclosure meets two primary criteria: (1) the person's permission to disclose is obtained in writing, and (2) the need to disclose can be justified in terms of benefit to the person. Two types of information thus are protected: (1) that provided by individuals in the processes of seeking and receiving human services (for example, health, education, welfare, employment, legal, and pastoral services), and (2) information generated by service providers (for example, medical diagnoses, treatment/service plans, nursing notes, welfare memoranda, counseling progress notes, and psychological reports). The first type of information offers few conceptual problems. It is deeply ingrained in the general culture that one should not gossip about confidences, however well one adheres to the principle in practice. On the other hand, for reasons relating to professional insecurity, fear of lawsuits or personal danger, and beliefs that people (especially "patients") could be harmed by facts/opinions about their own conditions/situations, the second type of information came to be withheld from the service recipients themselves! This meant that recorded opinions—to which they were not privy—about patients, clients, students, or otherwise designated service recipients would influence the opinions and decisions of all providers with access to the files. It also meant that when they signed release forms permitting information of record to be disclosed to other agencies, this situation would follow them.

People insistent on taking charge of their own lives traditionally have found ways to gain access to their medical charts, school records, and/or other agency file materials. Many have been surprised and angered by what they found: entries they considered inaccurate, prejudicial, or otherwise detrimental to them. An expanding volume of complaints led to the creation of "right-to-know" legislation: the federal Freedom of Information Act of 1966, the federal Privacy Act of 1975, and comparable state laws/executive orders and local ordinances. All of these now enunciate the right of individuals to know what has been written about them in agency records.

Initially, professionals from virtually every human service discipline had difficulty accepting this turn of events; and serious concern lingers, especially when psychological information is at issue. A psychologist lamented, "Our reports will be watered down and useless if we have to write them so the patient or client can read them." A psychiatrist added

> We daren't say anything that might offend the patient. But how can you avoid offending patients who are denying that they have psychiatric disorders? If you say they have them, they're offended and might sue. Then some judge, who is not a

qualified diagnostician and who'll be working from persuasive rather than objective information will end up deciding whether your diagnosis is correct!

Here, however, is a more positive view of the effects of writing psychological reports (or other reports containing psychological material) with the knowledge that the subjects may, sooner or later, read them. Although it was written at a time when direct patient access to charts was uncommon, the principles that this psychologist discovered are still worth repeating.

The psychology staff at a Veterans Administration Domiciliary learned quickly that certain Dom members made a regular practice of going into the chart rooms every evening to review entries made in their charts during the day. We knew the policing required to put a stop to the midnight chart review would be more damaging than permitting it, so we learned to write our reports so we felt comfortable with the fact that the subjects of those reports would probably read them sooner or later.

It took little time to learn that we could say everything we needed to say to the colleagues to whom the reports were ostensibly addressed deleting no concept of substance—when we wrote "as if" to the member whom they described. The rules were simple. Sadly, the first turned out to be "Don't get cute." When cleverly sardonic or other witty ways of describing a patient or client occur to you, suppress them. Experience in dealing with legal representatives over this issue in programs I've administered shows the primary type of material clients object to falls in the category of "unkind witticisms and insulting broadsides."

The second rule was "Describe the subject in behavioral terms." We learned to avoid the use of high level abstractions, particularly those which have crept into lay usage with inflammatory overtones (such as "paranoia") and those controversial as to their meaningfulness within the psychological community (such as "schizophrenia"). This was a particularly good lesson. As a result of disciplining ourselves to think through the actual, behavioral substrates of a diagnostic label or trait name we had accepted as describing the person, we came to understand him better as a human being, and to make sharper distinctions about both his problems and strengths. We saw, for example, how damaging it is for people to be labeled "hostile" or "passive" as if those labels encompassed their total beings. Once such a label "sticks," others stop looking for, or seeing, the moments when the person is loving, not hostile, or assertive, not passive. If lovingness or assertiveness are the qualities you want the person to develop, you won't reinforce them if you fail to notice when they happen.

I began to write my reports as if they were summaries of progress to the Dom member himself. I recorded my views of where he was making gains and where he was resisting change and what I thought that was doing to him. It was within this climate of honesty—with members about members—that more effective counseling techniques for aiding their transitions to the outside were developed.

The third rule was "Make sure your own motivations/emotions toward the subject are helpful/caring before you start to write." If you are feeling angry or disrespectful toward the person, you will have to rewrite twenty times to keep it from showing.

If you take time to get yourself centered first, you can save nineteen rewrites. If you are motivated to caution other professionals about what a difficult son of a gun this person can be, the first order of business is to deal with your feelings about that. Probably, if this rule were followed, there would be no need for rules one and two. A caring mode tends to block witticisms, broadsides, and jargonistic labels.

From more recent experience in a large bureaucracy comes a fourth rule. "Don't include undocumented, third party 'hearsay' material in reports or file notes"— especially if it could be construed as damaging to the person's reputation. To illustrate, drawing from an actual case, if a worker from a sister agency tells you by phone that a mutual client frightened her to the point that she felt her safety was endangered when he came to her office, don't put it in the record unless she is willing to put it in writing. You can't count on her being around later to testify if the client files a grievance. If she is, she might decide in retrospect that it wasn't so serious; and fail to recall feeling actually endangered. You, then, will have blemished the client's reputation by putting undocumented gossip in the chart. (Vash, 1977, p. 446)

Thus, while there are necessary rules to observe, the overall effect of writing reports to conform with realities such as those created by right-to-know legislation can be viewed in a favorable light. The potential for tightening clinical thinking, and the incentive for careful adherence to principles most professionals endorse anyway, combine to render this new type of demand more an opportunity than an imposition.

The Right to a Fair Trial

The ADA has broken down two previously troublesome barriers for people with disabilities: (1) the rights of deaf individuals to interpreter services during court proceedings, and (2) the rights of all disabled individuals to have their cases tried by juries of their peers. People with disabilities have the right to interpreter services, whether they are plaintiffs, defendants, or jurors, and the court pays the fee. Further, courtrooms must be accessible, and people with disabilities cannot automatically be excluded from service on juries.

The Right to Appropriate Treatment by Police

People with disabilities have occasionally reported mistreatment by law enforcement officers who did not recognize or refused to believe they were disabled. These accounts have included deaf people being shot or nearly shot for failing to comply with "halt" commands, people with cerebral palsy or multiple sclerosis arrested for public drunkenness, paralyzed individuals pulled out of cars onto the ground, and retarded people physically abused for failing to respond correctly.

An investigation of the extent and nature of training within state police academies (McAfee & Musso, 1995) revealed that 36 states included some required information about disabilities, and four others provided some optional training. The specific content varied, but most included training about mental illness. Few included specific information about physical disability, mental retardation, or learning disabilities. Disability-related advisory groups to mayors, city councils, and county governing bodies appear to be potentially helpful intermediaries in bridging the knowledge gap and encouraging more appropriate behavior. Their ability to draw the attention of both elected officials and the media to such dramatic problems has led to some "self-policing," that is, attempts by scattered law enforcement agencies to provide their officers with needed education and attitudinal reshaping.

Prisoners with disabilities still face special problems. One senior clinical psychologist in the prison system (Eisenmann, 1995) described cruel treatment meted out to young men with learning disabilities and emotional disturbance. He said they were often screamed at and were sometimes shackled to a marble slab in the nude. Another article (Perske, 1997) compared today's treatment of prisoners with mental disabilities to that dispensed in 1692 Salem. He and other writers (Brinded, 1998; Clare & Gudjonsson, 1995) have described prisoners' vulnerability to forced confessions during police interrogation, even without any physical evidence. They may not fully understand their legal rights or the warnings provided to them, and they may be susceptible to compliance, suggestibility, and confabulation.

Mistreatment by law enforcement officers—whether due to failures of discernment or angry assumptions that claims of disability are attempts to flout their authority—happens to a relatively small segment of the disabled population. To those to whom it happens, however, it can be devastating. The fear and anger or depression resulting from such episodes can take a long time to resolve. The opportunity to have one's experience and complaints aired before an official body with no vested interest in protecting the law enforcement agency, can ameliorate these aftereffects somewhat, whether or not correction/apologies can be secured.

The Right To Be a Parent

This issue was introduced in Chapter 4, where instances of nonvoluntary sterilization of disabled women and wresting of child custody from disabled parents were mentioned. Disabled activist groups all over the country have taken a keen interest in situations such as these, and although these occurrences are becoming less frequent, they are not extinct. Pfeiffer (1999) provided a summary of eugenics and disability discrimination. In 1994, 22 states allowed for involuntary sterilization upon the recommendation of the supervisor of a county institution or a county director of social services. The defense of the practice is *parens patriae*, which means that biological or legal fathers know what is best for a child, even if the child is an adult with a disability. Pfeiffer wrote "Even in the absence of a law authorizing sterilization, courts can and do compel persons with disabilities to undergo compulsory sterilization with no regard of the disabled person's view of his or her 'best' interest" (p. 16).

The picture is brighter with respect to marriage and parenting, thanks to the ADA and other legislation. Pfeiffer (1999) cited a study by Wells, done in 1983, which indicated that 38 states and the District of Columbia had laws on the books either banning or closely restricting the right of a person with mental retardation to marry. Most of these laws have been eliminated. A situation arose in Michigan in 2001 in which two people with developmental disabilities were refused a marriage license, based upon a 1949 law. The event was so unusual as to warrant coverage in the national news. At the time this text is going to print, both houses of the Michigan legislature have acted to remove this anachronism, and a new law awaits the governor's signature.

Another welcome change involves the recognition of the rights of individuals with disabilities, including mental disabilities, to procreate and parent (Kerr, 2000). Whereas it was once standard practice for courts to terminate the parental rights of individuals who were labeled mentally disabled, this would now be recognized as discriminatory and in violation of Title II of the ADA. Reasonable accommodations must be made in the form of training for the parents and provision of appropriate support services. Only if there is clear evidence that the welfare of the child is in jeopardy, despite the accommodations, would there be justification for removing the child from the parents.

Historically child-custody suits almost always have ended with custody being awarded to the nondisabled parent, regardless of whether affectional and socioeconomic advantages could have been offered by the disabled parent. A decision by the Supreme Court of the State of California in the case of *Carney v. Carney* (L.A. 31064, Superior Court Number SDD 68540, August 7, 1979) marked a turning point, however. In a unanimous decision, Justice Mosk stated

> We are called upon to resolve an apparent conflict between two strong public policies: the requirement that a custody award serve the best interests of the child, and the moral and legal obligations of society to respect the civil rights of its physically handicapped members, including their right not to be deprived of their children because of their disability. As will appear, we hold that, upon a realistic appraisal of the present-day capabilities of the physically handicapped, these policies can both be accommodated. The trial court herein failed to make such an appraisal, and instead premised its ruling on outdated stereotypes of both the parental role and the ability of the handicapped to fill that role. Such stereotypes have no place in our law. (pp. 1–2)

In the area of adoptions, important changes also have taken place. Title III of the ADA, which mandates nondiscrimination in public accommodations, applies to private adoption agencies (Freundlich, 1998). The principles of "equal opportunity to participate" and "equal opportunity to benefit" prohibit agencies from using criteria that screen out an individual or a class of individuals from enjoying the services unless they result in a direct threat to safety. It is perhaps too early to say whether discrimination can be eliminated, but at least it has become more difficult to perpetrate.

The Right to Redress

The final type of legislation to be considered here takes us back to the topic of legislatively created benefits and services. Provisions for redress when applicants/recipients are dissatisfied with administering agencies' decisions sometimes are built into the original legislation and sometimes must be added later. The decisions grieved usually involve eligibility, amount of allowable benefits, or appropriateness of services. The grievance systems generally are composed of an internal subsystem of administrative remedies—reviews and hearings at escalating levels of supervision—and an external appeals system to turn to if resolution cannot be achieved through administrative review.

In the main, such systems probably are well used and offer benefits to both aggrieved parties and agencies; however, problems exist at two extremes. For reasons of temperament and personality, a few people overuse such systems in ways that are costly and impair their credibility, not only with the involved agencies, but with the disinterested adjudicators as well. For the same reasons, many more are afraid to use the system at all. It takes a great deal of courage for most people to say to an agency worker, "I am dissatisfied with your decision and I want to talk with your supervisor." If the supervisor supports the worker, it takes even more courage to confront that person, too. For people who feel oppressed and hopeless, it takes a measure of courage that often simply doesn't exist.

For this reason, many agencies have developed ombudsman programs that allow greater anonymity to aggrieved parties and provide practical/emotional support during redress procedures. The Rehabilitation Act of 1973 mandated the creation of Client Assistance Programs (CAPs) to help individuals with disabilities who are applying for vocational rehabilitation services, who may have been denied desired services, or for another reason were dissatisfied with services. Each state has developed a CAP, and it may also cover other public programs, such as independent living centers. Services may include information and referral, advocacy, technical assistance, and litigation.

Self-Policing

Since the 1960s, dozens of disabled people's "bills of rights" have been published, each specific to some particular group of consumers of rehabilitation services. Some of the better-known examples are "A Bill of Rights for the Handicapped," developed by the United Cerebral Palsy Association; "A Bill of Rights for the Rehabilitation Client," displayed in many offices of the state-federal rehabilitation program; the "Declaration of General and Special Rights of the Mentally Retarded," composed by the International League of Societies for the Mentally Handicapped; and the "Patient's Bill of Rights," put forward by the American Hospital Association.

Commonly included elements of these examples relate to the issues examined in the foregoing sections of this chapter, namely, rights to (1) timely and accurate eligibility determination, (2) knowledge of what is being said about one to other service providers, (3) information being used for decision-making about one, or needed to make intelligent decisions for oneself, (4) confidentiality of sensitive information, (5) timely and responsive services, (6) respect, (7) consideration, and (8) avenues of redress when reasonable expectations seem not to have been met. Most of these bills of rights avoid guaranteeing any right to expect effective or competent services. Those displaying them are divided with respect to whether that "goes without saying" or "would be impossible." Despite any shortcomings, however, consumers' bills of rights reflect good-conscience efforts on the parts of service providers to hold themselves accountable for correcting errors made in the past. The age of accountability also has created a new form of "market research."

Client Evaluations of Services

First, college professors had to get used to receiving report cards from their students at the end of each quarter/semester. Student evaluations of instructor effectiveness have by now become the rule rather than the exception and, in most places, are considered a valuable source of feedback by teaching staff. Similar evaluations of service providers by agency clients are commonly being solicited by all kinds of service providers, including vocational rehabilitation agencies. Their purpose is to help agency managers determine how agency effectiveness and methods are perceived by their customers. The information from such program evaluation efforts is meant to be fed into program planning, where deficiencies would be corrected through policy or procedural changes, in-service training, or whatever seems to respond best to the kinds of criticisms received.

The path from such theory to actual correction is tortuous, partly because change tends to occur slowly and partly because the credibility of the client evaluators frequently is impugned. The threat to the evaluees is enormous, posing a sensitive test to the solidity of their outward attitudes toward service recipients. Thin veneers may be stripped away, exposing negative beliefs just under the surface, such as, "Clients can't realistically evaluate professionals, they don't understand the complexities we face"; or "If you give them the store you'll get a high rating, but if you deny them something they want, watch out." Instructors, as a group, went through a similar period of doubting whether they would be evaluated fairly, and, as the system matured, their fears leveled out. In time, the same probably will occur in this newer area. Regardless of whether corrections follow rapidly or slowly, the opportunity for clients to voice their frustrations and advice to agencies yields significant benefits.

Voluntary Affirmative Action

Not only service agencies are involved in self-policing. The last form to be mentioned here concerns employers throughout the country who are going far beyond what any law requires in the way of affirmative action for disabled workers. Local government and private employers alike are responding to the spirit, not the letter, of the law by developing outreach programs to recruit disabled applicants for job vacancies. Some participate in Projects With Industry (see Chapter 6) to train and help secure job placements for vocational rehabilitation clients. Others are extending themselves in the process of accommodating disabled workers through rehabilitation engineering and personnel policies designed to reduce job barriers.

An outstanding example has been set by the California State Department of Rehabilitation. This government agency employs over 2000 individuals. Long before the ADA, it had an explicit policy stating that it would provide the equipment and support services necessary to allow its employees to perform their duties satisfactorily, including special items needed to accommodate disabling conditions. This might include such equipment as electronic reading aids and motorized wheelchairs, or such assistance as interpreter, attendant, reader, or driver services. The underlying philosophy assumes that "If individuals offer sufficient potential to cause the agency to want to hire them, then adequate support must be given."

As Congress realized during the ADA hearings, it costs the taxpayers far less in the long run to provide even expensive equipment and support services permitting talented, severely disabled persons to make work contributions to society than it would to fund the likely alternative of paying for their total support through the SSI program and receiving no work in exchange for the much greater expenditure. Acknowledging that such operating principles apply only when both the employment and welfare costs are tax supported (pass-through costs in the free enterprise sector create, as yet, unresolved problems), this agency encourages other government agencies to adopt similar approaches.

One Step Beyond

In the Spring of 1978, hordes of severely disabled individuals descended upon the federal office of the secretary of the (then) Department of Health, Education, and Welfare (DHEW) in Washington, D.C. A smaller, still impressive number followed suit at the regional office in San Francisco. They were using their right to assemble in an effort to pressure the secretary to sign the long-delayed regulations promulgated by his agency to implement Section 504 of the 1973 Rehabilitation Act. Although they were the targets of the demonstrations, DHEW staff interviewed later reported staying long into the night to provide emergency attendant care and ensure sufficient food supplies for the demonstrators. One indicated that "It was a mess. We wish they could have found another way, but we were in sympathy with what they wanted and saw the demonstration as a big step toward the independence we've tried to help them achieve."

Another example of collaboration occurred prior to the passage of the ADA. In March, 1990, members of the National Rehabilitation Association, who were meeting in Washington on that day, joined ADAPT members for their "Wheels of Justice" march that moved from the White House to the Capitol. The demonstration, arrests, and related confrontations with legislative officials contributed to the progress of the ADA through Congress. These actions go a step beyond "self-policing" to show the commitment that rehabilitation professionals can have to the spirit of civil rights for people with disabilities. It also demonstrates what many consider the most appropriate style of partnership between disabled people and nondisabled professionals/ advocates: the former taking the lead to achieve their goals and the latter using their expertise/resources to help—not a reversal wherein the professionals try to do the job for their "constituents." The following section will explore other aspects of the utilization of protective laws.

Utilization of the Law

Becoming Informed

For protective laws to be of practical consequence, the target populations must be informed of their existence, strengths, and limitations. For example, the utilization potential of the right to assemble came into sharpened focus during the antiwar demonstrations of the 1960s and has been employed regularly by protesters ever since. In the case at hand, disabled people, rehabilitation professionals, and other advocates must get, and stay, informed about a wide range of laws, plus court tests and precedents that affect their applicability. These same groups of people also are responsible for overseeing the enforcement of such laws, because they almost certainly will not be enforced without "watchdogging" by concerned citizens.

Overseeing Enforcement

Across the decades since the disability rights movement began, the responsibility for enforcement oversight has expanded from being assumed by a few individuals and informal committees, through formalized organizations of disabled people and rehabilitation professionals, to lawyers in large bureaucracies and attorneys general. In the early 1970s, none of the state rehabilitation agencies had full-time attorneys on their staffs; now, many do. The Protection and Advocacy System is a powerful participant in ensuring that the community integration mandate of ADA is enforced as well as the other provisions of ADA and the Rehabilitation Act. Independent living centers work in tandem with consumers to identify infractions and seek redress.

The field of law is attracting increasing numbers of disabled individuals, many of whom eventually devote some portion of their practices to disability law, often without expectation of compensation. Others establish or go to work for the similarly increasing number of disability law centers devoted to helping disabled people who can neither afford nor elsewhere find qualified attorneys to pursue their unique kinds of cases. The existence of such resources is both a practical and psychological boon to the many individuals who otherwise would be unable to use legal avenues of redress.

A Closing Note

As the foregoing illustrates, legislation has proved to be an important "psychological intervention strategy," by offering improved quality of life and access to opportunity. It becomes clear how Hohmann's words (see Chapter 2), "disability isn't as depressing anymore," relate as much to the bettered politico-legal status of disabled people as to the advances in health science and technology. In addition to these tangible improvements, individual and collective advocacy serves to fight that pernicious creator of depression, learned helplessness (Seligman, 1975). Speaking out and producing change, individually and especially through collective advocacy, can lead to a sense of empowerment. Realizing that one has some control over the circumstances that affect one's life can make the difference between silent suffering and action. We began the chapter by indicating that legislation is a nonpsychological tool for improving the lives of people with disabilities. It is clear, however, that advocacy for legislative change is also a powerful psychological tool for internal as well as external change.

The next four chapters will examine intervention strategies more typically construed as psychological in nature. Such strategies use psychological research findings and clinical experience to help disabled people enhance their psychosocial functioning and, concomitantly, their subjective states of psychological well-being. The next chapter will discuss issues relating to psychological evaluation, and the following three chapters will turn to "treatment" or psychological service approaches.

10

Individual Differences

An implicit message of this chapter is that, contrary to the manifest attitudes of the general public, people with disabilities are not all alike. It is not possible to describe "the handicapped" or "the disabled" as a homogeneous group. As is true of people in general, the human traits of this subpopulation tend to be more or less normally distributed, and individual differences are marked. For reasons to be set forth in a following section, it becomes necessary to measure these differences from time to time. The process is called "assessment" or "evaluation." This chapter will discuss issues relating to psychosocial/vocational (PSV) evaluation in particular and the psychological aspects of evaluative processes in general.

Although the terms "psychological testing" and "psychological assessment" often are used interchangeably, there is an important distinction between them (Meyer et al., 2001). "Testing" connotes measurement and nothing more. Testing yields data reflecting the presence, absence, or relative standing of a measured variable or set of variables. On the other hand, "assessment" implies that a clinician works to understand a person by applying multiple test methods and interpreting the results in the context of observed behavior, interview information, the person's history and referral materials. Meyer also includes communication of findings to the individual, family, and referral sources as an essential component of assessment. The term "evaluation" is similar to this broad definition of assessment, although it is often applied in the context of vocational services and may rely more extensively on observational or functional approaches than on psychological testing. Both terms will be used in this book to describe any process in which a clinical judging process is entailed.

The ensuing pages will explore the fundamental issues associated with the evaluation process: why we evaluate, whom and what we evaluate, when and where it is done, and how it is done. In addition, certain ethical issues, problems, and pitfalls will be examined.

Approaches to Evaluation

Within medical and vocational rehabilitation programs, the essential purposes of evaluation include obtaining a complete and multifaceted understanding of an individual to aid in setting goals, helping to determine what services might be useful in achieving those goals, and measuring progress toward the goals. Assessment helps to make services more sensitive to individual needs and preferences. Before the development of good assessment tools, rehabilitation service approaches typically were oriented around a disability rather than the whole person (Frey & Nieuwenjuijsen, 1990). For example, a vocational counselor might have attempted to identify jobs that would be "suitable" for an individual with a particular disability and then help the person to choose among them. Needless to say, this approach could have neglected some critical dimensions such as the person's interests and values as primary determinants of an appropriate choice. Further, it would have overlooked the possibility of assistive technology and other accommodations in broadening the vocational horizon.

Three broad approaches to evaluation are interviewing, psychometric testing, and situational or functional assessment. The lines between them are permeable, and they are often used in combination with one another. Each approach has advantages and limitations, and each requires a skilled and sensitive evaluator as well as an involved participant to be effective. Because interviewing is the oldest and most universally applied technique, we will begin there.

Interviewing

Rehabilitation services typically aim to help a person make choices or changes in life after disability. As a foundation for many other more specific purposes, interviewing may be undertaken to shed light on an individual's personality, mood, and life situation as well as his or her feelings about being in rehabilitation.

The interview is generally regarded as the most powerful single tool available to the PSV evaluator because of its potential for depth, sensitivity, and face validity. No psychometric test can measure the subtle information transmitted through body language or tone and cadence of voice. Thus, despite impressive test technology, skillful interviewers attuned to their own affective reactions remain among the best "instruments" available. Interviews provide the ultimate flexibility to follow individual leads and to probe for deeper understanding of a comment.

Despite these advantages, research has repeatedly shown that tests are superior to even highly skilled clinicians when it comes to predicting behavior (Dawes, Faust, & Meehl, 1993; Grove, Zald, Lebow, Snitz, & Nelson, 2000).

One way to enhance validity is to use two or more interviewers and "triangulate" between their observations and conclusions to arrive at consensual validation. This strategy is costly, however, so it is reserved for such critical situations as hiring decisions or the assessment of potentially dangerous individuals.

Interviewing is particularly important in assessing people with disabilities because many standardized tests and inventories have uncertain reliability and validity when used with a disabled population (to be discussed later). Equally vital, no single assessment method can provide a complete picture of a person—the representation is inevitably incomplete (Meyer et al., 2001).

The strength of the interview is directly related to the skill and sensitivity of the interviewer. It stands to reason that if the interviewer lacks these qualities or is operating from a biased perspective the interview will be an ineffective evaluation tool. We have discussed in Chapter 2 the fact that many people in the society carry stereotyped views of people with disabilities, and so they may be led to asking certain questions (or avoiding others) that confirm their expectations. This is a strong reason for utilizing other more formal methods to supplement information gained through interviewing.

Psychometric Testing

Historically, rehabilitation psychologists and other service providers made extensive use of psychometric testing for service planning and decision making. Psychometric tests present an individual with standardized questions or other stimuli in order to elicit responses. Test validation involves determining the extent to which those responses correlate with other important outcomes, such as the ability to live independently or to succeed in school or a job. When highly valid tests are used by skilled examiners under the right circumstances, they can provide a useful, cost-effective alternative to trial-and-error decisions. Meyer and colleagues (2001) reported on a study of more than 125 meta-analyses of test validity and provided clear evidence of test usefulness across a wide variety of instruments and referral questions. They also demonstrated that the validity of psychological tests is comparable to that of medical tests, such as screening mammogram tests for predicting cancer within two years or dexamethasone suppression test scores for predicting response to depression treatment. At the same time, the best of assessment procedures are imperfect predictors. People and their functioning in the world are too complex to be fully measured, even at a single point in time. There are many other reasons why it is so difficult to consistently achieve univariate correlations much above .30 (Meyer et al., 2001). For one thing, tests typically measure only the personal side of the behavioral equation and do not take into account the way in which different environmental conditions may affect the individual's performance. Sometimes the assessment process attempts to predict rare events, and this reduces the chances for success. But even variables that seem easy to predict do not necessarily result in high correlations. For example, the correlation between weight and height for U.S. adults is .44 (U.S. Department of Health and Human Services National Center for Statistics, 1996, as cited in Meyer et al., 2001).

There are some particular challenges in the use of psychometric tests in rehabilitation. Few tests have been developed and normed on people with disabilities, so the results they produce may lead to erroneous interpretations. Furthermore, standardized tests require that administration be done according to strict guidelines, and a disability may require changes in procedures. For example, questions from a printed test booklet may need to be read aloud to a person who is blind. If the test is timed, such an individual may be significantly disadvantaged. If the questions are long, the person needs to hold a lot of information in memory in order to access the right answer, making the task more difficult than it would be for someone who can refer easily to the question and to alternative responses.

Few, if any, tests are good instruments in and of themselves. Most become good tests only in the hands of gifted examiners who can combine the maximum possible adherence to standard procedure with optimal innovation and skilled interpretation, thus generating an accurate picture of the test taker's present status and future probabilities. Even a test such as the Strong Interest Inventory, which is widely considered one of the best psychological instruments ever developed (research shows it accurately predicts very long-range behavior), is of little value when used mechanically by practitioners who are only superficially familiar with its construction and potential.

Situational or Community-Based Assessment

An evaluative approach that has moved from the nontraditional area to the traditional and is commanding increasing attention is that of performance sampling (Pancsofar & Steere, 1997). Here, the field of rehabilitation has pioneered for more than just the disabled population. Simulated and actual work-sampling techniques were developed as means of solving reliability and validity problems by narrowing the generalization gap when predicting disabled workers' job performance. It was reasoned that the more like the actual work situation the testing was, the less likely it became that predictions would go wrong. Nearly two decades after this was standard operating procedure in vocational rehabilitation, the civil rights movement created changes that required similar generalization-gap narrowing in assessing ethnic minority job applicants. Thus, the substitution of performance sampling for (poorly predictive) standardized tests—"old hat" in rehabilitation—became the "new thing" in mainstream job-selection screening. It is unquestionably a better way; now efforts need to be directed toward reducing the time required to obtain adequate samples to a cost-effective level.

To add perspective, rehabilitation counselors have practiced one type of performance sampling for years, requiring clients seeking artistic training to submit portfolios of their work to agreed-upon experts for talent evaluation. As another example, videotape feedback offers performance sampling to clients for self-appraisal of job interview and other interpersonal skills. This places the evaluative responsibility on the clients themselves. Situational assessment has been demonstrated in at least one study (Scroggin, Kosciulek, Sweiven, & Enright, 1999) to enhance participants' career awareness, vocational decision-making ability, and their expected ability to find employment.

Nontraditional Evaluation

On the borderline between traditional and nontraditional evaluative techniques are little-used instruments that measure traits considered nontraditional using traditional tests or inventory methods. Tests of creativity, operationally defined as "divergent thinking ability," for example, have been shown to predict vocational productiveness (Kemp & Vash, 1971). In addition, measures of sensation seeking, including boredom susceptibility (Zuckerman, 1978), and motivation to find purpose in life (Crumbaugh, 1977) have suggestive promise for rehabilitation. As research and clinical experience show particular traits to be useful predictors, they may move into the mainstream and become regarded as traditional. Of the three examples cited, only the first has made noticeable headway in that direction, and a review of research up to 2001 failed to show new revelations, even in that area. Problems associated with boredom and the will to meaning strike the authors as potentially powerful predictor variables and bases for treatment efforts. Each reader probably will think of one or two other traits that seem equally worthy of research and clinical attention.

A rich source of ideas for assessment research is arising from the field of positive psychology. Positive psychology is a growing force, as evidenced by the January, 2000 special issue of the American Psychologist. Shortly after World War II, the empirical attention of psychology narrowed to a focus on assessing and curing human suffering (Seligman & Csikszentmihalyi, 2000). For all of the benefits this work produced, the cost was an eclipse of interest in optimal functioning. Seligman has been leading its resurrection and the development of a major research program in the area of positive psychology, which has been defined in the following way:

> The field of positive psychology at the subjective level is about valued subjective experiences: well-being, contentment, and satisfaction (in the past); hope and optimism (for the future); and flow and happiness (in the present). At the individual level, it is about positive individual traits; the capacity for love and vocation, courage, interpersonal skill, aesthetic sensibility, perseverance, forgiveness, originality, future mindedness, spirituality, high talent, and wisdom. (Seligman & Csikszentmihalyi, 2000, p. 5)

Much of the assessment done with people who have disabilities has been focused on problems and limitations. The time has come to give serious attention to the strength and creativity that may be engendered by the challenges of disability. Such work could not only provide a more complete understanding of individual clients but also expand our theoretical understanding of human capacities.

The Evolution of Assessment

There have been substantial changes in the frequency, types, and extent of assessments used in both medical and vocational rehabilitation settings during recent years. In hospitals, both the time and the resources available for assessment have been squeezed by the changes in the health care system. Years ago, people with serious disabilities might spend months on an inpatient rehabilitation unit, and the usual treatment protocol allowed for substantial psychological and vocational services. Both testing and counseling were often covered by the overall "per diem" reimbursement rate or else were readily reimbursed by the insurers. Now, under managed care, the focus in hospitals is often almost exclusively on medical services, and people are typically discharged as soon as they reach the point of physical stability. PSV evaluation is therefore boiled down to a minimum or eliminated entirely. An exception to this trend involves individuals with brain injury. Neuropsychological testing is often carried out to determine the extent of functional impairments and their implications for discharge planning. Even in this area, the use of extensive, multifaceted, and expensive batteries has declined.

Substantial changes also have occurred with respect to assessment in vocational rehabilitation. The frequency of psychometric assessment has been reduced, replaced in part by less formal "situational assessment" that takes place out in the community or on the job. In deference to the right of consumers to make their own decisions regarding goals, rehabilitation counselors also may forgo assessment in favor of just giving a training program or job a try to see if it works out. Feasibility of a rehabilitation plan thus may be assumed rather than tested prior to initiation. If a person's initial capacity for work is insufficient, it may be built up through accommodations or coaching. Formal assessment may be saved for instances in which the individual with a disability is searching for direction or those in which an initial plan was discarded.

Just as the model for provision of counseling has changed in recent years from paternalistic to collaborative, so has the use of assessment in psychological and vocational settings. Instead of an expert selecting and applying instruments to generate knowledge for service planning, the accepted approach involves mutual decision-making by the professional and the customer/client/patient about how to obtain information that will enable the individual to make the best choices for the future. The extent to which this ideal is achieved varies depending upon the setting and individual contributions to the process. In acute medical settings, where the assessed individual is in the role of patient, professionals are more likely to select instruments to answer referral questions. Even in hospitals, however, informed consent is required for treatment, and patients have the right to refuse testing. In independent living and vocational settings, on the other hand, full customer participation is essential. Even people who once were thought to be incapable of understanding alternatives and making decisions are the focus of "person centered planning" approaches that empower the individual and his or her family advocates to make substantive decisions about the assessment and service process.

Although the practice of evaluation in rehabilitation has changed substantially, it continues to have many important functions, including the following: prediction of behavior; understanding the individual and his or her support system; assessment of functional capacities; service planning; decision making; assessment of progress and outcomes; screening and adjudication; and research.

Purposes and Uses of Evaluation

Behavioral Prediction

The overriding theme common to all purposes and uses of evaluation is the prediction of behavior. Assessment, coupled with knowledge of the findings' implications, enables one to predict such future behavior as responses to disability-related events, facts, and situations. According to Lewin (1935), behavior is a function of the person and the environment, thus, $B = f(P,E)$. Once the appropriate values of the relevant person and environment variables are inserted into the equation, and the nature of the mathematical relationship is known, the probability of occurrence of a given behavior (or set of behaviors—a behavior pattern) can be predicted. This is a simple statement of the basis of behavioral science research, and in theory, it is equally applicable to individual clinical prediction.

Personal variables are all those descriptors used to identify/characterize individuals or groups of individuals: demographic data, traits, historic variables, and so forth. These person variables are the objects of most clinical assessment procedures. Lewin (1935) separated environment variables into "proximal" and "distal" subvarieties. Proximal (nearby) variables influence the person directly, and distal (remote) variables exert their influences indirectly. Examples of proximal environment variables, with relevance to rehabilitation, are family support and community service availability. Examples of distal environment variables that influence behavior are federal funding trends and the first lady's interest in rehabilitation. Measurement of environment variables is primarily a research activity, but certain proximal environment variables, whose importance has been demonstrated, also may be assessed in the clinical situation.

Some people find efforts to predict human behavior objectionable, in the mistaken belief that prediction always implies a corollary will to control the behavior predicted. Typically, two arguments are offered to counter this. The more frequently used one admits to a control corollary but justifies it on the basis of benefit to the individual and society. In other words, the control potential is seen as morally neutral, and its use for good or ill is regarded as a separate concern to be monitored by ethical and legal systems rather than science itself. The less frequently used argument seems more to the point: prediction does not always imply the potential for control. For example, our ability to predict planetary movement in our own solar system is virtually perfect, but no one fancies that we will ever alter or control it. The predictive knowledge is used in other ways to make our lives more comfortable.

The same is true for much of the information gathered during clinical assessment. While it is true that efforts to change (control) maladaptive behavior patterns are sometimes intended, in many other instances the information is used only to alert the person to pertinent environmental stress conditions he or she may wish to avoid, or to point out hitherto unrecognized inner resources he or she may wish to exploit through training or job choice.

In the area of rehabilitation, several kinds of behavioral prediction may be important. For people who have sustained brain injury or another neurological impairment that affects cognition, planning for discharge from a rehabilitation hospital requires an understanding of the person's ability to make appropriate decisions, to solve problems, and to live safely, with or without supervision. Assessment can help to answer these and other questions, such as ability to drive or to handle money. Interviews, observation, mental status exams, and neurobehavioral screening tests all might contribute to answering these questions.

Coping inventories might help to predict an individual's approach to meeting and facing life problems. Some people tend to avoid engaging with stressors, if possible, whereas others attack them directly and try to solve them. Some people turn to prayer, some weep or become angry, and some look for help from friends or relatives. Predicting how a person will cope may help to anticipate problems or suggest alternative strategies.

Understanding Personality and Support Systems

Many tests are used in clinical settings to assess personality functioning. For more than 50 years the Minnesota Multiphasic Personality Inventory or its revisions have been used to provide complex descriptions of an individual's functioning and predict his or her response to disability and treatment. Other frequently used instruments range from the complex (e.g., Millon Clinical Multiaxial Inventory) to the straightforward (e.g., the Sickness Impact Profile). Depression is a frequent concern in rehabilitation settings, and instruments such as the Beck Depression Inventory may provide a means for calibrating a person's mood state. Anxiety is another symptom that may call for administration of a test such as the Hamilton Anxiety Scale.

The number of personality instruments in existence runs into the thousands, and even a brief description of the most popular ones is beyond the scope of this book (see Bolton, 2001 and Cushman & Scherer, 1995) for more information about assessment in rehabilitation). Some of the issues surrounding their use should be noted, however. Criticisms of these instruments include the fact that they usually are pathology-oriented and may not be appropriate for the many rehabilitation participants who are psychologically healthy individuals caught up in abnormal circumstances. In addition, most of the inventories have not been validated on individuals with physical disabilities, so the meaning of the scores they render is open to question. Some of the items contained in these scales would be answered in the "scored" direction as the result of neurological, sensory, or muscular changes (e.g., 'parts of my body are numb,' or 'I am tired and short of energy') rather than reflecting the concept (for example, depression) that is supposedly being measured. As a result, a psychological diagnosis could be inappropriately bestowed.

Some newer personality measures are oriented toward healthy functioning rather than pathology. For example, self-efficacy measures evaluate the degree of confidence an individual has in his or her ability to carry out certain behaviors that will produce a desired outcome. Self-efficacy has been shown to be negatively related to depression (Shnek, Foley, LaRocca, Smith, et al., 1995) and positively related to quality of life among a sample of people with spinal cord injury in China (Hampton, 2000). Self-efficacy also has been found to be an important predictor of positive change following rehabilitation interventions among people with fibromyalgia (Buckelew et al., 1998; Buckelew, Huyser, Hewett, Parker, et al., 1996; Buckelew, Parker, Keefe, Deuser, et al., 1994), multiple sclerosis (Wingerson & Wineman, 2000), and low back pain (Levin, Lofland, Cassisi, Poreh, & Blonsky, 1996). Self-efficacy also was found to be a predictor of employment outcomes among a sample of individuals with psychiatric disabilities who were provided with supported employment services (Regenold, Sherman, & Fenzel, 1999).

Social support has the potential to affect the way that a person responds to the onset of a disability, perhaps by providing direct assistance, and perhaps by mitigating the stressful concomitants of disability. Although social support may appear to be a straightforward concept, its complexity is apparent in the many ways it has been interpreted. Vaux (1988) suggested that it actually includes three broad dimensions: support network resources (which can expand an individual's functional capacities), supportive behaviors (efforts made to help a person), and support appraisals (the individual's perception of the quantity and quality of support available). Research in this area dates back at least to the 1970s, yet a scholarly review of the progress to date (Chwalisz & Vaux, 2000) indicates that the overall results have been inconclusive. It is not hard to think of some of the reasons for divergent findings; for example, although having a supportive family is generally an advantage, a doting family could actually interfere with an individual's progression toward relative self-sufficiency. Another source of inconsistency is that social support has been defined in varied ways from study to study, and it has often been thrown together with many variables in studies attempting to predict disability.

Some studies have turned their lens in the other direction, looking at social support as the dependent rather than the independent variable. Differing conclusions have been reached about effects of disability on social support systems. At times the occurrence of disability brings family members closer together, whereas in other cases the system splinters. It seems likely that the relationship between disability and support networks is moderated by other factors such as the individual's personality and the extent to which he or she conforms to expected behavior (Chwalisz & Vaux, 2000). Needless to say, the characteristics of other family members would also be significant determinants of the relationship.

Regardless of the limitations in our knowledge, however, the PSV evaluator should assess the support system available to an individual with a disability and also may do some assessment of family members to see how they are dealing with the changes that disability has imposed on their lives. By carefully evaluating the responses and coping strategies of all of the family, rehabilitation providers can improve the prospects for a successful outcome for everyone.

Spirituality is an essential part of a person that is often overlooked in the evaluation process. Only recently has it been receiving attention from rehabilitation professionals. It will be discussed further in Chapter 14.

Assessment of Functional Abilities

The functional abilities that would be assessed typically in medical rehabilitation settings include the ability to eat independently, to bathe, groom, use the toilet, and other kinds of daily living skills. In independent living settings, these same areas might be assessed, along with the ability to carry out community-based activities such as using public transportation. In vocational rehabilitation, an even wider range of functional abilities is relevant.

The following assessment model, originally designed to help allied health staff in a rehabilitation hospital to make appropriate referrals to the hospital's vocational rehabilitation program, will illustrate (1) a compact and comprehensive array of variables that must be evaluated in the process of moving disabled people from the medical to the vocational stage of rehabilitation, and (2) some of their important interrelationships.

Drawing from the job demands described in the Dictionary of Occupational Titles, it is reasoned that for a worker to have something to offer an employer, he or she must have capabilities in one of the five following "worker resource" areas:

1. Brawn—the ability to use one's body as a "power machine" or a mover of material. This includes such subcomponents as strength, endurance, and agility (coordination plus speed).

2. Brain—the ability to use one's intellect to perform operations on information and ideas. This includes such subcomponents as intelligence, creativity, special aptitudes, and learned knowledge.
3. Hands—the ability to use one's hands to create or manipulate objects. This includes such subcomponents as dexterity, special talents, and learned skills.
4. Personality—the ability to use one's personality to influence the attitudes and behavior of others. This includes such subcomponents as dominance, energy level, and learned interpersonal skills. (It should be stressed that this dimension is limited to that aspect of personality used as a work tool, much as we use our bodies, brains, and hands. Some jobs demand high levels of it—psychotherapist, teacher, trial attorney, receptionist, manager—and some require little or none—statistical clerk, laborer, bench assembler. It does not include aspects of personality that relate to getting or keeping jobs in general, such as poise, adaptability, and grooming habits.)

It is acknowledged that communication skills can be viewed as a subcomponent of the combined brain and personality dimensions. However, because the receptive losses of blind and deaf workers and the transmission deficits of persons with speech disorders affect communication in ways that do not fit with our usual concepts of "brain" and "personality," this has been factored out to form a separate dimension.

5. Communication—the ability to receive and transmit information accurately and efficiently. This breaks down into the subcomponents of visual/auditory reception, and vocal/written transmission. Comprehension and other "data processing" abilities are considered brain resources. Persuasive effect of communications is considered a personality resource. This variable is defined solely in terms of receiving/transmitting abilities.

In addition to the worker resource variables, "emotional stability" must also be considered as a necessary support or background variable in making oneself desirable to an employer. Therefore, this sixth and last variable is added to the list.

6. Emotional stability—the ability to perform a job adequately in the face of stress, and behave appropriately on the job.

These six variables can also form a basis for defining both type and severity of disability. "Type" here refers only to the job-relevant aspect of function that is impaired. For example, individuals can be rated "high," "moderate," "low," or "very low" in each area, compared with the workforce population. The functional limitations of a quadriplegic, for example, would always be reflected in "very low" ratings on "brawn" and "hands." Those of mentally retarded persons would reflect "low" or "very low" ratings on "brain" resources. Disabling mental illness would be reflected on the "emotional stability" scale, sensory disabilities on the "communication" scale, and so forth. If a disability reduces a person's reservoir of worker resources, it is reflected in this system. If it does not, it belongs in another part of the predictive equation—perhaps that which treats proximal environment variables affecting the likelihood of a person's working at all, such as social reactions to disability.

It can be seen from the foregoing that whereas "disability" is operationally defined by ratings on one or more of the individual scales, "vocational handicap" (or its obverse, "vocational potential") is defined by the total profile of all the scales. The lack of isomorphism between disability and vocational handicap also becomes readily apparent. For example, quadriplegia would be defined by "very low" ratings on brawn and hands. However, if the individual also had "high" ratings on brain, personality, communication, and emotional stability, his or her vocational potential would be very good (and, conversely, the vocational handicap could be considered mild).

Another example of a system designed to organize and clarify a counselor's understanding of an individual's vocational capacities is the Functional Assessment Inventory (FAI) (Crewe & Athelstan, 1981, 1984). This instrument is more detailed than the typology we have just described, and it incorporates some of the social and environmental characteristics that are important to achieving employment. The FAI consists of 30 behaviorally anchored rating scales of functional limitations and a checklist of 10 special strengths. It has been shown to be reliable and valid for the prediction of vocational outcomes among people with many kinds of disabilities. Factor analyses carried out with large and varied samples of rehabilitation clients have shown substantial consistency with regard to the broad dimensions of function that comprise potential for employment. Figure 10.1 shows the individual items from the FAI, grouped according to their associated factors (Neath, Bellini, & Bolton, 1997).

The FAI is unusual among approaches to functional assessment in that it has a companion instrument, The Personal Capacities Questionnaire (Crewe & Athelstan, 1981) that allows the individual with a disability to evaluate himself

Factor 1: Adaptive Behavior
  Judgment
  Congruence with rehabilitation goals
  Problem solving
  Interaction with coworkers
  Work habits
  Perception of limitations
  Social support
  Attractiveness
  Economic disincentives

Factor 2: Cognition
  Learning ability
  Ability to read and write in English
  Form perception
  Memory
  Vision

Factor 3: Physical capacity
  Endurance
  Capacity for exertion
  Mobility
  Motor speed
  Loss of time from work
  Stability of condition

Factor 4: Motor functioning
  Hand functioning
  Upper extremity functioning

Factor 5: Communication
  Speech
  Language functioning
  Hearing

Factor 6: Vocational qualifications
  Skills
  Special working conditions
  Acceptability to employers
  Access to job opportunities
  Work history

FIGURE 10.1   FAI items associated with six factors for a sample of 5,741 vocational rehabilitation clients.

Note: From "Dimensions of the Functional Assessment Inventory for Five Disability Groups," by J. Neath, J. Bellini, and B. Bolton, 1997, *Rehabilitation Psychology, 42*(3), pp. 183–207. Reprinted with permission.

or herself on the same items that the PSV evaluator has rated on the FAI. This allows more complete collaboration between them as they try to accomplish the goals of evaluation. No doubt, the combination of "insider" and "outsider" perspectives results in a composite picture that is nearer the truth than either of them could produce individually.

Neuropsychological Assessment

Neuropsychological assessment can be viewed as a special kind of functional evaluation. It is used most often in medical settings, and it is also of value in vocational rehabilitation. Originally, the field was oriented toward pinpointing the location of brain lesions so that surgeons could open the skull in the right place. Magnetic resonance imaging and other sophisticated imaging techniques obviated that need, so neuropsychology developed new missions. Now its primary purposes include: delineating a person's cognitive limitations as well as areas of strength; identifying problems that need to be addressed; determining the most effective ways to approach treatment with a particular individual; measuring progress resulting from recovery and services; and evaluating capacity for living alone, driving, and handling tasks of daily living.

Neuropsychologists have developed an impressive array of tests that evaluate intellectual abilities, attention and concentration, memory, problem solving and planning abilities, visual and spatial perception, and language functioning. They are able to go beyond simple measurement and collection of test scores. The "process approach" allows the psychologist to examine in detail how an individual approaches new tasks, what kinds of difficulties are encountered, and what kinds of compensatory strategies are usable. Such insights can be very important in determining the kinds of accommodations that could help an individual with neurological problems to master the challenges of school or work.

Service Planning

As we have just noted, a good functional assessment can lead directly into the process of planning for services. Assessment is relevant to service planning in other ways, as well. A key example is screening for problems that may not be apparent immediately but would require services if present. For example, some individuals who sustain quadriplegia in acceleration/deceleration injuries also incur mild brain injuries with long-lasting consequences (Cullum & Thompson, 1997). If the sequelae of brain injury are not recognized and dealt with, they could have significant repercussions during rehabilitation and especially later when the individual attempts to return to work.

Another kind of screening that was overlooked for years in most medical rehabilitation units was the issue of substance abuse. Among people with traumatic head injuries or spinal cord injuries, for example, the physical problems were so prepotent that they commanded most of the team's attention. Alcohol was not an option on the inpatient dietary menu, so the issue did not reach the radar screen. Even when behavioral evidence of misuse appeared, such as when an individual came back from pass inebriated or was found to have smuggled some marijuana into the ward, many staff shrugged it off as expected for young people who had been cooped up for a time and who were dealing with losses that may have been precipitated by the onset of disability. When research began to challenge this denial, it became apparent that more than half of people who sustain serious traumatic injuries have preexisting alcohol and drug abuse problems (Heinemann, Goranson, Ginsburg, & Schnoll, 1989), and that people with other disabilities (e.g., blindness, hidden disabilities, and mental illness) may also be at increased risk when compared with the general population (Wolkstein, 2002).

Screening for emotional problems, such as depression, anxiety, and other issues is another useful application of assessment techniques. Again, these concerns may either go unrecognized or may be accepted as unremarkable under the circumstances. Psychologists (Kemp, Kahan, Krause, Adkins, & Nava, 2002) undertook a study involving the use of cognitive therapy and medications to treat depression among individuals with spinal cord injury. Their intervention was successful, but more surprising was the fact that they could find no accounts in the literature of previous similar efforts. Again, deliberate screening may lead to recognition of the need for interventions.

Other kinds of targeted assessment may follow the request of physicians and members of the rehabilitation team for help in understanding and managing particular behavioral problems or answering specific questions. Assessment protocols have been developed, for example, to screen applicants for invasive or costly procedures such as transgender surgery, penile implants to correct impotence, or gastric banding to treat morbid obesity. In these situations, evaluation is intended to help identify those who would benefit from the procedures and to screen out those who have unrealistic expectations or psychological problems that would result in disappointment or disaster.

Decision Making

Assessment for decision making has much in common with functional assessment and service planning. The balance is shifted a bit, however, from the collection of information to be used by service providers to compilation of data that the individual with a disability will use directly to make choices. The variety of evaluation that developed for predicting work behavior and improving a client's employability is known as "vocational evaluation." Consonant with the theme of change that has been mentioned elsewhere in this chapter, the field of vocational evaluation is not what it was in years past.

During the 1960s, 1970s, and 1980s a thriving enterprise known as "work evaluation" developed, actually becoming a separate, specialized discipline with its own training and credentialing procedures. Its mission was to evaluate the potential of rehabilitation clients to become workers and to develop individualized vocational objectives along with plans for achieving them. The field encompassed many types of evaluative procedures, from psychometric testing of interests and aptitudes to sampling of actual work performance. Clients from the public vocational rehabilitation program were often referred for a period of weeks or months to undergo comprehensive assessment and return with a plan that the counselor could then help to implement.

During the 1990s the number of referrals for vocational evaluation decreased to the point where some believed that it had lost its relevance and was dying (Hilyer, 1997). One important reason for the situation was the shift from freestanding rehabilitation facilities and sheltered workshops to community-based services. Related to this shift was a dramatic change in the idea of how to prepare people with disabilities for employment. Whereas the old model of rehabilitation relied on a pattern of assessment, followed by training, culminating in placement on a job, the new model turned this sequence upside-down. People now are frequently placed directly on a job and provided with whatever supports they need in order to learn and master the work. Rather than requiring a lot of psychometric data to be collected from an individual operating in a simulated environment, less structured assessment began to take place, with the individual carrying out real tasks in real work settings. The expectation for reasonable accommodations, mandated by the ADA, also contributed to an increasing recognition that assessment of individuals in isolation from the work context was of limited value. Empowerment of rehabilitation clients for making their own choices about vocational goals is another element that led to declines in vocational evaluation referrals.

Thomas (1999) has painted a picture of vocational evaluation in the 21st century. He predicts that given the consumer-driven emphasis in rehabilitation services, vocational evaluation will be marketed directly to persons with disabilities and to other individuals who desire expert consultation to aid in their vocational planning. Evaluators will work with the general public and also will have specialized expertise for understanding the issues of people with disabilities. Community-based assessment will become the method of choice for individuals who have severe disabilities and many barriers to employment. Online evaluations will make services available to a wider population. A particularly intriguing aspect of Thomas's vision is that he sees the broadening of evaluation to encompass other aspects of quality of life in addition to work.

Tools for Counseling and Stimulation of Self-Evaluation

The evaluation process itself sometimes can have a "therapeutic" effect apart from the uses to which the findings are put. Most notable is the cathartic effect of describing one's history, situation, and problems to an interested interviewer, but responding to psychometric test or questionnaire items can fulfill similar needs. Going a step further, simply learning the findings—before they are put to active use in counseling—is helpful to some people. A client of an alcoholism clinic humorously indicated:

> Somehow, it helped me to know what kind of a nut I am. I got a kind of peaceful feeling that if a picture of me emerged from those zig-zaggy lines on the profile sheets, somebody must have a handle on things. For the first time in years I had this surge of feeling, "Hey, everything's gonna be alright." That got me off to a good start in counseling.

Others, of course, have opposite reactions of fearful defensiveness. The difference is probably a function of both the evaluee's personality and the evaluator's manner of presentation.

During any kind of counseling process—from educational advisement through reconstructive psychotherapy—assessment findings may be used to guide the participants in a number of ways. The counselor will keep them in mind when choosing the techniques or style. Both will use them in making decisions about which services to seek or offer, and about life in general (what to do about identified problems). The client may continue to use gleaned knowledge of capabilities/limitations and awareness of personal needs/traits for many years after counseling has terminated, when critical life decisions must be made. Moreover, observing the fruitfulness of connecting life decisions to relevant evaluation data can stimulate habits of self-evaluation in introspectively inclined people, and this is often an explicit intent of the evaluator-counselor. Evaluation data not shared with clients—to the limits of their comprehension—constitute a serious waste of both the client's and the professional's time.

Assessment of Progress and Rehabilitation Outcomes

Vocational rehabilitation has always had the advantage of a relatively straightforward measure of success: getting a job. For psychosocial service providers in medical rehabilitation settings, however, proving their efficacy is more difficult. Another role of assessment, therefore, is to measure an individual's level of functioning at the time he or she enters a treatment program and at points along the way, especially upon discharge from the program and, when possible, at follow-up points.

The primary instrument currently being used to measure the outcomes of medical rehabilitation treatment is the Functional Independence Measure (FIM) (Granger & Hamilton, 1992). Only two of the 18 items on the scale touch upon psychological areas, and the rest involve basic life activities such as locomotion, eating, bathing, dressing, and toileting. This lopsided ratio reflects not only the greater value that hospitals place upon physical functioning and the relative ease with which physical outcomes can be measured, but also the fact that the benefits of psychological services may take months or years to become evident. If a practitioner serves well as therapist, counselor, teacher, guide, or guru, then the individual may be better prepared to deal with exigencies of his altered life, weeks, months, or years after he has left the hospital. That is the hope and intent. But the hospital staff, including the third-party payers who hold the purse strings, will never witness the "payoff." This dilemma makes outcome assessment an issue of critical importance to PSV providers, not only in medical rehabilitation but also in most programs that provide services to people with disabilities.

Screening and Adjudication

Evaluations help determine whether individuals should be screened in or out of programs or jobs, or judged eligible or ineligible for certain kinds of benefits. In these contexts, evaluators and evaluees often are working at cross purposes: evaluees want in, and evaluators are responsible for screening out all but the clearly suited or eligible. As a result, numerous problems, pitfalls, and legal-ethical issues arise. These types of evaluations carry enormous social responsibility for evaluators because the outcomes have critical influence on the lives of evaluees; for example, whether they are hired, permitted to attend college, granted social insurance/welfare allowing them to live outside of institutions, or assigned to public guardians who will control their finances.

For people with disabilities, two particularly significant screening areas involve eligibility for services from the public vocational rehabilitation program and eligibility for Social Security benefits. Hurdles in front of the former program have been lowered significantly, whereas breaking into the latter system is still a major challenge for many applicants.

Historically, the public vocational program required evidence to prove that individuals had a disability that affected their ability to work and that they also had the potential to benefit from services before deeming them eligible. Formal testing was often used by counselors in order to arrive at a determination of eligibility. A fabled (but true) story recounts the experiences of Ed Roberts, a man with quadriplegia from polio, who was refused services because he was thought to be unemployable. A few years later, he was appointed by the governor of California to head the agency that had denied him services. The 1992 Amendments to the Rehabilitation Act mandated that services be provided to the most severely disabled applicants and that their potential to profit from services be assumed to be present. This directive shifted the burden of proof from documenting that the applicant was eligible to the reverse. In many cases, this shift eliminated the need for PSV testing. Vocational rehabilitation still is not an entitlement program, so individuals must qualify for services, but the process is less stringent than before.

The Supplemental Security Disability Income (SSDI) program, on the other hand, involves a challenging application process with strict requirements. Many people are rejected upon first application, and many of them are rejected again upon appeal. I (the first author) had personal experience with this process, having seen my capacity for work gradually reduced from 10 hours a day to less than 2. I am appalled by the fact that at every level applicants are greeted with the assumption that they are not really disabled and they are out to defraud the government. I was treated shabbily, as are many others, and a person doesn't need that kind of stress at the point of realizing that you just can't keep up any longer.

Research

Research efforts in service delivery contexts provide direct benefits to scientists and service providers and indirect benefits to rehabilitation service consumers. We have cited a number of such studies elsewhere in this chapter. Program evaluation, demonstration projects, and other research pursuits—basic and applied—can require extensive assessment of personal variables to discover or document relationships between antecedent conditions and outcome variables. At times, the evaluative data do double duty, serving to guide clinical decision making as well as provide a basis for scientific prediction. At other times, research is the only purpose, and the subject benefits only when findings are translated into program improvements and enhanced techniques of service. In actuality, it is later generations of clients who most likely will be the beneficiaries.

Certain ethical issues arise when data are gathered solely, or even partially, for research purposes. The subjects must give consent to provide research data that will not directly benefit them, and they must be informed of the general purposes of the research project. When, in order to protect the soundness of the research design, full disclosure is withheld until after a project is completed, subjects must know and agree to this. Any research conducted within an institution or funded with grant monies must be scrutinized by an institutional review board (IRB), a mechanism that serves to clarify the responsibilities of researchers and helps to ensure that the rights of participants are protected.

Maximizing the Benefits of Assessment

When assessment accomplishes its ultimate purposes, individuals understand themselves more fully, providers are able to offer better services and support more appropriate choices, and people reach more satisfying outcomes. Sometimes the process falls short of these aspirations for unavoidable reasons, such as imperfect measuring tools. Other times, potentially avoidable problems sabotage the effort. Some of the most common unnecessary hazards include: (a) failure to sufficiently involve the person with a disability in the assessment process; (b) use of tests that are inappropriate in terms of content or normative date; (c) misusing or avoiding accommodations; and (d) failing to account for cultural issues in selecting and interpreting assessment tools.

Customer Involvement

As we have noted, assessment has the potential to either be therapeutic or to be threatening and unwelcome, and the value of the findings that result from the process are likely to be significantly affected by the client's perspective. The therapeutic value of assessment is enhanced when collaborative approaches are used at the beginning of an assessment process to engage and motivate the individual to put forth his or her best efforts. At the least, this should include an explanation of the need for evaluation and the ways in which it may be of value to the individual. When possible, he or she should also be a participant in selecting the approach to assessment.

Customer involvement is equally crucial at the other end of the assessment process, when the findings become available. As has been pointed out in many contexts, information is power. Whoever possesses the pertinent information also possesses the power advantage of being equipped to make critical decisions. This is poignantly true with respect to evaluative information. As long as the professionals possess, control, and guard the information yielded by evaluation procedures, they are in more favorable positions than clients to make decisions about clients' lives. The solution is simple: give the information to the evaluees. A way of doing this will be described briefly in the hope that some readers may find it worthy of trying.

This model is borrowed from a practice used by Milton Hahn in his career-counseling work with high-level executives. In a personal communication with the senior author, he indicated that he prepared a "know thyself" manual for every client, which contained all test protocols and profiles, and summaries of all interpretations and recommendations made to the client during consultation. He commented:

> You have to give clients like these a tangible product of what you've done for them. After all, they've paid you a handsome fee for a job of work [sic] and they expect something to show—literally—for it. They are highly competent people who don't turn their lives over to anyone else, even temporarily. You're just another consultant with the kind of expertise they need at that point to make their own decisions. Those decisions go on after counseling, and the manual can help in making them.

Knowing the different population the author worked with, he added wryly:

> It's a shame we don't treat welfare recipients with the same respect these executives force us to show them. Your clients need to be taught how to be as much in charge of their lives—and their own information—as my executives are.

From this remonstrance, a variation was developed for use by rehabilitation facilities that offer staged evaluation, work adjustment, and job placement programs. Ordinarily, work evaluators report their findings to the work adjustment staff, not the evaluees; and the work adjustment staff reports to the placement staff at the next transition. The professionals conscientiously transfer information from one to another while the customers wait, passively and powerlessly, for selected bits to be shared with them. It was decided that this situation would be changed by beginning a "know thyself" manual for each person at the outset of the process. Then they would be in charge of taking their own information folios to the next type of expert to be seen and would command the information sharing. (Everyone loses things sometimes, so file copies would be kept). Customers would be privy to all evaluative information about themselves; they would be in a position to query the experts about unclear or conflicting findings; they would feel far less than helpless pawns in a game with undeclared rules; and they would be better prepared to serve as their own case managers, a lifelong responsibility that will fall to them after leaving the facility.

In short, the advantages of designating customers as the prime repositors of their own evaluative information are considerable. At the end of services, they would have a software product, their "know thyself" manuals, to take with them and use after being trained to do so. Another power-related issue involves evaluees' fearing evaluation because the resultant labels might stigmatize them. Labels do have immense power to affect attitudes toward oneself and others; however, their value as shortcuts to understanding can be used, and the distressing aspects avoided, simply by conferring common-sense, neutral terms instead of diagnostic categories that sound clinical and frightening. The public does not resist labeling per se, as the prevalence of "Are you a Virgo? I'm a Leo!" attests. Clinicians can use people's attraction to labeling constructively, toward enhancing self-understanding, if they apply only terms that accentuate the positive. For example, Skip Heck, a psychologist specializing in problems of loneliness, assigns clients palatable "diagnoses" based partly on Native American typologies, which they use in the process of self-discovery. He points out, in a personal communication, that:

> To be called an "obsessional neurotic" is insulting, but to be called a "visual mouse" can entice you to find out more about what kind of a person you are. Neither term has any meaning to the uninitiated, but the more you know about what is meant by "obsessional neurotic," the less you want to be called one—because only pathology is mentioned. The more you learn about what it is to be a "visual mouse," however, the more you see both the positive and negative features of intense attraction to minute detail, and can intelligently sort what you want to expunge from what you want to keep. When the positive side is highlighted as well as the negative, you don't have to get defensive to keep from feeling like a fool.

Test Selection and Accommodations

In order to maximize the value of assessment, tests must be selected that are appropriate to the individual customer and to the population that he or she represents. In some cases, a disability precludes the use of certain tests altogether. At the extreme, a blind person cannot respond to Rorschach cards, nor can a person with paralyzed arms respond to the Purdue Pegboard. In these cases, the exclusion is unequivocal. More subtly, it is necessary to recognize that certain tests may be inappropriate because the inferences that may be generated from test results presume a set of experiences that do not apply to people with varied disabling conditions. We have already mentioned the fact that some psychological tests include items that suggest emotional pathology when, in fact, responses may reflect realistic physical symptoms of a disability (Heinrich & Tate, 1996). Another important example involves assessment of people who are deaf. Olkin (1999), citing many studies that show problems in using ability testing with deaf people, concluded that "the clinician is generally safer in assuming that a test will be invalid with this population" (p. 213).

In situations where assessment is potentially appropriate, however, the manner of testing may still be discriminatory unless adjustments are made in the manner of administration. Section 504 of the 1973 Rehabilitation Act mandated nondiscrimination in activities funded by the federal government, and the ADA extended that prohibition to the private sector. The legislation calls for reasonable accommodations for disability, including "appropriate adjustment or modification of examinations." Employment criteria that tend to screen out people with disabilities are prohibited unless they have been demonstrated to be job-related and no other alternative measure exist that would be less discriminatory. The purpose is to open doors to people who could do a job if they had reasonable accommodations. The guidelines to the EEOC regulations specify that tests may not be given in formats that require the use of an impaired skill unless it is job-related and that skill is intentionally being measured.

In 1985 the *Standards for Educational and Psychological Testing* (American Educational Research Association, American Psychological Association, and National Council on Measurement in Education) first included a chapter on "Testing People Who Have Handicapping Conditions" (1993). It encouraged the development of tests for people with disabilities, and it also urged caution when interpreting tests that had been given under modified conditions.

Nester (1993) describes three kinds of testing accommodations that are mentioned as appropriate in the EEOC's regulations for Title I of the ADA: changes in the testing medium, extending time limits, and altering the content of the test. For tests that are printed in English, presenting the questions in Braille, audiotape, large print, or through a reader would all be examples of changes in format. Graphic material presents particular challenges in these cases, as does extended verbal material that must be held in memory prior to responding. Nester also points out that translating a test into sign language is not just a change in format, but actually involves a change in language. If the examiner can sign, the problems are reduced, but the effect of translating is still unknown. The presence of an interpreter introduces yet another unmeasurable difference from standard procedure.

The third-party effect also must be considered when evaluees must speak, in order to have another person record, answers that usually are written. In personality testing, one may say no more than "true" or "false"; however, when that reflects an emotionally charged confession, there may be less tendency to speak it to another than to record it on paper when working alone. In ability testing, an examiner is more likely to give extra clues to the test-taker under these circumstances, leading to an elevated score. On the other hand, anxiety about "performing" for a listener could operate to lower scores. In short, nonstandard forces are tugging on the scores, and their ultimate direction of movement is unknown.

Extending the time limits for a test, which is usually necessary in accommodated testing (Nester, 1993), raises questions about how the results can be interpreted. Most tests of intelligence, aptitude, and achievement are timed although a few are untimed ("power") tests. Studies by the U.S. Office of Personnel Management have found that people with visual impairments required at least twice as much time to respond to questions involving short paragraphs or mathematical problems when they were presented in any alternative format (Nester & Colberg, 1984). Clearly, changing the format alone would not be a sufficient accommodation without also changing the time available. The problem is sometimes handled by administering a test in both ways; that is, the number of items completed by the time limit is recorded, but the examinee is allowed to continue for an additional number of minutes, until either the test is completed or he or she appears to be making no correct responses. Thus, both "time" and "power" scores are obtained, and the examiner estimates from the difference what an accurate score might be. A highly subjective method at best, it may be more useful than a single score that almost certainly is spuriously depressed. Empirical studies to establish the reliability and validity of tests that have been given under altered conditions are rare because they are possible only when large samples of test-takers can be found.

The issue of appropriate norms also arises with respect to ability testing, because it has been observed that rehabilitation client populations tend to score lower on aptitude tests than other indicators would predict. From time to time, clinical settings attempt to create "local norms" to compare their disabled clients with other disabled individuals on such tests. However, since aptitude tests are used largely to guide people in the competitive world of work, it is well that most such projects never come to fruition. In this case, it is more useful to know how one scores against actual competitors—most of whom will be nondisabled—than to enjoy more favorable comparisons with peers who also might be at a competitive disadvantage.

Circumstances of Testing

The attempted use of standardized tests too soon after catastrophic disablement may result in bizarre and meaningless patterns reflecting only the acute state of turmoil the individual is in. The disabled psychologist quoted several times in Part I describes, from personal experience, what can happen later in the adjustment process:

> A few months after I was up in a wheelchair, the high-school psychologist gave me a battery of tests for vocational guidance. The personality tests looked as normal as apple pie because I desperately wanted to impress everyone with how well I was handling things. I "faked good" without even being conscious of it . . . sort of "Oh, that's the healthy response, that's gotta be me," and I knew better than to "bite" on the faking-detector questions. My IQ, however, unaccountably dropped about twenty points from my ninth-grade scores (which I wasn't supposed to know). Since the psychologist didn't have those tests for comparison, and my score was still good college material stuff, he figured I was in fine shape. However, my personality test scores reflected my intelligence, and my IQ score showed how depressed I was.

Even after a disabled person has stabilized emotionally, certain personality-test findings may have altered significance. An example comes from the Minnesota Multiphasic Personality Inventory (MMPI), where physical symptom responses scored on the Hysteria (Hy) and Hypochondriasis (Hs) scales do not take into account the fact that people with certain disabilities report many critical symptoms for physiologic, not neurotic, reasons. Thus, scores on these two scales may be spuriously elevated. The problem relates to the appropriateness of the normative comparison sample. To get a more accurate appraisal of hysterical or hypochondriacal tendencies in, say, paraplegics, one would need to compare their responses with those of other paraplegics.

Cultural Issues

Any discussion of assessment issues for people with disabilities would be incomplete without acknowledging that multicultural issues are also crucial in selecting approaches and interpreting findings. Cultural awareness and understanding are essential to avoiding unintentional bias. For example, a client's willingness to comply with the assessment process may be compromised by the impersonal, task-oriented style that is typical of European-American evaluation (Dana, 2000). Dana described a multicultural assessment-intervention model that demonstrates how cultural issues affect each step of the evaluation process and how bias can be corrected. He notes that people from racial and ethnic minorities relate to the dominant culture along a continuum that ranges from assimilated at one end to bicultural, marginal, transitional and traditional at the other end. The farther the individual is from full assimilation, the more crucial it becomes that the appropriateness of standardized tests and typical procedures not be assumed to be satisfactory. Tests that measure universal characteristics across cultures may be possible in the future. In the meantime, we have generally used Anglo-American tests as a standard.

Dana (2000) specifies a number of parameters that can promote competence in multicultural assessment of people with disabilities. First, he recommends adoption of Malgady's (1996) mandate to reverse the usual null hypothesis of no cultural bias to instead operate from the assumption that cultural bias does exist throughout the evaluation process. Evaluators need to recognize that disability is, in part, a cultural construction and that different cultures construe it in different ways. Evaluators need to routinely provide accommodations in interviewing and test format to account for the individual's degree of acculturation. The professional's service-delivery style (for example pace and emotional tone) will convey a sense of being understood that will affect the person's motivation to become engaged and to perform as well as possible. Assessment should be done in the individual's preferred language. If that is not possible, the results must be interpreted with extreme caution.

I (the second author) was called upon to do a neuropsychological evaluation of a visiting professor from China who had been involved in a motor vehicle accident. Working with an interpreter, and using tests that had questionable relevance to his culture and no appropriate norms, I made some very circumspect attempts to provide information about his functioning to the rehabilitation team. My goal was to ferret out as much information as possible about capacities that could be utilized in treatment. I drew no conclusions about areas of dysfunction since there was no way to tell whether limitations were the result of his impairments or of the evaluation procedure. This was strictly a strength-oriented assessment.

Working with Americans from multicultural backgrounds, it is not always so obvious that assessment must be tailored to their situation. Nevertheless, evaluating each person's degree of acculturation can lead to interventions that are more likely to succeed (Dana, 2000).

Unbiased Interpretations

A further potential problem area shared by all disciplines in their evaluative functions is that of individual practitioner distortions in drawing conclusions from assessment data. The sources are basically two: theoretical bias and unresolved personal problems. To illustrate the first, the Freudian may see sexual concerns, or the Adlerian, power striving, where others would not. To illustrate the second, the practitioner with strong unmet needs in a given area may overstress or avoid that area in evaluating clients. The first source may be the more difficult to deal with, since one person's bias may be another's ultimate truth, and no court exists to prove one of them right. The latter may be correctable, given a practitioner who is open to nondefensive self-examination and, perhaps, a supervisor who is sensitive to the issues and skilled in helping subordinates recognize and correct such problems.

Somewhat akin to evaluative biases is the tendency to prolong the evaluation phase because of professional insecurity about initiating and conducting treatment. Interminable evaluation can be used as a stalling device and is very common among neophyte practicum students and interns. The stall is "covered" by a belief that additional information will make the existing data fall into place, make sense, and provide clear treatment direction. The magical thinking in this usually is obvious to everyone but the uncertain soul caught in the process.

A final bias, also of a behavioral rather than perceptual sort, should be mentioned. Many PSV professionals choose their lives' work partly out of fascination with the intricate interworkings of human nature. Thus, in evaluating, and especially in the interview situation, there is a tendency to gather personal information far afield from what is needed for the treatment program at hand, simply because it is of clinical or scientific (hopefully not prurient) interest. A subtle matter not yet a frequent target of civil rights concern, it may be in the future, as consumer sophistication increases about what information is really needed to plan, say, a vocational rehabilitation program. Civil rights attorneys consider it an invasion of privacy, and psychologists regard it as a counterproductive form of voyeurism that diverts attention from critical issues and wastes client and professional time. Although attended to regularly in psychologists' and social workers' training programs, the problem exists among rehabilitation counselors, too. Thus, this discipline also may need to focus on minimizing it during preservice training.

The use of evaluative procedures as integral parts of treatment serves as a fitting transition to the following chapters. In them, we will begin to examine the ways in which people work with peers and professionals to strengthen their skills and resources for staying healthy—psychologically, socially, and vocationally—despite the "slings and arrows" that may accompany disablement.

11

Psychogogic Approaches

Once a rehabilitation client has been evaluated with respect to psychosocial vocational functioning, the next step is to select the appropriate training, treatment, or other PSV interventions that will aid the adjustment process and enhance rehabilitation success. This and the following two chapters will be devoted to surveying some of the issues and techniques considered most important. Although there are countless ways to categorize the welter of techniques currently in use, a simple dichotomy between psychogogic and psychotherapeutic approaches seems most appropriate, especially to reemphasize the point that the psychology of disability is largely the psychology of ordinary people responding normatively to abnormal stimulus situations.

In case the term "psychogogy" is not familiar to all readers, it is a word coined by Abraham Maslow (1965) to denote psychosocial intervention strategies based on an educational, not a medical, model. The suffix "-gogy" denotes teaching, or leading, as in the more familiar "pedagogy." He developed the construct in contradistinction to "psychotherapy," where "-therapy" denotes serving in a curative role. The crux of the distinction can be stated as prevention versus cure. Psychogogic approaches strive to strengthen the individual against the onslaughts of stress, in order to avoid or prevent mental/ emotional/behavioral disorder. On the other hand, psychotherapeutic approaches strive to redress or correct disorders that have come about already.

This distinction, like much of Maslow's theoretical work, was influenced by extensive study of Eastern psychology, philosophy, and religious thought. Maslow, like Carl Jung, was responsible for transporting a treasury of ancient Eastern concepts to spark "new" ways of thinking in the West. The report that in ancient China a physician was paid to keep the "patient" well, and that payment ceased if illness occurred since he obviously hadn't done his job, is cited frequently by people disenchanted with modern Western medical care, or angry about iatrogenic illnesses induced by curative attempts that backfire. Western health care has developed primarily as a corrective mode, with preventive medicine a tiny subspecialty still practiced en masse (for example, through public health agencies) far more than with individuals who go to see their doctors.

Maslow's infusion of the preventive orientation into Western psychological intervention carried with it two important implications. First, the "patient" has a great deal of responsibility for active follow-through on what the physician teaches and, conversely, the physician does not so much administer treatment as inform and guide. Second, integral to these Eastern philosophical underpinnings of health care is a holistic conception of human nature that emphasizes the spiritual as much as, if not more than, the bodily and mental components. This contrasts with Western body-mind dualism that either denies spirituality or relegates it to an aspect of mind. Historically, Western psychotherapeutic techniques grew out of this dualistic conception of human nature.

Some general distinctions also can be made between the kinds of clients and practitioners most commonly associated with the two approaches. In the main, clients who receive psychogogic services are psychologically well individuals with severe enough situational problems to need help. Those who receive psychotherapeutic services are experiencing psychological symptoms severe enough to motivate them (or someone else) to seek cure of the symptoms and (it is hoped) their underlying causes. Accordingly, the specialties of practitioners serving the two groups vary somewhat. Counseling and rehabilitation psychologists, rehabilitation counselors, and other counseling specialists provide mainly psychogogic services. Psychiatrists and psychiatric social workers provide mainly psychotherapeutic services. Clinical psychologists and medical social workers may provide either or both, depending on work settings and personal predilections. A summary of these distinctions is presented in Table 11.1.

It is important to bear in mind that no absolute demarcations exist. As the advantages of holism, attention to spirit, an educative orientation, and patient/client responsibility become recognized as important to cure as well as prevention, psychogogic styles are being adopted by psychotherapists. At the same time, such corrective techniques as behavior modification are taking important places in service to people who are not psychologically ill but who have habitual response patterns that interfere with their lives. Despite the overlap, the distinction may help clarify some of the conceptual polarities involved in PSV service techniques.

This chapter focuses on approaches that are predominantly psychogogic, i.e., the techniques most likely to be appropriate for people with bodily disabilities that create difficult situational adjustment demands and problems. We will look at ways in which traditional counseling specialties are, or can be, applied. We also will examine an array of special techniques: those drawing from the transcendent arts; such Eastern techniques as the martial

TABLE 11.1 Comparison of Educationally and Therapeutically Oriented Counseling Services

Orientation	
Psychogogy	Psychotherapy
Educational Model	Medical Model
Prevent	Cure
Teach	Treat
Strengthen	Correct
Inform and guide	Administer to
Strong Eastern influence	Strong Western influence
Holistic	Dualistic
Stress client/customer responsibility	Stress physician responsibility
Psychologically well clientele	Psychologically unwell clientele
Practitioners	
Counseling and rehabilitation psychologists	Psychiatrists
Rehabilitation counselors	Psychiatric social workers
Other counseling specialists	
Clinical psychologists	Clinical psychologists
Medical social workers	Medical social workers

arts, yoga, and meditation; and bodywork techniques that seem particularly suitable for a disabled clientele. Finally, we will examine the blending of all of these into rehabilitation-related PSV approaches.

The chapter immediately following will continue to examine psychogogic techniques, but as they are applied by peer, rather than professional, providers. Then, Chapter 13 will discuss psychotherapeutic approaches oriented toward people whose primary disabilities are characterized as mental, emotional, or behavioral, or who have developed serious mental-health problems secondary to bodily disablement.

Traditional, Mainstream Counseling Specialties

For many years there has been a debate about how to best offer counseling and other services to people with disabilities. Special programs have grown because people's needs were not being met in mainstream programs. Professionals were sometimes blithely unaware of these populations or else imagined that they could not work with them because they were not rehabilitation experts. Many counseling offices, substance abuse treatment programs, and the like were architecturally inaccessible, creating the illusion among mainstream providers that potential clients with disabilities were scarce to nonexistent. The disability rights movement and the legislation of the 1990s have all supported a shift toward providing services in integrated community settings rather than in segregated programs. As an example, the Workforce Investment Act of 1998 was designed to create a "no wrong door" access that will help any person, with or without a disability, who is seeking employment. The Olmstead decision, offered by the Supreme Court in 1999, required states to provide community living services in the least restrictive environment. It may also call into question the use of segregated services in other areas, such as employment (Kiernan, 2000).

Transition is underway, although the old biases linger among providers and create serious gaps in mental health services for disabled people. Nonetheless, generic services often may be the most appropriate resources for disabled people, particularly if the counseling need is unrelated or only tangentially related to the disability. Although it seems obvious, this likelihood apparently needs to be stressed: disabled people do experience problems in psychosocial and vocational areas that have little to do with their disabilities. Consequently, mainstream counselors only need to be prepared to take a disability in stride and not let it become an artificial focus in their counseling efforts. Olkin (1999) provides an excellent introduction for psychotherapists who need to better understand their occasional clients with disabilities. She lays out the issues, particularly those that stem from environmental and social barriers, that affect the lives of people with disabilities and influence their psychological adjustment. As more counselors and therapists become familiar with these issues, mainstream services will become increasingly useful.

Assuming disabled clients can gain access to them, four basic counseling traditions can be identified: (1) educational/vocational counseling; (2) personal or psychological counseling; (3) social casework; and (4) marriage, family, and child counseling. Although some social workers might object to having casework labeled a counseling approach, it is included here for completeness in surveying traditional psychogogic approaches. As noted earlier, some social casework would be grouped with psychotherapeutic techniques under this two-way classification.

Educational/Vocational Counseling

This is the one type of counseling that a large number of people from the general population have experienced. Most people who attend school into the secondary level have at least a passing acquaintance with a school coun-selor who helps students choose elective courses in line with future goals, such as college versus trade school or immediate employment. This function usually is called "advisement" rather than "counseling." Because school budgets typically allow for a very small number of counselors to help a very large number of students, the service seldom is recalled with much appreciation. Often, course advisement is all there is time for, and even that is likely to be "mass produced" and mechanical. When genuine counseling and guidance are available, students may get testing, interpretation, and useful consultation on future educational and career choices.

It would be hard to say whether school counseling for disabled students is worse or better than for others. In general, this society has not valued the function enough to provide funding for it. Disabled students probably get a bit more than others, but they need much more because of disability-related career barriers. Schools, both segregated and mainstream, usually have liaison arrangements with the local office of their state-federal vocational rehabilitation (VR) program, whereas no comparable counseling resource is available to nondisabled students. In recent years, "transition services" have become a priority for many schools and rehabilitation agencies. The Individuals With Disabilities in Education Act (IDEA) requires that students with disabilities and their families participate in the development of an individualized educa-tion plan, which specifies services that will be provided to the student, along with a plan for the transition from school to the broader community. Planning for transition needs to begin by the time of junior high school or earlier, not when the student is about to graduate or drop out of school. This allows for more deliberate and useful consideration of alternatives.

The higher you go in school, the richer the counseling and guidance offerings become. Most colleges and universities have counseling centers for their students, offering personal as well as career counseling. Some have more extensive counseling resources for disabled than nondisabled students because stronger funding pressures have been brought to bear. Resource centers for students with disabilities are common. Besides providing counsel-ing services, they facilitate provision of reasonable classroom accommoda-tions to students who need them. They consult with faculty and often advocate on behalf of students. Liaison with the state VR program usually exists. They also may be linked with on-campus consumer organizations devoted to mutual help, advocacy, and related missions (discussed further in Chapter 12).

Personal or Psychological Counseling

College counseling center staff members observe that many students seek educational/vocational counseling when it is actually personal counseling or psychotherapy they need or want. The former simply offers a less threatening entry into the personal-help service system. Such services are likely to be available in either the counseling center or the student health service; thus, college students enjoy better-than-average access to personal counseling. Few practitioners are available in the private sector because few insurance carriers are willing to pay for preventive (construed as nonessential) services. Individuals generally share this reluctance or simply are unable to pay for them. Because of the strong link between disability and poverty, only a few disabled people can afford the hourly rates asked.

Forward-looking employers sometimes have personal counselors on staff or contract to work with employees whose personal problems seem to interfere with work productivity. Also, a number of churches offer pastoral counseling for members, and community counseling centers and free clinics (usually sponsored by local government and/or a charitable fund) exist in some areas. Most often, personal counseling is available to people involved in some other service system (for example, school, work, or social agency) when the need becomes manifest. Still, even when services are available, people often are reluctant to admit they need help, seeing such as a sign of "weakness." As will be seen later, transforming/repackaging similar processes and relabeling them "personal growth" has removed this barrier for many people. Further, Americans have come to have increasingly high expectations for the degree of happiness that they deserve to have in their lives, and this may have led to greater willingness to accept counseling. An interesting new reflection of this trend is the proliferation of people who are earning their living as "life coaches." They may or may not have specialized training in psychology or another helping field. They aim to help people live more effective and satisfying lives through heightened motivation, organization, and self-discipline, so their services clearly fit into the realm of psychogogy. Their clients tend to be high-achieving people with complex lives who are seeking to maximize their level of functioning.

Sexual counseling is a particularly important aspect of personal counseling for a disabled clientele, for all of the reasons cited in Chapter 5. It is rare, however, for staff in mainstream counseling centers to have the specialized knowledge required to distinguish disability-related dysfunctions from those with psychogenic origins; thus, they are not well prepared to determine when sexual counseling is all that is needed, or when a more intensive, psychotherapeutic approach should be taken. Ordinarily, it is the authors' impression that a psychological practitioner who is good with people in general also is good with people who happen to have disabilities. Part of why they are good is their ability to take a host of human differences in stride, and disability is just one of many they will confront. It is only because of the rather esoteric neurophysiological information base that may be involved that sexual counseling presents a few problems. Most physically disabled clients can tell a psychological counselor all he or she needs to know about the disability; but in the emotionally-charged sexual area, the counselor may not really know or may "scapegoat" the disability. The counselor may not recognize this unless he or she seeks out "instant training" on the relationships between sexual functioning and (a given client's) specific disease process or injury residuals. If he or she is wise enough to know to do this, and willing to make the effort, a mainstream counselor can do sexual counseling with disabled clients as well as anyone else.

Some years ago, Annon (1976) proposed the acronym PLISSIT to distinguish between four levels of involvement in the provision of sexual counseling. The most basic level, P, stands for permission. Every counselor, and for that matter every person who is in a helping relationship with people who have disabilities, should be comfortable conveying permission to have sexual interests and concerns. They should be able to respond to comments or questions without embarrassment or confusion. If their level of knowledge and the boundaries of their job allow them to do so, they may go on to provide some counseling. Otherwise, they may listen respectfully and provide a referral to someone who is in a better position to help. The second level, LI, stands for limited information. Here, helpers may offer some targeted information from their store of knowledge or may offer books, films, or other resources that could be useful to the person with concerns. At the next level, SS, helpers would need to be skilled enough to take on responsibility for offering "specific suggestions" that may help to resolve the concerns. In doing so, they would need to take a sexual history so they would understand the issues and the measures that had already been taken to try to resolve them. They would also need to understand a range of treatment options in order to suggest strategies that would have the best likelihood of success. Finally, the IT (intensive therapy) level is reserved for counselors and therapists who have high levels of skill and training in sexual therapy.

The PLISSIT system seems particularly useful in that it provides a place for every counselor to engage at an appropriate level in meeting needs for sexual counseling. At the same time, it sanctions referral to more specially trained helpers as soon as the counselor feels a need, whether because of skill limitations or because sexual counseling falls outside of his or her job responsibilities.

Social Casework

Social workers operating in a psychogogic mode may use a style of service that is little different from the counseling offered by psychologists and other counseling specialists. It seems that the nature of the client's problems and the personality or temperament of the service provider have more to do with what actually takes place in the counseling room—and its effectiveness—than theoretical orientation or training background. Nonetheless, such experience does influence style, and the caseworker may be more prone to deal with the client as part of a larger social system—taking into account socioeconomic and related factors—than the psychologist-counselor. The latter is more apt to use methods evolving from psychological research, such as behavior modification or biofeedback. The social worker also is less likely to be found in employment settings, but more likely to serve in community counseling centers and free clinics.

Virtually the same barriers to utilization exist as were cited earlier regarding personal counseling. These barriers seem to be reduced, however, when a child, rather than an adult, shows evidence of psychological service need especially when pressure from school authorities is applied. When the disturbance is attributed to family relationships, a fourth variety of counseling may be sought.

Marriage, Family, and Child Counseling

Marriage and family therapy (MFT) is a distinct mental health field that addresses problems within the context of couples and family systems. Their practitioners believe that psychological treatment needs to address the relationships in which a person is embedded, not just the individual alone. Their national organization, the American Association for Marriage and Family Therapy (AAMFT) (http://www.aamft.org), describes their approach as brief, solution-focused, and specific, with attainable therapeutic goals. The same Web site claims that research indicates that this approach is more effective than standard and/or individual treatment for a variety of conditions including chronic physical illness in adults and children. Since the research is not specifically cited, it is not possible to evaluate the claim. Nevertheless, the field has grown, with a 50-fold increase in the number of marriage and family therapists since 1970 (AAMFT, 2002). Practitioners have graduate training at the master's or doctoral level and are licensed in most states.

Perhaps the most significant stimulus to the development of MFT as a distinct discipline is growing societal concern over the threatened dissolution of the American family. Because few pressures can wreck the homeostatic balance and psychological well-being of a family more effectively than disability (Jackson & Haverkamp, 1991; Rolland, 1994, 1999), these three interrelated areas of counseling are supremely important to disabled people and their loved ones. Medical family therapy has been described as a biopsychosocial model that can be helpful for families that include a member with disability or chronic illness (Doherty, McDaniel, & Hepworth, 1994). The authors believe that the field of family therapy has defined itself too narrowly as a mental health field, and that a more holistic model could help families achieve greater feelings of agency and communion. A particularly outstanding example of psychogogically-oriented family services is evident in the work of Through the Looking Glass (Kirshbaum, 1995). Their professional staff, most of whom have personal experience with disability, apply a family systems approach that avoids assumptions of pathology. Instead, through support, education, and provision of resources including adaptive equipment, they help parents who have disabilities to cope with the challenges of raising their children.

As indicated in Chapter 4, the disabled individual has a better chance of getting counseling services than his or her affected family members. The person with a disability is likely to have access to personal counseling through the rehabilitation service system (discussed below), but the spouse, parents, or children are just as likely to be excluded or nearly so. Theoretically, such help might be available through the state VR program, if marriage or family problems were construed as impediments to the vocational rehabilitation of the identified client. Practically, however, agency demands for production of rehabilitation plans and successful closures discourage most rehabilitation counselors from offering time-consuming family services (Accordino, 1999; Herbert, 1989), even when domestic problems are known to be sabotaging rehabilitation progress. They are reluctant, too, because they have no more training for it than the other practitioners and far fewer incentives and opportunities to learn by experience.

Awareness of the problem is by no means absent, however. The literature contains many descriptions of services that have been provided to families with disabilities (Feuerstein, 1995; Seligman & Darling, 1997; Singer & Powers, 1993). Nevertheless, research on families and disability is limited (Buck, 1993; Herbert, 1989; Kirshbaum, 1996) and ties between research and service programs are weak (Quittner & DiGirolamo, 1998). Years ago, two counselors in a large state VR agency (Connell & Berkowitz, 1976) proposed and conducted a family-centered program for a severely disabled SSI-recipient population with an extremely low acceptance-for-service rate. They found that by working with the families, instead of solely the disabled individuals, they increased the number of such clients accepted and served by several hundred percent compared with offices not involved in the project.

Figures on rehabilitation outcomes are unavailable because the project was not continued past the originally agreed-upon time period for demonstrating changes in acceptance rate. Longitudinal follow-up and support for more studies of this kind would be of value to the field.

So far, we have focused on the need for family counseling as an adjunct to rehabilitating a disabled family member. However, as stated in Chapter 4, counseling also is needed for the disabled family members themselves, so they do not become "casualties" of another's disability. Kevin (see Chapter 4) described the kinds of interventions he believed would have helped his mother:

> She needed to be *trained* to take care of herself as well as me. She needed *counseling* to eradicate the guilt feelings that led to excessive self-sacrifice. She needed *advocacy*, someone to get across to her that mothers have rights, too; that I wasn't the only one suffering. I didn't have to be protected from the fact that my care was a drag. If she knew that I knew and accepted that, she wouldn't have had to work so hard to pretend it was "no problem" when her ass was dragging, just so I wouldn't feel bad. She also needed a different kind of *counseling for me*, to clarify my supportive responsibility toward her. That would have helped me, too, because my role was all taking and I felt guilty and unworthy. That led me to a very crazy conclusion "I've used up my dependency quota in the physical area; therefore, I must never expect or accept any emotional support." Naturally, no one can live without it, so every time I sopped up a little emotional support from someone, I felt I was stealing. Suffice it to say, counseling could have avoided unnecessary self-sacrifice on her part and a long-lasting neurotic error on mine. [Emphasis added.]

Clearly, all four traditional counseling varieties have much, potentially, to offer disabled people and their families if the barriers can be broken down. The next section will discuss an approach that has lowered one barrier successfully—that of reluctance to admit the need for help.

Human Potential Development

The human potential development movement was a product of the 1960s—a time when psychologically well individuals began to look inward to cope with unease about a future-shocked world taunted by a war with little meaning to them. Esalen, a resort setting in Big Sur, California, became "Mecca," and dozens of similar "growth centers" emerged throughout the country. No admission of psychological or interpersonal incompetence was necessary; participants had only to acknowledge desire to maximize their inner resources and enhance fulfillment in their lives. They flocked to the centers for training experiences designed to do both. Those who labeled it a passing fad note, with satisfaction, that only a few centers still survive, and their popularity has waned. However, the philosophy, the goals, and the methods have by no means disappeared or even abated. They simply have transformed and continuously reemerge in newer forms—often itinerant rather than center-based—and exert enormous influence on traditional psychological and bodily health-care practices.

As indicated in Chapter 8, the disability experience can be a powerful stimulus to developing a coherent philosophy of life that imparts meaning to a source of considerable pain. For this reason, the philosophy of human potential development (HPD) may be uniquely appropriate for people with disabilities; HPD is a wholesome approach because it minimizes the "pathology error," and disabled people often are overwhelmed by confrontations with their own pathology—real or exaggerated. The philosophy of accepting oneself "as is" and growing from there is a helpful counterfoil to previous overemphasis on deficits, limitations, and liabilities, coupled with enjoinders to "try to overcome them." Trying to overcome what you are isn't easy for anyone; it is particularly defeating when part of what you are is permanently disabled. The mass media nevertheless loves stories of how exceptional individuals with severe disabilities manage to accomplish things that they have been told would be utterly impossible. Zola (1991) pointed out that the hidden message behind these stories is that the vast majority of people with disabilities (whose accomplishments involve meeting the mundane challenges of daily living over and over again) can be blamed for personal weakness in failing to "overcome." So whether these perspectives exaggerate limitations or inflate expectations, they fail to convey the genuine acceptance promoted by HPD.

The human potential development movement has been shaped significantly by the importation of philosophy and technique from the Far East. The ancient philosophical, psychological, medical, and religious writings from China and India have had the most notable influence, although Japan and other Asian countries also are represented. Let us look next at some of the specific Eastern approaches that have been adopted in the West, and consider their applicability to a disabled clientele.

Eastern Influences

The martial arts have been familiar in the West for many decades. First jiu jitsu appeared on the Western scene, followed by judo, karate, and now a vast array including tai chi, aikido, and others too numerous to mention.

Sometimes they have shown up in customized training for special-interest groups, sometimes in public parlors. The emphasis generally is placed on self-defense, whether for vulnerable clients such as women, senior citizens, or disabled people, or for strong, young, agile males.

Human potential development (HPD) practitioners have been interested in the additional benefits of martial-arts training—those relating to self-discipline, energy utilization, and the enhancement of physical and psychological well-being. The martial arts require development and integration of bodily, mental, and spiritual energies for correct execution. In short, they are holistic. Individuals who never find it necessary to use their arts for self-defense report sometimes minor, sometimes major improvement in the sense of well-being. Terms such as "centered" and "balanced" convey to others who've shared similar experiences what is meant by their claims. Part of it may result from the vigorous exercise plus improved confidence or reduced feelings of vulnerability. An additional part seems to emanate directly from the processes of learning the necessary self-discipline and methods for synchronizing bodily, mental, and spiritual energies.

Yoga has been familiar in the West perhaps even longer than the martial arts, but to a less diverse audience. (One still sees no yoga parlors interspersed among the fast-food stands as is currently true for karate.) Hatha yoga and mantra yoga are the most commonly taught systems. Hatha yoga focuses on body and breath control. Mantra yoga tends to be referred to in the West as "meditation," and the trademarked Transcendental Meditation (TM) became a widely practiced variant.

Hatha yoga training is fairly widely available: on television, in HPD programs, in university extension courses, exercise gyms, and health spas. A major difference from Western exercise approaches is that stretching, rather than contracting, of muscles is emphasized because the goal is fluidity of motion rather than muscle-mass development or increasing muscle strength. Pranayama (breath control) training is less widely available, generally only within HPD programs. This is unfortunate for people with such severe disabilities that most of the bodily postures of hatha yoga are impossible for them to attain. Breath control exercises, even for people with sharply limited vital capacities, would be a feasible form of yogic practice to use to attain the effects of calming, relaxing, and quieting anxieties. These are the primary purposes and benefits of hatha yoga (Rama, Ballentine, & Ajaya, 1976).

Mantra yoga training is very widely available, at least in the form of TM. It is not only available privately, it sometimes is provided by employers who are convinced it will enhance productivity. It also is available to the clients of some rehabilitation agencies; a few private rehabilitation facilities arrange for such training for their clients, and a few state VR agency counselors have managed to procure such training for theirs. As is true for hatha yoga, the most palpable psychological benefits relate to calming, relaxation, and reduction of anxieties, and it is commonly incorporated into stress management programs. Some individuals also report such sequelae as increased creativity, improved insights about themselves and others, and clearer thinking abilities. Mantra yoga is coming to be suggested or even prescribed by physicians treating people with such conditions as hypertension, in efforts to avoid use of medications with unpleasant or unknown future side effects. Kabat-Zinn (1991) developed a widely-recognized program of mindfulness meditation for pain control and stress reduction at the University of Massachusetts Medical Center.

Trieschmann (1995, 2001), who worked for many years as a traditional rehabilitation psychologist, became disenchanted with the contemporary health care system and its nearly exclusive focus on physical functioning and illness. She pursued intensive study in eastern spiritual practices, especially qi gong, and began to propound an energy model of health and wellness that integrates mind, body, emotions, and soul. She teaches people with disabilities to meditate as a first step toward spiritual practice. Unless the customer initiates discussion of religion, that topic is not raised in counseling. Instead, the combination of meditation and counseling serve to assist the individual toward deepening self-understanding and acceptance.

Complementary and Alternative Health Care

The holistic health-care movement evolved out of the human potential development movement, probably as a result of the involvement of health-care professionals in HPD activities. The two movements merged, with the encompassing goal of fostering total mind-body-spirit health in a self-actualizing person. It is to the totality and inseparability of the mind-body-spirit that the term "holistic" refers. The health of one component cannot be achieved or maintained in the absence of attention to the other two. The Eastern influence is as apparent at this basic philosophical level (the inclusion of spirit along with mind and body) as it is when the actual healthcare techniques are examined. Three aspects of the holistic approach are particularly salient to the PSV rehabilitation of disabled people: (1) the emphasis on self-responsibility, (2) the emphasis on nutrition, and (3) the addition of "body work" to the "talk therapy" tradition in counseling and psychotherapy. Although the validity of the three elements remains undiminished, the term "holistic" has gradually evolved to mean "alternative" health. Perhaps "the H word" came to imply acceptance of ideas and practices that are unacceptable to the scientific community. At the same time, the traditional medical establishment has opened significantly to subjects that previously would have been rejected out of hand. The strongest evidence of this shift has been the establishment of the National Center for Complementary and Alternative Medicine within the National Institutes of Health. This center, while holding to the strict scientific standards of the NIH, is encouraging research on alternative techniques such as manual therapies, herbalism, and mind-body therapies.

After leaving the rehabilitation hospital, many disabled people have been forced to assume more self-responsibility in health care than the average person because so few practitioners in mainstream medical practice know how to deal with disabled individual. For example, a quadriplegic person who finds it necessary to use a community hospital needs to explain her or his personal care needs to all levels of staff as thoroughly as to an inexperienced applicant for a job as a personal-care provider. Unfortunately, not all are prepared to do so, and others have found their efforts to inform health providers to be resented and ignored. Hopefully, the emerging emphasis on self-responsibility will lead to more consistent preparation of disabled people in this respect, and more receptiveness on the parts of health practitioners to being instructed by them.

In 1988 the Office on Disability and Health ODH) of the Centers for Disease Control and Prevention was established to promote the health and quality of life of individuals with disabilities (Thierry, 1998). The office has identified many barriers to health services, especially for women with disabilities, including physical, attitudinal, and policy barriers. Research has shown that many women with disabilities report receiving less routine health care than general populations and even being refused health care because of their disabilities (Nosek, Howland, Rintala, Young, & Chanpong, 2001). A major concern of the ODH is the prevention of secondary conditions in people with disabilities. The recognition of secondary conditions is relatively new and is still frequently misunderstood (Gonzales, 1999). Some common examples include weight gain, pain, depression, fatigue, and problems specific to particular disabilities, such as pressure sores among people with spinal cord injury. Secondary conditions comprise any physical or mental health condition that occurs with increased frequency among people who have a primary disabling condition (Thierry, 1998). They are often preventable, or else they can significantly complicate life with a disability.

Increased concern over the nutritional quality of food consumed is particularly important among people whose disabilities lower their energy reserves and their caloric needs. A severely paralyzed individual, for example, who needs only 1200 calories per day, can less afford to waste any on junk food than a person who needs twice that number to maintain an ideal weight. When energy is depleted by the nature of a disability, or by inordinate effort required to function in spite of it, good nutrition is essential to body-mind-spirit health. A mild case of hypoglycemia might go almost unnoticed by a nondisabled person, yet keep a severely disabled person from making it through the day. The margin of error is too narrow. Few rehabilitation programs give nutrition the emphasis it deserves. Hopefully, the growing social awareness of the relationships between inadequate nutrition and psychological as well as physical symptoms will filter into more rehabilitation programs in the coming decade.

Traditionally, psychogogy and psychotherapy have been limited, virtually, to "talk treatment." Psychiatrists might prescribe drugs or arrange for psychosurgery, but psychologists, counselors, and social workers only talked. The HPD movement brought with it enormously increased interest in exercise and other body work, particularly varieties designed to improve psychological functioning. Intensive efforts to reunite mind and body began and have exerted considerable influence on mainstream psychological services. The reasons for this are diverse. Because of the noted failure of psychological services to "work" for people who are not verbally oriented, it was finally recognized that the "talk treatment" bias emanated from tendencies of people who enter the involved professions to solve their own problems through rational and verbal explorations, but that other, equally valid ways also exist.

During the 1970s and 1980s, specific Eastern techniques incorporating bodywork (such as the martial arts, yoga, and movement meditations), along with the general, working philosophy of mind-body-spirit holism, were being integrated into Western approaches. It was acknowledged that bodywork was not just an alternative for nonverbally oriented people; it was a needed corrective for people who were too verbally oriented and had neglected their bodies, failing to recognize the impact of bodily habits on their psychological well-being. Naturally, the impact of Western medical sorties to China in the early 1970s, and the ensuing reports that acupuncture "works" although no one could explain how in terms of Western physiological conceptions, was also a great contributor to the wakening realization that at least one path to psychological health is through the body. Countless varieties of bodywork now have emerged: Eastern and Western, structured and unstructured, aerobic and anaerobic, active and passive, athletic and aesthetic. Currently, however, most mainstream rehabilitation psychologists avoid approaches that incorporate physical touch because of concerns about the ethical and legal boundaries of their practice and because few have been trained in these areas. Many utilize biofeedback, hypnosis, and guided imagery in addition to talk therapy, but there are virtually no reports in the professional literature of the application of other kinds of bodywork in clinical practice. The falling off may reflect the increasing conservatism within the society as a whole as well as increased pressures to engage only in activities that are likely to be reimbursed by third-party payers. It is entirely possible, however, that people with disabilities may be participating in bodywork activities through other channels such as health clubs, retreat centers, or even community education. Research has indicated that a higher proportion of individuals with physical disabilities used alternative therapies (a general term for health practices that have not gained widespread acceptance by the medical establishment) and consulted providers of those therapies than did a randomized national sample (Krauss, Godfrey, Kirk, & Eisenberg, 1998).

The Influence of the Transcendent Arts

The fields of recreation and psychology are turning virtually every artistic discipline known to humankind into "therapies," most notably, music and the visual, performing, and writing arts. Sometimes they are therapies in the corrective sense used here; at other times they might be classed better as psychogogy. Central purposes in all such approaches are relaxation and renewal; facilitation of self-expression; enhancement of self-understanding; and the improvement of mental focusing, self-esteem, and feelings of psychological well-being. The discovery of substantial creative talent and drive is generally a peripheral concern.

As reflected in the familiar quotation from William Congreve's *The Mourning Bride*, "Music hath charm to soothe a savage breast, to soften rocks, or bend a knotted oak," music therapy is used often with people who need to have intense or pervasive fears quelled but find other relaxation methods threatening. Thus, it is used most widely in psychotherapeutic settings, but it has psychogogic applicability as well. Music therapy usually implies listening, or music appreciation, rather than singing or playing instruments. Accordingly, the latter activities are grouped here with the performing arts.

Traditionally, the visual arts have formed an important basis of occupational therapy activities in both psychiatric and medical rehabilitation settings, with crafts and painting the most commonly employed. When budgeting allows, sculpture and various graphics techniques also may be used. It seems to the authors that sculpture offers greater potential for psychogogic work with blind individuals than has been exploited. Also, life-history murals—a technique created at SAGE, a highly progressive senior citizens' program in Berkeley, California (Luce, 1979)—might be used profitably with people who are coping with life changes imposed by disability, as well as aging.

Among the performing arts approaches, psychodrama now has a long-established history in psychotherapeutic settings. The minidrama techniques associated with Gestalt therapy and transactional analysis, for example, are included here, generically, as psychodrama. They are used fairly widely with psychogogy clients, disabled and nondisabled. An unusual form of psychodrama has clients become the "directors" and professionals do the "acting." Professionals and students are sometimes exposed to role-playing opportunities in which they learn something of what it is like to be disabled. Spending a day or a week blindfolded or using a wheelchair are the most common simulations. These techniques, aim to give nondisabled providers better understanding of the frustrations encountered and the trust that must be developed by people whose disabilities generate and demand them. The disabled participants in such programs may gain greater confidence in the empathy of those who serve them, plus a sense of mastery, of having something important to teach or share. Others have raised sharp criticism of the practice, however, pointing out that simulation does not really replicate the experience of disability, and it may lead participants to exaggerate feelings of frustration and helplessness that they assume people with disabilities must feel (Olkin, 1999; Wright, 1983). Olkin also points out that the focus of simulations is on the physical experience of disability and it largely overlooks the social and environmental barriers that are major components of the experience. Wright urges that any time simulations are used they incorporate effective compensatory strategies and coping techniques so that participants come away with appropriately positive understanding rather than a more distorted view of the disability experience.

Dance and movement therapies are being recognized as part of the disability culture that has emerged in Britain and the United States (Corbett, 1999), and it provides a source of pride and a method of self-identity for people with disabilities. Although the number of dance groups seems, by informal observation, to be growing, virtually no descriptions or studies are yet being reported in the professional literature.

Singing, especially group singing, and playing musical instruments, such as small stringed instruments and recorders, are used occasionally in psychogogic or psychotherapeutic work but have not been developed systematically. This may be more a function of their auditory intrusiveness than lack of psychological service potential. Singing is used sometimes as a means of improving breath control, but it is regarded more often as a physical or inhalation therapy than as a psychological technique. Music has also been used with traumatically brain-injured individuals to help develop functional and social skills (Barker & Brunk, 1991; Gervin, 1991; Knox & Jutai, 1996; Nayak, Wheeler, Shiflett, & Agostinelli, 2000). Mime has been explored as a means of encouraging self-expression among people with mental or speech disabilities, but no systematic programs are known to have been reported. Each of these areas seems worthy of additional investigation, especially singing, because of the apparent relationship between breath control and control of anxieties. Lowered vital capacity and poor breath control are found among people with numerous physical disabilities.

The writing arts have long been used in psychological services, both in the passive (reading) and active (writing) modes. Bibliotherapy is being elevated to a high level of importance in pain-management programs, where well-stocked libraries of self-help books on stress management, meditation techniques, spiritual development, and related subjects are often part of the service offerings for clients and patients learning to manage their own pain. Autobiography writing, for the dual purposes of diagnosis and treatment, has long been recognized for its treatment potential and relevance for psychogogy clients. Poetry writing is a relative newcomer but already has been the object of considerable theoretical development and technical systematization. Information about these techniques is spread through conferences and informal channels, but they are rarely the subject of scientific studies or papers.

All of these techniques based on the transcendent arts should be considered for disabled clienteles because of their potential for supplying new mechanisms for emotional discharge and new sources of reward and pleasure after familiar mechanisms and sources have been lost. These are just two of many special issues PSV practitioners must consider in serving clients with disabilities.

Special Issues in Counseling People With Disabilities

Three clusters of special issues will be discussed here: common problems, common skill-training needs, and the applicability of selected group counseling approaches.

Common Problems

Very early in the recovery process, emotional support is needed to cope with the shock, fear, and anger experienced after what has taken place. People born with disabilities, or acquiring them while still very young, need similar support when they begin to realize that they are disadvantaged, compared with others, by their disablements. The central theme of the support needed in either case is assurance of unimpaired self-worth and hope for a gratifying future. If these assurances are offered by individuals who sincerely believe that disablement in no way reduces a person's human worth or obviates chances for a fulfilling life, it may matter very little how they are delivered. When permanence of disability is known to be likely before the affected individual is ready to acknowledge that, the holding out of false hopes regarding prognosis can be avoided, somewhat, when the assuring messages suggest, "Sure, it's conceivable that you could recover; but whatever the outcome in that regard, your human worth is unchanged and opportunities for fulfillment will be many."

Many disabled people who have attained outstanding success in life say this was the consistent message they got from their loved ones, often nonexplicitly. It was felt, and it was transmitted in one way or another. This has important implications for hospital and other rehabilitation personnel. However disability is viewed, it is likely to be communicated to the individual; thus, more important than learning techniques for providing emotional support is gaining personal perspective so that a sense of tragedy, the belief that irreparable damage to human worth has occurred, or feelings of dread will not be conveyed, because they do not exist.

Somewhat later in the adjustment process, more specific aspects of loss must be dealt with. Three highly significant areas confronted by people with the full range of disabilities are: (1) the loss of emotional discharge mechanisms, (2) the loss of reward or pleasure sources, and (3) the loss of physical and economic independence. These frequently lead to what might be termed "secondary losses" in self-esteem and the sense of meaning, or purpose, in life. They also may lead to such secondary disabling conditions as alcoholism or boredom-induced amotivation syndrome. For example, the loss of emotional discharge mechanisms appears to be a frequent contributing factor to excessive drinking among people with disabilities, a problem that elicits great concern from both peer and professional providers. An individual who has relied on vigorous activity to discharge emotional/physical tensions may resort to dulling their impact with alcohol when such physical "exhaust" methods become impossible.

The supports needed to counteract such maladaptive behavior patterns are practical help and consultation in finding more effective, less debilitating ways of coping, laced liberally with the kind of emotional support described previously. First, information is needed in the form of exposure to other ways of discharging tension, other sources of reward and pleasure, and available opportunities for gaining/regaining economic independence. Second, consultation is needed on how to use the new information, coupled with "supervised practice" opportunities for action and self-expression, followed by accurate feedback on the effectiveness of such efforts in developing constructive insights and responses to altered circumstances. Third, cognitive/attitudinal restructuring is needed to (a) help the person separate real losses from imputed but unnecessary ones; (b) avoid equating physical dependency with total dependency; and (c) understand that temporary confusion does not mean life-long disruption of purposes, meaning, values, and goals.

An achievement-oriented society such as ours stresses goals of accomplishment, and goals of acquisition are associated with materialism. Such biases can be defeating to people with disabilities that limit their potential for success along these dimensions. It is particularly important, therefore, for them to know that other kinds of goals, at least as worthy, also exist and are reachable. Life goals can be grouped roughly into three general categories: goals of doing, goals of getting, and goals of being.

Goals of doing relate to activities, achievements, and accomplishments. The person says, "This is what I want to do in life to achieve or accomplish." He or she might conceive it in terms of an epitaph: "I want it to say I did such and such well." The specific goals might be as common as wanting to do a good job of child rearing or as unusual as wanting to devise a testable theory of the origin of the universe.

Goals of getting relate to acquiring, gathering, and accumulating. The targets of striving may be material or nonmaterial. Material goals range from garnering the barest survival basics of adequate food and shelter to enjoying opulence that requires vast accumulations of wealth. Examples of nonmaterial goals are reputation, prestige, status, power, and fame. They are externals to acquire in that their existence lies in the perceptions of others. The material and nonmaterial aspects of "getting" goals are interdependent; attainment in one aids attainment in the other.

Goals of being related to developing attributes of character, which reside within. Here, the individual says, "I want to be a certain kind of person, one who is (honest, tough, spontaneous, firm, loving, fiery, fair, critical, sensible, reverent, wise, courageous, or countless other valued qualities)." The characteristics sought for may be unrelated to reputation; the individual strives for an inner surety that the prized attributes are being attained.

Most people set goals in each of the three areas—sometimes without realizing it—but concentrate on one or two. To illustrate, individuals who move quickly to the top of the corporate ladder focus heavily on goals of doing and getting. Creative artists who pursue painting or writing despite poverty and ignominy may disdain the executives' goals of getting while sharing with them a deep commitment to goals of doing. Spiritual aspirants and leaders may concentrate mainly on goals of being.

It is important to help people realize that disabilities need not interfere with attaining goals of being. A totally paralyzed person with impaired vision, hearing, and speech could succeed as well in this realm as anyone else. As pointed out in Chapter 8, the disability experience can block this type of goal seeking, but it can catalyze and foster it equally well. In order to facilitate the latter, skill training in the goal-setting process may be required.

Personal and Interpersonal Skill Training

At some point in the course of adjustment, either the disabled person or a rehabilitation consultant may realize that formalized training in specific personal/interpersonal skill areas is needed. Disability creates unusually heavy demands for assertiveness, decision making and goal setting, and life- and family-management skills. Training programs have been developed in each of these areas for the general population, and for disabled people in particular. Assertiveness training is perhaps the best known, but all of the mentioned varieties are offered widely by rehabilitation facilities and individual practitioners.

The subject of enhancing physical attractiveness is rarely addressed in rehabilitation settings. Kammerer-Quayle (2002) explains the omission in a couple of ways, one being the discomfort that many health professionals feel about society's superficial value system, which places such emphasis on appearance. Further, health professionals seldom have the training or skills to advise people who have disfigurement or other visible disabilities. Nevertheless, a strong case can be made regarding the need for programs to enhance physical attractiveness, ranging from basic grooming tips, at the simplest level, to cosmetic surgery, at the far extreme. Variations on the "charm school" theme are a frequent middle ground. This seems to be a hard area to address without tempers flaring. The "pros" indicate improved attractiveness and poise will better a disabled person's chances for success and it is thus irresponsible to ignore the matter. The "cons" want to avoid emphasizing shallow concerns better left unstressed in society at large, as well as any implication that disability makes one less attractive. Conversely, they point out that disabled people could be hurt by being tempted to compete in an attractiveness market where they are predetermined to come out second best.

The "pros" counter that if a person gets a job within a month after attending "attractiveness school," following two years of previous turn-downs, that speaks for itself. By the very fact of providing service, counselors tacitly acknowledge an opinion that clients could profit from behavior change. The controversy over confronting clients with the possibility that changes in grooming behavior or social presentation also might yield rewards seems deeply ingrained in our own insecurities about whether we make the grade as beautiful people. Any issue powerful enough to generate so much discomfort and resistance must be important to deal with in counseling!

People whose disabilities interfere with communication and, therefore, interpersonal relationships have uniquely important skills to learn. First, they must learn to transmit and receive messages as accurately and rapidly as possible. For this, speech therapy or training, sign language and lip reading training, and the use of sensory/communication aids represent three major approaches for people with speech, hearing, and vision disabilities. Beyond such basic assistance, subtler aspects of interpersonal communication must be attended to. For example, nonhearing speakers must learn to use others' facial responses in monitoring their voice modulation. Blind individuals must learn to discern, from auditory cues, all those nuances of interpersonal and group dynamics that others deduce from body language. People with extremely slow or labored speech must learn to capture their listeners' attention and patience and also put them at ease. Actually, speech therapy or training could be construed as an additional psychogogic variety in view of the central use made of psychological principles and counseling methods. The feelings, especially anxieties, of speech therapy clients are as important in their speech training as the physiological difficulties presented. For this reason, relaxation training techniques are being adopted by speech practitioners as quickly as those more typically considered "counselors."

Members of the University of Kansas Research and Training Center on Independent Living have published several relevant accounts, including one in which people with disabilities were taught how to effectively recruit personal care assistants (Balcazar, Fawcett, & Seekins, 1991) and another in which members of an advocacy organization were trained to participate more effectively in action-oriented meetings (Balcazar, Seekins, Fawcett, & Hopkins, 1990; Seekins, Mathews, & Fawcett, 1984). Their outcome measures confirmed the effectiveness of their training, both immediately and upon follow-up several months later.

"Patient education" is another commonly used psychogogic approach in hospital and rehabilitation settings. It grew along with the recognition that poor life-style choices are responsible for much of the illness in our society, and self-responsibility is a critical component in maintaining health. Explanatory leaflets now typically accompany prescription bottles, and individuals are often provided with educational programs on video or in person (individually or in groups) before being discharged from treatment facilities. The effectiveness of patient education has been documented in the management of conditions including asthma (Soondergaard, Davidsen, Kirkeby, Rasmussen, & Hey, 1992), HIV infection (Chaisson, Keruly, McAvinue, Gallant, & Moore, 1996), osteoarthritis (Edworthy & Devins, 1999), ankylosing spondylitis (Barlow & Barefoot, 1996), and diabetes (Brown & Hanis, 1995). In the authors' experience, patient education groups offer distinct advantages in addition to efficiency. Most importantly, they may reach people who resist involvement in counseling, especially when the programs deal with sensitive topics such as sexuality, family issues, substance abuse, or depression.

Group Versus Individual Approaches

Regardless of the type of counseling or skill training involved, the question arises: Can it be done more effectively with individuals or in groups? Group techniques are popular because of their apparent cost effectiveness, but it is important to determine whether sacrifices in quality will be made or whether a group approach will produce equal or enhanced effectiveness.

In the authors' opinion, group approaches are frequently the modality of choice for psychogogic work, for several interrelated reasons. First, by comparison, one of the primary reasons for choosing to work privately with individuals in psychotherapy is that their ability to trust other human beings is often so impaired that it is more feasible to begin rebuilding it with one other person (who is professionally skilled in nurturing trust) than with a group of several people (some of whom may have attacking tendencies). In psychogogy, severely damaged trust is not at issue. Second, both a mechanism and goal of psychogogy with disabled people is augmenting their understanding that they are not alone; others are experiencing similar facts and feelings, others have useful insights they can share, and others can profit from their insights—they are helpful persons as well as persons needing help.

The literature contains a few accounts of group approaches developed specifically for use with disabled clients (Barber, Jenkins, & Jones, 2000; Fow & Rockey, 1995; McDaniel, 1991; Saarijaervi, Rytoekoski, & Alanen, 1991; Salmon & Abell, 1996). One early example is Structured Experiential Therapy in Rehabilitation (SETR) (Lasky, Dell Orto, & Marinelli, 1977). Although labeled a "therapy" by its creators, it is more akin to what is classified here as psychogogy, because of the target clientele and the nature of the problems addressed. Its central theme is the reduction of interpersonal stress between disabled and nondisabled people, especially that arising from disability-related stigmatization.

The structured group format highlights goal orientation, accountability, mutual help, and the development of coping skills. Sessions consistently include about half disabled and half nondisabled members, all of whom are striving toward more effective problem solving, better use of their resources, psychological growth, and satisfactory living. Two coleaders work with eight to ten members and attempt to establish strong group cohesiveness and mutual concern. The job of the members is to identify, explore, evaluate, and act on specific problems. Written contracts are used to facilitate the process, as are such other practical approaches as establishing contact with resource people, organizations, events, and articles. Members are exposed to role models, and the value of incidental learning from each other is stressed. The process is seen as comprising three fairly distinct phases. The first is individualistically oriented and includes goal identification, exploration, and evaluation, with some didactic interventions such as recording behavioral base rates. The second phase is group oriented, utilizing the group cohesion and felt mutual responsibility to help the members attain their goals. This phase also includes feedback from the group to help members assess their levels of goal attainment. The final phase stresses generalization of what has been learned to other (or future) problem areas, consolidation of learning, and recapitulation of learning in follow-up sessions after the group has formally ended. "Booster" sessions can be planned if the members wish.

Individual counseling's greatest value may be its potential for spontaneity. When someone needs help immediately, an ad hoc counseling session can be invaluable, whereas convening a group would be farcical or impossible. Counselors, like therapists and medical practitioners, are in the habit of scheduling standard periods of time for working with clients. It has been done that way for so long that everyone imagines it should be done that way; alteration may even be seen as reflecting faulty professionalism. A more flexible and responsive approach to services should be considered when the setting allows it, however. The concept of dealing with issues while they're "hot" has considerable common-sense appeal. Moreover, demand-responsive service systems, such as crisis intervention hotlines, have proved to be effective in the treatment of drug abuse and suicidal compulsions. In these situations, the inadequacy of a delayed response becomes immediately obvious. In less dramatic situations, the need for immediate reckoning may be just as great, although the consequences, when no help is available, are less public.

Thus, programs that make counselors available as needed, who can respond with alacrity when a client's issue is hot, may be as vital to effectively helping people adjust to disability as in preventing drug recidivism or suicide.

The PSV Melting Pot

Any combination of the psychogogic approaches and techniques discussed so far may be brought together in the highly eclectic field of PSV rehabilitation. Rehabilitation psychologists and counselors must help disabled people deal with the full array of ordinary human problems, as well as the special issues related to disabilities.

Influences of the Rehabilitation Milieu

Regardless of the specific type of rehabilitation setting being considered, the psychological impact of the milieu is of foremost importance. This is not a statement about milieu therapy for people in rehabilitation hospitals (see, for example, Kutner, 1977); it is a statement about the quality of the ordinary social environments in which disabled people find themselves when needing services.

The importance of emotional support has been cited many times already and is appropriately reiterated here. Capacity for emotional supportiveness is not only important for professional staff, it should be a screening variable for every person hired to work in a rehabilitation setting. Clients spend considerable periods of time with secretarial, attendant, and housekeeping personnel, too. An indication of the shift in emphasis and attitude within vocational rehabilitation offices is the use of the term "customer" to identify individuals receiving services. Customers are in a setting by choice, and the staff exists to meet their needs.

One aspect deserving special mention because it is so often underemphasized is the need for massive support when disabilities impair cognitive functioning. For example, patients with traumatic head injuries, strokes, or multiple sclerosis frequently mention that their physical (motor or sensory) losses are less frightening to them than the realization that their mental (intellectual or emotional) abilities are "out of control" to some degree.

The infusion of certain language habits into the rehabilitation milieu is almost as basic as creating an emotionally supportive environment; and they are the same language habits that should be stressed in public education designed to reduce disability stereotyping. Countless discussions and arguments about appropriate language have taken place during the past couple of decades. Words that were acceptable at one time (e.g., crippled or handicapped) have become taboo. Others (e.g., physically challenged) are preferred by some and abhorred by others. The following five provisos, although more relaxed than politically correct, can set the stage for more positive ways of thinking about and reacting to people with disabilities. The earlier a person is exposed to such "cleaned up" language, the less undoing of destructive attitudes will be required later on.

1. Avoid the shorthand terms "the handicapped" and "the disabled." These phrases are prized for their brevity, but they carry the hidden cost of summarizing the individual(s) described as nothing more than one of their many characteristics, one that conjures a negative image in the minds of most. They also may be republicans, democrats, lawyers, homemakers, Catholics, Buddhists, beautiful, homely, or play any number of other roles and possess any number of other traits. All that is lost and forgotten when they are "collapsed" into the sole category of "the handicapped/disabled."

2. Avoid the imprecision of describing a person as "handicapped" when what is meant is "disabled." As pointed out in the introduction to this book, it makes sense to refer to "a disabled person" when that is a consistent, permanent condition for him/her; however, it does not make sense to speak of "a handicapped person" because virtually no one is handicapped by a disability in every activity. References to handicaps always should make clear in what pursuits the individual is handicapped.

3. As often as possible, avoid use of the verb "to be" and its conjugations in discussing people with disabilities or handicapping conditions. For example, "Sally has arthritis" is preferable to "Sally's an arthritic," when the subtleties of language-induced stereotyping are examined. The latter construction, like "the handicapped," summarizes Sally as nothing more than her arthritis; the former implies that she is more, that Sally, among other things, has arthritis. The "name calling" quality of using the verb "to be" becomes very evident in speaking of people with disabilities that arouse social disapproval. For example, some people who have maladaptive drinking patterns resist being labeled "alcoholic" because they fear being reduced to nothing more than this in the conceptions of others. Their preference for admitting to "having a drinking problem" is derided in some quarters as denial of the

problem, but it may equally well be a sensible avoidance of socially destructive stereotyping.

4. Whenever possible, put the person before the disability in sentence construction. "Person with a disability" is preferable to "disabled person. "The first thing to stress is the personhood of the subject (or object) of the sentence. After that basic mental image has been set, the modifying adjectival clause "with a disability" is less likely to dominate the conveyed concept of the person.

5. Abjure passive constructions such as "person in or confined to a wheelchair" in favor of such active constructions as "person who uses a wheelchair." The former conveys an image of passive sitting and victimization. The latter suggests a person who is actively using a wheelchair as a tool for living life. The difference is that between the "helpless invalid" of fifty years ago and the "consumer activist" of today.

The rehabilitation milieu also should provide support for customers to develop their inner resources. For this reason, the pathology bias must be overcome so that staff will be alert to discerning existing or potential resources. Very important in this is to avoid misdiagnosing resources as pathology! A commonly acknowledged area in which this can happen involves aggressiveness and uncooperativeness, which are signs in some people of their determination to stay in charge of their own destinies, even while institutionalized. It may be troublesome to the staff while it's happening, but the same traits may harbinger better adjustment later on.

Another resource often misconstrued as pathology in institutional or agency settings is manipulativeness. When it is noted that a customer attempts to manipulate others, staff are resentful and quickly focus their efforts on blocking the individual from successfully manipulating them. This is self-(ego-) serving rather than client serving. Alternatives are possible. First, severely disabled people who are unable to manipulate the physical world have no other way to operate in it except through other people. It may be neither reasonable nor kind to try to block their only avenue toward mastery. Second, if manipulativeness is noticed, then part of the problem is that the manipulator's not doing it right. A good manipulator doesn't get labeled; part of the skill is escaping detection.

If manipulating other people is the only path toward mastery, and if a skill level that avoids offending others is possible, perhaps part of PSV rehabilitation is teaching clumsy manipulators to be more adept. Manipulating does not necessarily imply exploiting or harming those manipulated. Manipulation of others' feelings, perceptions, and behavior is central to an immense array of respectable occupations: psychology, teaching, trial law, counseling, the ministry, management, fundraising, sales, and the entire entertainment industry. If manipulation training for disabled people stressed the importance of being fair to the targets of manipulation and of offering them rewards for what they do (as much as occurs in the just-mentioned occupations), perhaps it would become an acceptable alternative to extinguishing one of the most useful survival traits a severely disabled person might have.

Special Issues in Vocational Rehabilitation

When an adult with a physical disability leaves the hospital or rehabilitation center, two service systems are most often available to meet PSV needs: the state-federal VR program and/or independent living centers (ILCs). In the ideal situation, referrals are made seamlessly between the systems and the individual receives the needed services. This does not always occur, but independent living centers can play an important role in addressing personal and social concerns by means of peer counseling, group programs, and advocacy. Rehabilitation counselors have the training and often the interest to provide personal, sexual, or family counseling, but they frequently are constrained by their mandates from devoting the requisite time or case-service funds to these services.

One reason for this is the peculiarly diverse role of the rehabilitation counselor. Their responsibilities vary depending upon the setting in which they work as well as the degree to which they specialize in serving particular populations. Leahy (1997, pp. 96–97), summarized the fundamental responsibilities of rehabilitation counselors across settings as including the following: "(a) assess client needs, (b) work with the client to develop goals and individualized plans to meet identified needs, and (c) provide or arrange for the therapeutic services and interventions (e.g., psychological, medical, social, behavioral) needed by the client, including placement and follow-up services." Counseling skills are fundamental to all aspects of the work, but rehabilitation counselors in the state-federal system and those in the private sector also have substantial demands for case management and administrative activities that compete for time and require distinctly different skills and temperament.

Complicating the basic problems of interfering demands and too little time and money to expend on psychological services is the fact that VR agency counselors have case-service funds—to expend on behalf of clients or to withhold—and this strains counselor-client relationships in ways not confronted by others who do personal counseling. Counselors seldom are prepared for the impact of this in their preservice graduate training. They are in unique power positions. They can choose to be "good guys" and spend large amounts of case-service funds for private training, personal vehicles, monthly maintenance allowances, or whatever is needed/desired by their clients; or they can choose to be "bad guys," conserving agency funds and requiring clients to find other ways to meet these economic needs. Because of their fiscal discretion, they can choose to be "good guys" with some clients and "bad guys" with others. Then, because of the ethical constraints against discussing one client's situation with another, they may be unable to explain their professional rationales for differential treatment. Thus, the potential for their fiscal role eclipsing their counseling function in the eyes of the clients and for being seen as autocratic, parental authorities, rather than helping persons, is introduced and must be dealt with directly before a rapport conducive to personal counseling can develop.

The agency role also involves a philosophical dilemma for many counselors. They may wonder, "Whose agent am I? Do I work for the taxpayers/state, or do I work for the client? Am I here to reduce the welfare rolls and increase the number of disabled people paying taxes, or am I here to help disabled people achieve equity, dignity, and improved quality of life?" The dilemma is even more acute for rehabilitation counselors in the private sector whose clients are often injured workers. In some cases the desires and best interests of the client may be at odds with those of the insurance company that is hiring and paying the counselor. Fortunately, as the field has matured, the answer to these dilemmas has been directly addressed in the Code of Professional Ethics for Rehabilitation Counselors (CORC, 2001, p. 1). Standard A.1.a reads as follows:

> Definition of Client: The primary obligation of rehabilitation counselors will be to their clients, defined as individuals with disabilities who are receiving services from rehabilitation counselors.

Although the stress of multiple responsibilities may not fully disappear, at least the directive is clear and the counselor has support in standing up to systems, when necessary.

Two client-service developments provided some relief for these interrelated problems. First, the burgeoning of independent living rehabilitation has led to many new resources for meeting the psychological as well as social/survival needs of clients. For ILCs, these needs are the primary focus of interest, not secondary issues behind vocational goals.

Second, job clubs—an approach to job finding developed by behavioral psychologist Nathan Azrin in the early 1970s—are widely used in vocational rehabilitation, to the psychosocial as well as vocational benefit of both clients and counselors. Job clubs combine job-search training with mutual help, much of which is composed of motivational/emotional/moral support, as well as job-lead sharing and other practical assistance. A series of side benefits emanate from this approach. Counselors who fear and avoid doing job placement can work in teams, with other counselors and job-club members, thereby receiving the support they need to confront this difficult part of their jobs. Their active involvement in helping with job search then alters the clients' perceptions of them; they come to be seen as more genuinely helpful. This, in turn, has a positive effect on the likelihood that clients will seek their counsel when they need to, and are ready to, deal with personal problems. When clients initiate such services, they are unlikely to be withheld.

The Self-Help Philosophy

Job clubs and consumer-run independent living programs are but two highly significant manifestations of the self-help philosophy that is spreading rapidly throughout the industrialized world. Others mentioned earlier are the holistic health movement, pain-management clinics and, of course, Alcoholics Anonymous, the prototype organization for mutual helping among people who share similar problems. Futurists (Cornish, 1982; Toffler, 1980) trace the pattern by which the same social forces—notably skyrocketing advances in electronics technology, with a resultant explosion of data-processing and telecommunications capabilities—are giving impetus to both the "self-help" and "do-it-yourself" movements. They predict that future society will reunite production with consumption at the individual level; that is, each of us will tend to produce more for our own consumption, and less for the market or for consumption by others.

Within the broadly conceived health-and-human-service field, we are seeing already that the watchwords are, "know thyself" and "heal (serve) thyself"; we all are becoming our own "physicians." Mutual-help approaches can be seen as barter-economy variations on the self-help theme, and the following chapter will examine the self- and mutual-help phenomena that now loom large in rehabilitation. Specifically, peer-provided psychogogic services and the psychological impact of other peer-provided service approaches will be reviewed.

12

Peer Counseling and Related Services

Like several other human-service innovations mentioned earlier in this volume, a prototype for organizations operated "by the disabled, for the disabled" germinated in the fertile social soil of Berkeley, California. The Center for Independent Living (CIL) came into being when a number of severely disabled graduates of the University of California at Berkeley (UCB) discovered that college degrees had not made them independent. Unable to find jobs even as college graduates, they had to find ways to survive in the community if they were to avoid custodial institutions or returning to their parental homes. Thus, in the early 1970s, CIL was essentially a community extension of the Physically Disabled Students Program on the UCB campus. Partly because there are so many more disabled people struggling to survive out in the community than on college campuses, it was destined to outgrow the size and fame of its parent organization within five years.

The zeitgeist was right. The same phenomenon was beginning to appear elsewhere at about the same time. Massachusetts, Texas, Ohio, and gradually, other states developed independent living programs operated by and for the disabled. In California, they multiplied quickly after the Berkeley CIL's prime mover was appointed by the governor to head the State Department of Rehabilitation. The new director encouraged the development of similar centers throughout the state by funding grants and giving technical assistance. Other states began equivalent campaigns. In 1978 the Rehabilitation Act was amended to provide for independent living as well as vocational rehabilitation, and a new era in rehabilitation was underway.

A highly significant aspect of the new era is the provision of some rehabilitation services by people who have experienced disability themselves. The embracing of this concept by rehabilitation professionals represents a greater shift in values and attitudes than some veteran providers care to remember. Well into the 1960s, disabled applicants to many academic programs for professional training in rehabilitation disciplines were not welcomed by screening committees unless they demonstrated unusual ability to avoid "identification" with clients' or patients' problems. Nondisabled professionals feared disabled providers would be unable to separate their own problems (and resulting emotions) from those of their clients, reducing their objectivity and helpfulness. The largely unrecognized assumption underlying this prejudice was that a person who is disabled must be so pervasively damaged by it psychologically, that recovery of objectivity and emotional control, when the subject is raised, is virtually impossible. This attitude was tempered first by the increasing realization, within the entire psychosocial/behavioral helping field, that "identification" is neither so rare nor so deadly as previously imagined. Second, it was quelled by the rising voice of an increasingly political disabled constituency. People with disabilities began to insist that they could do the job better, in some respects, and they demanded the right to try. The Centers for Independent Living (CILs) provided a mechanism for them to do so. They demonstrated their capability so well that legislation now requires that a majority of both CIL staff and their boards of directors be people with disabilities.

Peer Services

To the extent that CIL staff members have disabilities, often their rehabilitative offerings are construed as peer services, regardless of their professional backgrounds. Here, peer status is defined clearly in terms of disability. In other contexts, the term "peer" provider connotes the absence of professional training; it is used in contradistinction to "professional" provider. Thus, peer status sometimes relates to professionalism. It may be helpful to keep this dual nature of peership in mind when considering peer-provided services. In this chapter, the terms "peer provider," "peer service," and similar variants will connote "personal experience with disability with or without professional training for providing services." This definition allows for disabled professionals to do peer counseling when to relate as a peer rather than as a professional seems more appropriate. It also allows for peer-helping relationships among family members of disabled people, as well as the disabled individuals themselves.

The Coaching Concept

Psychogogy relies on teaching methods, and coaching is one of them. Typically, coaches are or have been players in a given game, and their teaching power resides in their deeply ingrained understanding of both the game's demands and the players' needs. This holds true whether the "game" is athletic competition, artistic performance, or virtually any other activity. It is important to distinguish coaching from tutoring. A tutor may not have learned through experience; in fact, the subject matter is often didactic rather than experiential. Also, tutoring is a one-to-one process. While coaching may be, it is not limited in this respect. Group (most likely team) coaching may be combined with adjunctive individual coaching.

Coaches employ a vast array of teaching methods. They instruct; that is, they provide factual information. They advise; that is, they offer judgments and make recommendations based on the facts. They counsel; that is, they attempt to motivate and provide emotional support. They do role modeling; that is, they demonstrate how given activities should be performed.

Coaches also provide ongoing feedback during and after the learner's performance. They don't deliver lectures and leave the performer to incorporate suggestions and correct errors without further guidance. They stay with the learner, instructing, advising, encouraging, demonstrating, and supporting as the performance unfolds. This aspect of coaching makes it time consuming and therefore expensive. As a result, it has been used mainly in the sports world, which society is willing to subsidize, and the performing arts, which highly motivated individuals will scrimp and save to finance. It has not been considered feasible for PSV rehabilitation providers.

The advent of CILs staffed with volunteers or modestly paid workers has made the cost of coaching feasible in PSV rehabilitation. As a result, its unique power in preparing disabled people for independent living has come to light. People who themselves have adjusted emotionally and practically to disability can coach others, using both their abilities to "identify" and their parallel experiential bases. They coach sometimes as effectively and sometimes more effectively than professionals whose knowledge is "secondhand." The importance of peer counseling is evident in its designation as one of the four mandated core services that must be provided by all CILs. The other required services are advocacy, independent living skills training, and information and referral.

Varieties of Peer Service

Peer counseling is explicitly psychogogic in nature. It has become ubiquitous in recent years, with the growth of the independent living movement and its identification as one of the four key services that must be provided by all

CILs. Peer counseling is a term that encompasses and overlaps with many related activities, however, so it would be well to explore the varied connotations of the term. To begin, some peer services carry "counseling" in their titles but are actually more akin to ombudsman services. That is, they combine coaching (instruction, advisement, role modeling) with advocacy (agency intervention). Examples include financial advice, personal assistance, and housing counseling. On the other hand, some counseling activities go by alternative names. Some CILs have chosen to discontinue using the term "peer counseling," preferring "peer support" to describe the sharing of life experiences that occurs between participants in the process (Brown, 1999). Another common term, which describes a process that may cross over between counseling, advocacy, instruction, and friendship is "peer mentoring." Because these terms overlap and are used in inconsistent ways, this chapter will not attempt to distinguish between them.

An essential element in peer counseling is that it is offered by someone who shares the experience of living with a disability or chronic illness (hence, the individual is a peer). In that respect, peer counseling is part of the wider self-help movement, which dates back, at least, to the founding of Alcoholics Anonymous in the 1930s. Saxton (1983) estimated that 500,000 mutual-aid or self-help organizations were operative in the United States, involving millions of people. Two decades later, that number has increased, but to an unknown degree. Peer counseling may occur in groups or one on one. The peers may be volunteers or paid staff members, but the sine qua non is that they bring their own life experiences into the process.

The term "counseling" implies the establishment of a relationship between people that aims to facilitate the personal growth of at least one of the participants. Traditionally, the counseling process depends primarily on verbal interaction, but other kinds of peer activities can have psychogogic effects. Psychological growth is enhanced in part through the process of incidental learning; clients observe that disabled people can learn to solve their practical problems and then teach others how to do it. This message alone can contribute to a client's growing self-confidence.

It also must be recognized that the facts of resolving financial, personal assistance, and housing problems have enormous impact on psychological well-being; even having an aware person to talk with about them can be helpful. None of these benefits were readily available to disabled people in the community before CILs and their peer-provided services came into being. In the hospital, there were social workers to help with such matters; but once home again, unguided trial and error coupled with unchanneled worry soon eroded any previously acquired sense of well-being. Now, peer providers are attending to psychological health, both in these indirect ways and directly through the medium of peer counseling.

Peer Counseling

Selection of Peer Counselors

Although the professionals of an earlier era may have misjudged both the degree to which "identification" interferes with good counseling and the degree to which counselors with disabilities might project their own problems onto customers, they were attuned to a real, potential pitfall, that is, having experienced disability is not, in itself, sufficient qualification for functioning competently as a peer counselor. Just as the best football, drama, and other coaches typically have been good performers, the best peer counselors ("living-with-disability coaches") perform well in their own lives with respect to emotional and practical adjustment to disability. No one wants as a coach the player who couldn't make the team; and no one needs a counselor who is bitter, ineffectual, and unfulfilled.

Selection of peer counselor candidates, by programs that use them, is made even more difficult than ordinary employee selection by two factors. First, unlike the situation in hiring professionals, there is no long and arduous preparatory process that can be relied on to either correct problematical habits or eliminate individuals clearly unsuited for the work. Often, decisions must be made on immediately available data plus, at most, a very brief period of preservice training. Since the peer counselor will be drawing mainly from effective life experiences and good personal adjustment, methods for quickly and correctly assessing such notoriously hard-to-assess matters must be developed.

Second, sometimes people offering to work on a voluntary basis have to be rejected. It is doubly hard to turn away free services when the "employer" knows the applicant is searching for a way to be and feel useful; no one wants to be responsible for aborting such efforts. Nonetheless, if the requisite personal qualities are absent, other ways to encourage such an applicant must be found if harm to that individual and those he or she would attempt to help is to be avoided.

Selecting one or a few peer counselors who will be working regular hours within an organization is quite a different process from selecting volunteers who will be seeing their counselees out in the community under less direct supervision. The Arizona Bridge to Independent Living has a very large peer mentoring program, with approximately 50 volunteers contributing thousands of hours annually (Redford & Whitaker-Lee, 1999). Because mentors are typically active for only about a year, recruitment is a year-around effort. They use an application form that includes questions about work history, counseling experience, affiliations with community service agencies, what the applicant hopes to gain from volunteering, and how they believe they can be effective as a mentor. They also check character references, even for people who are known to their CIL. They ask about alcohol and drug use, criminal history, dependability, concern for and respect for others, punctuality, cleanliness, trustworthiness, and other matters. Finally, the selection process requires applicants to sign a list of guidelines wherein they agree to maintain confidentiality, to report any consumer's suicidal or homicidal thoughts (or suspicions thereof), to maintain proper boundaries with the mentees, to maintain regular contact with mentees, and to participate in continuing training and oversight. This careful selection process is followed with an ongoing evaluation process.

Settings

Like the CILs themselves, peer counseling as a service entity took root on college campuses. When disabled students joined forces for mutual aid and political amplification, informal counseling among peers was a natural result of their coming together. Today, campus programs for students with disabilities and community-based CILs are the major settings in which formalized peer counseling services can be found. Undoubtedly, the reason is that both tend to be operated by and for the disabled. The genre seems to be here to stay and has, in fact, generated several subvarieties.

At the same time, a significant number of traditional, professionally-operated rehabilitation settings such as hospitals, centers, and agencies have added peer counseling to their own selections of service alternatives. While this reflects a view that peer counseling has something unique to offer, its addition has been met with mixed reviews from both sides. For example, some disabled activists charge "tokenism" and insist that disabled people with the talent for peer counseling should be encouraged instead to pursue full, professional training so they can reap the economic benefits of mainstream work. This does happen for some; for example, peer counseling experience gained as an advanced rehabilitant working with more recently admitted clients/patients has been a stepping stone toward professional training for a number of people. Another problem is that peer counselors in traditional settings tend to work under the supervision of largely nondisabled PSV professionals who reportedly treat them as "patients" rather than as "colleagues." This same complaint, however, is voiced by fully trained professionals with disabilities about nondisabled coworkers in rehabilitation settings.

The issue of pay is an important element in the controversy about the role of peer counselors. Being compensated for one's time conveys respect and signifies the value of the work. Furthermore, it is easier to hold paid workers accountable for their commitments, so they may be more dependable, especially about tasks like documentation of activity. For these reasons, Saxton (1983) concluded that, whenever possible, it seems advisable to pay peer counselors. The Arizona Bridge to Independent Living (ABIL), on the other hand, arrived at the opposite conclusion. They believed that it would mean more to mentees to be involved in a relationship with someone who had no incentive except the desire to be with them. They viewed the peer mentorship program as an extension of the community where friends simply choose to help friends. Their position was emphatically made as follows (Redford & Whitaker-Lee, 1999):

> Peer mentoring is at the heart of the independent living movement. Having paid staff persons in the role of providing "peer support" can unintentionally *dis*-empower persons with disabilities. No matter how hard we try, if we are getting paid to be there, then we are just one more service provider.

Training

Although the term "peer counselor" connotes "untrained," this reflects a matter of degree. Initially, training was resisted in the belief that "having been there" provided more salient preparation than the professionals had, and that professionals urging or offering training were acting out of self-interest. However, on finding that totally untrained peer counselors too often were unequipped to either help others or protect themselves in the demanding, emotionally charged relationships that sometimes developed, this resistance weakened. Later, most programs using peer counselors either combined screening/training methodologies or made concerted efforts to develop them. A survey of 123 independent living programs conducted by the University of Kansas Research and Training Center on Independent Living (Mathews, Mathews, & Pittman, 1985) found that nearly all of them offered training, usually in small groups. More recent professional literature is nearly devoid of references to training of peer counselors, however, and a staff member at the Kansas R & T Center confirmed that many personnel in CILs currently do little training and screening (White, 2001, personal communication).

A few centers use professionally-trained disabled counselors in the role of peer counselors, to maximize the quality of counseling; however, these people still retain the title "peer counselor" because of its greater customer acceptance.

As previously noted, candidates are screened primarily on the basis of personal qualities, that is, their apparent potential for learning rather than their possession of skills. This is partly because the pool of potential counselors needs to be continually replenished, and is partly a function of a design to give many disabled people opportunities to fill the role because of its power to aid their own growth. The truth of the maxim, "one learns best by teaching," is accepted here.

Available training ranges from structured, rather sophisticated programs that train groups of candidates and last for several weeks, to single orientation sessions conducted by volunteer professionals from such disciplines as social work, rehabilitation counseling, or psychology. An example of the former comes from ABIL. In 1990 they offered their first training program for 6 volunteers; it was 48 hours long. At present, volunteers are provided with a 50-page resource book and 12 hours of training. The topics that are covered include the following (Redford & Whitaker-Lee, 1999):

- ABIL programs
- Independent living philosophy
- Adaptation to disability and the grieving process
- Disability oppression
- Community resources
- Crisis intervention and the "duty to report" policy
- Goal setting
- ABIL program guidelines and procedures

The center also offers monthly continuing education meetings that provide education on such topics as peer counseling techniques, self and community advocacy, disability awareness, civil rights, and disability oppression and liberation.

Both peer counseling and the various professional counseling varieties are referred to regularly as "the art of forming helping friendships." The friendship entails the elements of relating with warmth, genuineness, and empathy, as well as having a usable reservoir of knowledge about community resources. While it is true that they share this characteristic, the ABIL training program highlights a significant difference in that it excludes coverage of principles and techniques relating to basic psychological intervention strategies (for example, behavior modification and nondirective counseling). It is possible that, in time, peer counselors will wish to upgrade their discipline to the paraprofessional or professional level. At that point, such material might be added profitably to their training.

Peer Cybercounseling

Discussion of the selection and training of peer counselors presumes the existence of an organizational structure such as a CIL or rehabilitation program within which the counseling activities occur. The World Wide Web offers a largely unregulated venue for peer counseling. Anyone with the means and desire can put up a Web site or set up a chat room or discussion board to provide peer counseling services, and it in up to the user to separate good counsel from poor. A usually reliable key indicator of quality, however, is that the site is sponsored by a reputable organization. DIMENET, for example, is a cooperative effort of the National Council on Independent Living, the Research and Training Center on Independent Living at ILRU, and several other major organizations. Besides offering public newsgroups on many topics, it sponsors the DIMENET Virtual CIL (Dimenet, 2000). The virtual CIL offers a group of chat rooms related to disability activism, family-friendly chat, and the disAB-café "where people from all over the world—whether disabled or able bodied—can chat in friendship and be supportive of one another."

The CyberCIL of Arizona (Benshoof, 2000) identifies itself as the first virtual Center for Independent Living, and a counter on the home page indicates the number of visitors since January, 2000. Among its offerings is a peer counseling area which is managed by Judy Benshoof, a person with hemiplegia who has been an independent living advocate for 10 years. The site includes a discussion board and a chat room as well as a link for sending personal messages to Ms. Benshoof. Given the ability of electronic communications to reach around the world without time or travel barriers, it seems likely that this approach to peer counseling will blossom in the years to come.

Peer Counseling as the Service of Choice

Although peer counseling often is relied on when professional staffers are in short supply or too expensive, there also are times when it is clearly the service of choice. A prime factor has been alluded to already: customer acceptance. Many customers, who do not acknowledge the need for professional psychological services (perhaps because the psychogogy-psychotherapy distinction has never been made clear to the general public), are very willing to admit that peer counseling might be useful. Coaching by a peer is bereft of the threat associated with accepting a psychologist's help, so at least some help is accepted.

It follows that peer counseling might be the service of choice for people who need to be prepared to accept more intensive psychological services. A peer counselor who has profited from professional help and can communicate this comfortably may have far greater credibility and influence than a professional. Also, disabled people who have had little opportunity to be with, and develop positive identification with, other disabled people can profit especially from helping friendships with disabled peers. For many such individuals, shared facts about coping possibilities come as revelations and have the power to alter motivation levels, belief systems, and behavior. Generally, peer counseling is the service of choice when a good-quality, helping friendship is all that is needed. There is no point in bringing out the "heavy artillery" of high-level professionals unless their sophisticated knowledge of psychological principles and their finely tuned skills are actually required.

Peer counselors carry a unique set of credentials: credibility as an ordinary person who has been able to "make it," special insights that come only through experience, a capacity for forming a special rapport that stems from shared experience, and a potential for role modeling that emanates from the first three. Each of these credentials deserves further examination. As Saxton (1983, p. 172) noted, "Peer counseling offers someone who understands."

Credibility as an ordinary person who is succeeding in life is extremely important to at least the middle two-thirds of any normally distributed population. For this reason, efforts to hold out the success of disabled professionals as inspirational examples often backfire, as illustrated in Part I. Only people in the top 10% of the population intellectually could hope to emulate them, and when such other requisites as drive and interpersonal support are taken into account, the percentage dwindles further. This suggests that the very best peer counselors might be part-timers who tread another occupational path during the rest of their working hours. This would expand the range and depth of feasible options to which counselees would be exposed.

The issues of special insights and the capacity for special rapport also must be viewed with a degree of caution. Counselor and counselee are two different people, and a valid charge still can be made that "You don't understand; you're not me." Peer counselors who invest a great deal of their feelings of confidence and competence in their capacities for special insights and rapport building may be particularly vulnerable when such charges come, as they inevitably do. Lowering peers' expectations for automatic rapport based on similar demography is an important part of the preservice orientation. It is equally important for peer counselors to learn when to share their own experiences and when not to. Those who are still reckoning actively with their own adjustments may be especially prone to "taking over," sharing too much too soon, in ways that inhibit rather than facilitate counselees' progress. It was overgeneralization of this realistic concern that led earlier professionals to discredit the concept of peer counseling.

Similar caveats attach to the matter of role modeling. Role models are chosen, not imposed. For example, able-bodied White males have had a vast array of potential role models to select from throughout history, but their own inner needs will determine whom they pick. Recent efforts to present potential role models to non-White, nonmale, or nonable-bodied individuals sometimes overlook this fact, assuming that the proffered role model is indeed a role model rather than only a potential one. Thus, peer counselors may or may not prove to be lifestyle role models for given counselees. However, at a more mundane and practical level, modeling—or demonstrating—effective techniques for, say, contacting agencies can be emulated whether or not clients wish to pattern their lifestyles broadly after the counselors'. It is this level of role modeling that can be striven for consciously.

Few studies have compared the effectiveness of professional and peer counseling. One series of studies compared the effectiveness of such individual counseling services for caregivers of frail elderly people (Toseland, Rossiter, Peak, & Hill, 1990; Toseland & Smith, 1990). Recipients benefited from both, and those receiving professional services appeared to improve to a somewhat greater extent. Another team of authors (Toseland, Rossiter, & Labrecque, 1989) also compared the effectiveness of group counseling by professional and peer leaders and concluded that both strategies helped people cope with the stress of caring for a frail parent. Obviously, this narrow range of studies cannot lead to conclusions about the comparative effectiveness of peer counseling in other circumstances. A few other studies could be located that discussed the value of combining professional and peer leadership in group counseling (Black & Weiss, 1990; Kostyk, Fuchs, Tabisz, & Jacyk, 1993).

Peer Counseling Approaches

Peer counseling is construed generally as a one-to-one interaction with psychogogic intent, and it often takes place in offices not unlike those used by professionals. However, it is no more limited to this than is professional counseling. Six major variations will be discussed.

Adventitious Peer Counseling

This occurs when psychogogic purposes are added to the practical goals of advisement on such matters as managing finances, procuring personal assistants, obtaining suitable housing, and meeting recreational needs. The natural dovetailing of personal-growth counseling into the context of such practical planning has advantages in terms of reaching people who might not ask explicitly for this kind of help, as well as in clarifying the importance of personal growth to success in day-to-day coping. Peer counseling can happen adventitiously in a less formal sense, too. People who learn how to form helping friendships can use their skills in ordinary contacts with disabled friends and acquaintances as well—and be better friends than before. Hopefully, this may have a cumulative effect akin to that which TM practitioners claim for their discipline; that is, as the number of practitioners increases, anxiety-induced social aberrations will decrease exponentially. It is reasonable to imagine that each disabled person skilled in helpfulness will transmit his or her ways of behaving to several others; thus, the effect would magnify. This is another reason for maximizing the number of individuals admitted to the field.

Of all the peer-service specialties focused on specific coping skills, personal assistant counseling creates the heaviest demands for psychogogic inputs. To be done effectively, the employer-employee relationship must be examined thoroughly. This is because assistant turnover problems are often the result of disabled employers' failures to (1) empathize with assistants' needs and frustrations, (2) create rewarding job situations to counterbalance the low pay levels, (3) maximize flexibility in procedures without becoming subject to exploitation, (4) communicate effectively about job demands and performance satisfactoriness, and/or (5) confront potential relationship problems in timely, effective ways. Peer counselors who display solid understanding and helpfulness initially may be called on to mediate if relationship problems arise after an assistant has been hired. The needed skills and conceptual framework have much in common with marriage counseling and conflict resolution among workers in organizational settings. Sometimes, professional intervention will be required, and it is important for the peer counselor to discern when this is true.

Support Groups

It is the intensity and complexity of interaction between (or among) individuals being counseled that determine whether professional skills are needed, not simply the fact of working with more than one person at a time. The success of support groups, for limited purposes, attests to this. The on-line counterpart, the chat room, serves similar needs for human interaction and encouragement. Peer counselors frequently conduct support groups as a central activity, with individual counseling sessions evolving from needs discerned in the groups. The term conveys "nothing heavy-duty going on here." Opportunities to ventilate, exchange ideas and experiences, obtain moral support, and other relatively nonthreatening interchange are cited in publicizing such groups. Support and relief may come from sharing "war stories" with people who can understand immediately the subtle ironies that often must be explained to nondisabled associates; shared belly laughs feel good. Because of this psychodynamic "lightness," the support group sometimes is disparaged as a psychogogic tool. However, while it may have little direct impact on serious psychological problems, Norman Cousins (1979) made a convincing case for the value of feeling good and happy in improving both bodily and mental health. It is easy to overlook the obvious. The psychological essence of Cousins' highly acclaimed book is that laughter is the best medicine. Many sophisticates have responded to this as if it were a revelation, although *Reader's Digest*, one of the country's most popular (but unsophisticated) periodicals, has carried a feature by this title for years. Thus, a group's greatest strength may lie in its ability to improve feelings of well-being temporarily, because this improved state of consciousness makes further, deeper changes more feasible.

Consciousness Raising

An important feature of some discussion groups is consciousness raising (CR). In addition, groups explicitly designed for this purpose may be conducted along the lines of CR groups for women. Here, emphasis is placed on helping participants enhance their self-concepts or feelings of self-esteem through clarified recognition of their rights as members of a given class of people. Individual frailties are separated conceptually from responses to externally imposed constraints, in the hope that participants then can perceive expanded vistas and greater degrees of freedom with which they can operate. The perspective fits well with the social political or minority view of disability, which holds that most of the problems experienced by people with disabilities stem from societal attitudes and barriers, not from the disabilities. Obviously, this relates to what was called "the other half of the psychology of disability—the politics of disability" in the introduction to this book. Accordingly, consciousness raising as a psychogogic modality is not confined to CR groups: it occurs as an integral part of advocacy by the disabled, for the disabled, as well.

Brown (1999) provided several examples of peer support becoming shared advocacy experiences. He described a one-day peer support training day organized by a CIL. The morning included training in communication skills, definitions of peer support, and development of peer support. Participants then broke into small groups and talked about issues of concern to them. Then a facilitator led each group into the community to advocate for changes relating to their issue.

Improved effects on participants can be equally important. It can help people become desensitized, in the sense of being less vulnerable to hurt, to uncontrollable words and actions on the parts of others. Once this is accomplished, vistas can be expanded "safely" because fewer fears remain of vulnerabilities that might take one by surprise and prompt withdrawal from other challenges.

Hotlines

Occasionally, in nearly everyone's life, the challenges of living threaten to overwhelm coping abilities. When this happens, still another peer counseling service, the hotline, may be used to help disabled people, especially those who are isolated or immobilized, to handle such crises. The use of the telephone for crisis intervention grew from programs designed for people in such serious trouble—psychologically and physically—that the telephone might be as far as they could reach out for help. The term "hotline" grew out of the urgency of these situations.

Alcoholics Anonymous has long offered "twelfth step" work: when tempted to drink, call another member and talk it out instead. Later, suicide prevention and drug rehabilitation programs developed techniques for telephone diagnostic screening, as well as refined methods for remote treatment intervention. Now, hotlines have been instituted in a wide range of programs for an increased range of purposes, from truly "hot" issues such as defusing urges to batter children, to such "cooler" needs as the dispelling of loneliness. A few CILs have hotlines operated by peer counselors, and others are working to establish them. When the counselors are willing to do so, residence numbers may be provided to give potential callers extended hours of telephone coverage.

Peer counseling by telephone is uniquely appropriate for people who have difficulties in arranging transportation. The potential of telephone counseling is not limited to that provided by peers, however. The senior author began using this method in the early 1960s when working as an outpatient psychologist with former patients of a rehabilitation hospital. No implication is intended that telephone counseling is superior or even equal to in-person contact; however, it is vastly superior to its very real alternative of nothing for people unable to get to a service location. As mentioned earlier, the rapid development of chat rooms and bulletin boards on the Internet may be rapidly replacing telephone hotlines, particularly for psychogogic rather than crisis intervention purposes. The medical and psychological communities are developing electronically delivered services under the name of "telehealth." This will be discussed in the following chapter

Peer-Provided Body Work

This area of peer service began years ago in a few CILs. Although it has not developed widely, the authors believe that the idea should not be allowed to slip away. Disabled staff members who have had martial-arts training may offer informal training in karate or other disciplines to program participants. Also, several centers have instituted movement and dance therapy programs. For example, in one, a staff member whose dance career was interrupted by mental illness provided a variety of dance and movement experiences for people with either physical or mental disabilities. Another program began with professionally-provided dance experiences aimed at opening up relationships among participants; it now has a cadre of experienced staff and clients who are passing the approach on to others.

A more fully developed approach came not from a CIL but from a conceptually similar program for senior citizens. Luce (1979) described the bodywork program that evolved at SAGE (Senior Actualizations and Growth Experiences) in Berkeley, California. In addition to martial arts and dance/movement offerings, the program established a highly valued program of massage administered by self, staff, or other participants. Although SAGE is described here as "conceptually similar" to CILs, it should be pointed out that, in a sense, it reversed the usual priorities of CILs; that is, practical survival and coping skills were placed second in importance compared with personal growth and inner development.

The goals are similar in all of the just-mentioned programs: (1) to learn that the body, even if it is disabled or aged, is a source of pleasure, beauty, and grace, and (2) to use body work as a means for improving one's psychological well-being and ability to connect with others. The SAGE program found that nude body work was particularly powerful as a means of helping participants unlearn the misconception that old bodies are no longer beautiful or a pleasure to touch. The same goal is clearly relevant to people who believe disabilities and/or deformities have rendered their bodies unbeautiful.

This illustration also brings out a desirable direction for peer services of a psychogogic nature—the potential inherent in a coalition between seniors and disabled people of all ages. Many of the needs and issues are the same, and more are at least comparable. A few programs are tapping this symbiotic potential, such as foster-grandparent programs for disabled (or nondisabled) children who lack loving families and for older people who need to give love, and programs wherein mentally retarded students make regular visits to convalescent hospitals to entertain and socialize with elderly disabled people. In another example, a small rehabilitation hospital found it necessary to discharge two young paraplegic men to a nursing home populated solely by elderly patients, because independent living situations in the community could not be arranged for them. Viewed as potentially catastrophic for them at first, it was later regarded as divinely inspired. One of the young men changed within a month from morose and apathetic to the self-ordained recreation director for the elderly. The other, following this lead, helped to conduct the activities. The morale of the elderly patients was affected similarly. In about three months, both had made their own independent living arrangements in the community and moved on.

13

Psychotherapeutic Approaches

This chapter provides an overview of psychotherapeutic services, primarily for rehabilitation professionals who are not fully familiar with their scope and purposes; and it will discuss concerns that often are addressed in psychotherapy for people with disabilities. Because a massive research and clinical literature exists in the field, a comprehensive synthesis would require more pages than have been allotted for this entire volume. The scope of the chapter will be clarified further, but first several definitional distinctions should be made.

The psychogogy-psychotherapy distinction was made earlier (see Chapter 11) in terms of whether the intent is preventive—to strengthen the person so psychological breakdown will not occur, or curative—to correct psychological disorders that have developed already. Whereas the term "psychogogy" might be applied to any methods employed in prevention, psychotherapy is but one of three paths that might be chosen for treating existing disorders. The other two are psychosurgery and the use of drugs or nutrients. Psychotherapy, like psychogogy, generally is mediated by a learning process, in contradistinction to surgery, medication, and nourishment, which operate directly on bodily tissues in the attempt to bring about psychological change. This does not mean that all psychotherapy is verbal. As recently as the 1960s, psychotherapy was referred to as "talk therapy" by its practitioners; however, since that time, many new techniques have been adopted, including an array of nonverbal body-work techniques. The line between the two is soft and permeable because psychological health is not a dichotomy (you have it or you don't), but rather is a continuum. In recent decades large segments of the general population have been seeking psychotherapy to deal with the baggage of imperfect childhood experiences and the disappointments of adult life. It is reasonable to assume that people with disabilities have similar rates of psychoses, neuroses, and personality disorders as the population at large. In addition, with or without mental illness, they often cope with the stresses that accompany stigma and physical limitations and may seek psychotherapy as a means to improve their lives.

Traditionally, psychotherapy has referred to a verbal interchange between a therapist and one or several individuals who want to make life changes. Increasingly, verbal therapy has been combined with the use of medications, especially for treatment of mood disorders. An array of nonverbal body-work techniques have been added to the therapeutic armamentarium. Exercise, massage, and other bodily procedures are used as media for teaching such behaviors as relaxation. Biofeedback training often is used in the cure of phobic reactions and maladaptive habit formation. Other behavior-modification procedures also may serve psychotherapeutic purposes.

In the past, a clear distinction was drawn between "talk therapy" and other approaches, reflecting an assumption of mind/body dualism. This perspective has changed as developments in neuroscience have shown that even talking and learning change brain chemistry and circuitry, just as physical changes can lead to new thought patterns. For simplicity in this chapter, however, our discussion of "psychotherapy" will include here any curative approach to psychobehavioral disorder that excludes surgery, drugs, and nutrients. No effort will be made to examine the latter approaches, leaving their discussion to authors with the appropriate medical or physiological training. The focus here will be on psychological approaches of either a verbal or nonverbal nature.

Psychotherapists rely on varied theories to guide their work: psychodynamic, cognitive-behavioral, existential, narrative, humanistic, reality, solution-focused, and many others. Theory helps the therapist to identify the source of an individual's problems and determine the kinds of intervention needed in order to help resolve them. Olkin (1999) has argued that when people with disabilities are clients these counseling theories interface with other theories (she calls them models) that therapists hold about disability, which also influence the kind of treatment they offer. Traditional models of disability (such as the medical or functional models) view problems as residing within the person. Therapeutic efforts, then, are directed toward resolving the intrapsychic conflicts, irrational thinking, damaging emotions, or destructive behavior patterns that are believed to be impeding the person's efforts to live a satisfying and productive life. Olkin suggests that a more appropriate model of disability is the "minority model," which holds that disability-related problems are substantially the result of discrimination and stigma that confront the individual at every hand. A psychotherapist who works from the minority model would strive to raise the client's awareness of the ways in which societal attitudes and behaviors conspire to create problems and suggest solutions such as political activism, peer support, and environmental changes.

Adherence to a minority model as presented by Olkin does not preclude attention to personal issues but rather requires an awareness of the pervasive social factors that create or amplify the person's concerns. This perspective represents a significant shift in the typical patterns of psychotherapeutic thought. Psychology has always focused on the individual, and this emphasis is consistent with the American culture's pervasive individualism. Contemporary understanding of disability, however, requires comparable recognition of the social dimensions of emotional distress.

Psychotherapeutic Services

In keeping with the general theme of this book, the discussion of psychotherapy will apply chiefly to individuals for whom emotional problems coexist with other kinds of disabilities. It will address several problems that have been identified as having special relevance to people with physical disabilities. A brief overview of psychosocial rehabilitation (sometimes also called psychiatric rehabilitation), which is provided to individuals with a primary diagnosis of mental illness, will follow.

Cognitive-Behavioral Therapies

Of all of the psychotherapeutic approaches that have been studied in their application to people with disabilities, cognitive-behavioral approaches have probably been the most frequently used and the most often demonstrated to have some beneficial effect. In simplest terms, this approach rests upon the assumption that people are continuously thinking, feeling, and acting. These processes occur simultaneously, they influence each other, and they strive for internal consistency, one with another. For example, when a person is frightened of a social situation such as going out in public and meeting new people, that fear is stoked by thoughts or beliefs like "no one will want to talk with me," or "I'll make a fool of myself." Then he or she will be motivated to avoid the situation, which, in turn, perpetuates the fear and leaves the negative beliefs to continue unchallenged.

Cognitive-behavioral psychotherapy strives to break into this counterproductive cycle, usually by helping the individual to challenge and reframe beliefs or by daring to change behavior patterns despite the fear and in so doing make it possible to change beliefs. Attempting to change emotions directly (for example, by telling someone to cheer up) is seldom effective, but if beliefs can be altered, congruent feelings are apt to follow.

Brewin (1989) reviewed many varieties of cognitive-behavioral therapies and identified three cognitive change processes that seemed to form the active ingredients in all of them. The first one involves correcting mistaken beliefs or providing new information. In some cases, therapy could be educational, providing details about a condition or information about what one could expect in the future. Followers of Rational Emotional Behavior Therapy (Ellis, 1997) look for blatantly irrational beliefs (for example, assumptions about the way that the world *should* be or how perfect their own behavior *must* be) and try to convince the individual to change them in therapy. "Reframing" is a cognitive change process that involves seeing a situation in a different light. For example, a person who sustained a lower extremity amputation as a result of a car crash might initially see the event as an unmitigated tragedy but later recognize it as a wake-up call that provides an opportunity to make major changes in life direction.

A second change process identified by Brewin (1989) involves reactions that are based in old and largely unconscious learning. Some individuals are highly anxious or reactive to certain situations, as a result of being sensitized to them by early experience. Even though the individual may not be consciously aware of these memories, cognitive-behavioral therapy may serve to help him or her recognize the way that certain disability-related concerns trigger excessive or problematic reactions.

The third change process in cognitive-behavioral therapies involves development of more effective coping strategies. One method of understanding the many ways that people deal with problems is to sort them into categories. Moos and Shaeffer (1984) described three major coping categories: appraisal-focused, problem-focused, and emotion-focused. Appraisal-focused strategies involve primarily cognitive changes, such as reframing the problem, finding meaning in the situation, and mentally analyzing the problem to find ways of making it more manageable. Problem-focused strategies are more externally oriented and include taking direct action to resolve the problem, finding information and social or professional support, or finding new sources of satisfaction to replace ones that have been lost. Emotion-focused coping includes emotional venting or developing increased emotional control, resigning oneself to the situation, or finding ways of avoiding the problem. A psychotherapist may help an individual understand the kinds of coping strategies he or she relies on most often and the effect they have on quality of life. Perhaps the person needs to create a larger repertoire of strategies or change from one that is not working well to another with more potential for success. Problem-focused coping is frequently considered more effective than emotion-focused coping, but the essential question is which brings the best results in a given situation. Sometimes, resignation may be the best way of coping with a problem that cannot be changed, but usually more active strategies provide the individual with a greater feeling of competence and offer some prospect for a better resolution of the difficulty.

Other Therapies

Solution-focused therapy is a relatively new therapeutic approach that seems particularly useful in many rehabilitation settings, where tangible issues need to be resolved within a limited amount of time. It suggests that instead of focusing on problems in their exquisite detail, the counselee and therapist should identify a desired solution and concentrate on how to achieve it. The individual is encouraged to notice times when the problem does not occur and find ways to extend that positive experience. For example, Sherry was discouraged about continual conflicts with her personal care assistant who seemed annoyed by Sherry's directives and unwilling to do more than an absolute minimum of work. Sherry considered firing the PA, but she had encountered similar problems before with other employees and was afraid that she would be no better off with a new person. The solution-focused therapist helped her to envision a relationship that would be mutually satisfying and to notice times when her interactions with the PA were good. By attending to and fostering these occasions, the dynamic of their relationship (and Sherry's level of personal distress) changed significantly. The solution-focused approach mirrors techniques taught in a range of western mystery school (spiritual) traditions.

Person-centered therapies emphasize the importance of the relationship between a therapist and the person receiving therapy. A trusting relationship in therapy can allow the individual to explore painful emotions and serve as a bridge to more effective personal relationships and psychological health. The therapeutic alliance is generally recognized as an important contributor to therapeutic gains, however, no matter what theory or strategy is the focus of treatment. It is the authors' view that psychotherapy, by whatever name, does and should include all three of these approaches.

Problems Frequently Requiring Psychotherapy

Depression

Depression is probably the emotional condition most often presumed to follow the onset of disability. Wright (1983) suggested that the general population expects (and virtually insists) that people who become disabled go through a significant period of grieving. She termed it the "requirement of mourning." Given that the culture places such a high value on health, beauty, and physical abilities, it seems to most people unthinkable that anyone who faces some degree of loss in these areas would not be distressed. Rather than question these cultural values, people find it easier to assume that a nondistressed individual is aberrant.

Traditional "stage" theories of adjustment to disability have posited depression to be one of the normal steps traversed by people as they come to terms with the changes in their lives. After the shock and an initial period of disbelief have passed, the newly disabled person is expected to recognize the implications and enduring nature of the condition, to grieve losses, and through the resolution of the sadness find his or her way back to a positive frame of mind.

The professional literature supports the likelihood that depression is a common problem among people with severe disabilities. For example, a study involving more than 1,300 people with spinal cord injury (Krause, Kemp, & Coker, 2000) found that 42% screened positive for some form of depression, and 21% had probable major depression. Many possible reasons for depression, in addition to the theoretical explanations just mentioned, can be suggested. Disability can bring multifaceted losses, such as the ability to participate in valued activities, changes in relationships, economic repercussions, pain, and social barriers and prejudices to contend with every day. Nevertheless, many people with disabilities do not become depressed, and many people without disabilities do suffer with depression, so disability alone cannot be the only explanation for a mood disorder.

A number of studies have attempted to answer the question of whether people with various disabilities have higher rates of depression than does the general population. This question is deceptively simple for many reasons, however, including discrepancies in terminology, measurement problems due to overlapping symptoms of depression and physical disabilities, the challenge of generalizing the results of small studies to broader populations, and the analytic limitations of correlational studies.

Looking first at the matter of consistent identification, the term depression has often been used interchangeably with distress, sadness, grief, depressed symptoms or mood, and similar terms (Elliott & Frank, 1996). Confusion about terminology makes comparison among studies difficult. Speaking precisely, depression is a clinically diagnosable condition that meets criteria specified in the DSM-IV (American Psychiatric Association, 1994). Even then, it is an umbrella term that includes several distinct conditions, i.e., major depressive disorder, dysthymic disorder, depressive disorder not otherwise specified, and bipolar disorder, each of which have unique characteristics. A number of widely used inventories have "depression" in their titles, such as the Beck Depression Inventory (Beck, Guth, Steer, & Ball, 1997) and the Center for Epidemiological Diseases Depression Scale (Radloff, 1977) but do not actually follow the criteria for assessing clinical depression. They could better be described as measures of general psychological distress (Coyne, Thompson, Palmer, Kagee, & Maunsell, 2000). As a result, drawing any conclusions about the relationship between disability and "depression" first requires that both terms be carefully specified.

Another complication with some inventories is that they contain items regarding sleep, appetite disturbance, or physical sensations that may be marked as true because of a neurological impairment rather than depression, affecting the interpretability of results (Grayson, Mackinnon, Jorm, Creasey, & Broe, 2000; Heinrich & Tate, 1996). Some writers have suggested that all of these items be removed when the inventories are used with people who have physical disabilities and that only items reflecting depressed mood be retained. On the other hand, there is little or no evidence available to indicate how such selective deletion would affect the predictive validity of the instruments. Even when the screening inventories are used with a sample of the general population (who do not have physical impairments that complicate item interpretation), drawing conclusions from the results is not a simple matter. A high proportion of the people whose scores suggest the presence of significant distress turn out not to have diagnosable depression (Coyne, Thompson, Palmer, Kajee, & Maumsell, 2000).

Interpretive challenges grow when varied methods are used to identify distressed affect. Bramston and Fogarty (Bramston & Fogarty, 2000) examined three ways by which emotional disorders, including depression, have been measured most often in research. They compared three approaches—self-ratings, ratings by a significant other, and clinical interviews—to evaluate stress, depression, and anger in a sample of 147 people with mild or moderate intellectual disabilities. They found little agreement among the methods. Perhaps the amount of agreement would be greater with people having other kinds of disabilities, but that remains to be tested.

Despite all of these methodological problems, can anything be said about the extent of depression among people with disabilities? A number of articles have asserted that people with varied conditions are at increased risk for emotional distress (Bruce, 2000; Carson, Ringbauer, MacKenzie, Warlow, & Sharpe, 2000; Cox, 1999; Guth, 2000; Kanner & Nieto, 1999). Occasionally a study appears in which participants do not have higher scores on symptom scales than the normative populations (Rabkin, 2000; Kemp, Krause, & Adkins, 1999; Kirk, 1999; Rybarczyk, Szymanski, & Nicholas, 2000; Schrag, Jahanshahi, & Quinn, 2001; Smith & Young, 2000; Stein, Gordon, Hibbard, & Sliwinski, 1992; Weigartz, 2000; Whyte & Niven, 2001). At the least, though, it seems safe to say that a significant number of people with physical disabilities also contend with depression or some form of emotional distress.

A question that cannot be answered based upon the typical correlational studies reported in the literature is whether disability causes depression or whether depression produces increased levels of disability. A high correlation between two variables demonstrates that they tend to go together, but it cannot tell which is the cause and which is the effect.

Occasionally studies are designed that allow for causal inference. Among a large sample of individuals 65 years and older, depression was found to increase the risk of mobility and other functional limitations (Penninx, Leveille, Ferrucci, van Eijk, & Guralnik, 1999). Individuals who did not have disabilities at the onset of the study were screened using the Center for Epidemiological Studies Depression (CESD) Scale and then were tested annually for disability over the course of six years. Individuals who initially scored at a level on the CESD that suggested depression were found to have higher rates of disability years later. The authors concluded that these people might have had lower rates of social interaction and physical activity, leading to more functional impairments.

In one study (Smith & Young, 2000) people with multiple sclerosis were asked to rate the severity of their disability, and those ratings were compared to the assessment made by their physicians. Individuals who had elevated scores on measures of depression were much more likely than nondepressed individuals to perceive their disability as more severe than did their physicians. On the other hand, a study of people with rheumatoid arthritis (Griffin, Friend, Kaell, Bennett, & Wadhwa, 1999) found that functional disability produced negative affect and symptom reporting; the same relationship did not hold for a sample with end-stage renal disease.

In all likelihood, the relationship between distressed mood and disability is reciprocal, with depression contributing to more impaired functioning, and higher levels of disability contributing to more depression. This position is also supported by epidemiological and clinical data (Bruce, 2000). Authors who reviewed the literature on depression among elderly people (Lenze, Rogers, Martire, Mulsant, & Rollman, 2001) concluded that depression puts people at risk for disability and vice versa, and that physical functioning improves when depression is treated. Gurland, Katz, and Pine (2000) examined the nature of the relationship theoretically. They asserted that depression and physical disorders are complexly interwoven phenomena, affected by multiple elements of the mind, body, and environment, and that there is no value to be gained from a search to determine which is a primary cause or effect.

Depression is considered to be a highly treatable condition. Several forms of psychotherapy have been found, through randomized controlled studies, to be effective with major depression (Chambless, 1998). Cognitive-behavioral therapy has most often been supported, and interpersonal therapy also has been found to be useful. Psychotherapy, in combination with medication, is probably the best alternative for treating serious depression. According to one study, anti-depressant medication alone is successful in about 60–70% of cases (Belanoff, DeBattista, & Schatzberg, 1998). Despite these encouraging results, very few (if any) empirical studies have attempted to measure the effects of treatment for depression among people with physical disabilities. Perhaps the findings that apply to the general population are equally valid for people with disabilities, but some careful research is needed. Just one study was located (King & Kennedy, 1999) that used a randomized design to test the effects a psychological intervention provided to people with disabilities (in this case, spinal cord injury). They documented greater reductions in levels of depression and anxiety among individuals who participated in a brief group counseling program.

It is interesting to speculate about why so few efforts apparently have been made to study the value of psychotherapy for people with disabilities. Perhaps it reflects the assumption, cited earlier, that such people are *expected* to be depressed and so nothing can be done about it. Practical issues such as transportation problems and lack of insurance coverage for services may also play a part. Alternatively, people with disabilities (like many other people) may be unwilling to acknowledge their psychological issues or need for psychotherapy. In Britain a study of 300 individuals who were newly-referred to general neurology outpatient clinics revealed that 47% met DSM criteria for one or more mental disorders (major depression being the most common), but only about one in five of those distressed individuals wanted psychological or psychiatric help (Carson, Ringbauer, MacKenzie, Warlow, & Sharpe, 2000).

Anxiety

Like depression, anxiety is a commonly used term that has both everyday meanings and specific diagnostic criteria, and it has often been linked to the presence of disability. In a colloquial sense, anxiety involves tension and worry, emotions that may be understandable concomitants of the onset of disability. Disabled people face uncertainties every time they enter new environments, meet new people, or take on new responsibilities. While some individuals take these challenges in stride, others experience anxiety to varying degrees.

The DSM-IV (American Psychiatric Association, 1994) sets out criteria for almost a dozen codable anxiety disorders, including acute stress disorder, generalized anxiety disorder, phobias, obsessive-compulsive disorder, and posttraumatic stress disorder. Taken together, they comprise the largest group of mental disorders (Morrison, 1995). They are also the mental conditions most often seen in primary care medical settings (Roy-Byrne & Katon, 2000).

A number of studies have reported a high incidence of anxiety disorders as well as depression among people with disabilities (Dersh, 2000; Diaz Olavarrieta, Cummings, Velazquez, & Garcia de al Cadena, 1999; Kanner & Nieto, 1999; Smith & Young, 2000). Among a sample of veterans with long-term spinal cord injury, over 40% screened positive for anxiety disorders (Weingardt, Hsu, & Dunn, 2001). All of the definitional and measurement issues described above with respect to depression also apply to anxiety. The lack of experimental studies regarding the value of psychotherapeutic intervention with people who have disabilities is similarly evident. Within the general population, however, medications and a number of treatments have proven effective in managing anxiety, including progressive relaxation, cognitive behavioral psychotherapy, systematic desensitization, and stress inoculation (Chambless, 1998). The development of virtual reality technology holds promise for increasingly effective treatment of phobias and other kinds of anxiety disorders (Rothbaum, Hodges, Ready, Graap, & Alarcon, 2001). A person could be exposed to a virtual situation that only slightly resembles a dreaded one, and after becoming accustomed to it could encounter incrementally more realistic situations. The final steps would involve switching from virtual exposure to real life.

Posttraumatic stress disorder (PTSD) is a special kind of anxiety disorder that sometimes occurs among people who have survived seriously shocking events, including spinal cord injury, extensive burns, heart attacks, and amputations (Martz & Cook, 2001). In PTSD, the individual repeatedly reexperiences the trauma through flashbacks or illusions. To escape the pain, the person attempts to avoid thinking about the event through suppression of related thoughts or the use of psychological defense mechanisms, including emotional numbing and repression of memories (Morrison, 1995).

A debate has occurred regarding whether people who sustain head injury and posttraumatic amnesia are ever subject to the development of PTSD symptoms. Some psychologists have argued that it is impossible to develop the syndrome if one is unable to remember the traumatic event (Sbordone, 1999). Cases have been reported, however, in which such individuals have developed PTSD (McNeil & Greenwood, 1996). A study of 47 active-duty service members in this condition (Warden, Labbate, Salazar, Nelson, Sheley, Staudenmeier, et al., 1997) revealed that although none of the participants met the full criteria for PTSD, 13% met the criteria of avoidance and hyperarousal, leading the authors to conclude that some patients with head injury may develop a form of PTSD, even though they do not reexperience the traumatic event. The risk seems to be particularly high among people with mild brain injury (Bontke, Rattok, & Boake, 1996; Wright & Telford, 1996).

According to the National Institute of Mental Health (NIMH, 1999) cognitive behavioral therapy, group therapy, systematic desensitization therapy, and medications have all proven to be helpful in dealing with the symptoms of PTSD.

Substance Abuse and Alcoholism

Disability can be caused or complicated by alcohol or other substance abuse. Substance abuse is a widespread problem in our society, and studies have indicated that the incidence among people with physical or mental disabilities is comparable to or higher than the incidence in the general population (Stude, 2002; Watson, Franklin, Ingram, & Eilenberg, 1998). More than 50% of some groups, such as those with traumatic injuries and young people with mental illness, may abuse alcohol or other substances. Many reasons could help to explain this situation. The substance may have been a contributor to the onset of the other disability in the first instance, and the urgency of the physical or mental problem might lead health workers to overlook the existence of substance issues. Conversely, life with a disability might increase the likelihood of substance abuse over the long run. Most people with disabilities are unemployed, meaning that they may be bored and have too few productive outlets. They may use substances as a way to defend against feelings of isolation and loneliness. Friends and family, feeling sympathy for the losses or deprivations that they perceive to be the individual's lot, may find drinking to be understandable. They are reluctant to take away what seems to be one of the person's few pleasures in life, so they avoid confronting abuse.

People with disabilities are often at risk for substance abuse for other reasons, too. They may have pain, which leads to self-medication with alcohol or street drugs. Alternatively, they may use prescription drugs such as opiates that are addictive over time. Of course, all of the reasons that lead anyone to abuse substances (pleasure, avoidance of problems, peer pressure, etc.) are equally applicable to people with disabilities.

The effects of substance abuse can be particularly problematic for people with disabilities (Watson, Franklin, Ingram, & Eilenberg, 1998). For those with learning disabilities or brain injuries, problems with memory, listening, and speaking can be increased. Alcohol and recreational drugs can interfere with the efficacy of many prescription medications. Furthermore, these substances can contribute to the development of secondary disabilities (for example, pressure sores among people with spinal cord injury) as a result of neglect or risky behaviors. Symptoms of mental illness are likely to be exacerbated by alcohol and other drugs as well.

If people with disabilities seek treatment for addiction, they may find it hard to locate services that are physically accessible or accommodating to other disabilities (e.g., ones that provide sign language interpreters for deaf people or ones that provide materials appropriate for those with cognitive disabilities). The ADA mandates accessibility in services, but reality is still far from that ideal. The Center for Substance Abuse Treatment, part of the Substance Abuse and Mental Health Services Administration (http://www.samhsa.gov) produced a Treatment Improvement Protocol, which outlines steps to be taken in order to make services accessible to those with coexisting disabilities. Other organizations such as the National Association for Alcohol, Drugs and Disability (NAADD) and the Rehabilitation Research and Training Center on Substance Abuse Resources and Disability Issues (SARDI) at Wright State University are among the organizations established during the 1990s to improve services and strengthen the knowledge base about this issue.

Psychiatric Rehabilitation

A chapter on psychotherapy would be incomplete without some discussion of services to people whose primary disability is mental illness. Paradoxically, however, psychiatric rehabilitation is distinct from treatment. Medication and psychotherapy are important to people with severe mental illness such as schizophrenia and mood disorders since they serve to reduce the severity of symptoms of illness. Psychiatric rehabilitation complements treatment by providing services to increase the level of functioning so that recipients are able to be as successful as possible in work and social roles within the community (Anthony, Cohen, Farkas, & Gagne, 2002).

According to the National Institute of Mental Health (NIMH, 1980) the population served by psychiatric rehabilitation includes those who have been hospitalized for psychiatric care or who have experienced continuous services for an extended period of time (at least two years). They also have impaired functioning in at least two major life areas such as work, personal relationships, and basic living skills, or have been involved with governmental welfare or legal systems. Anthony and colleagues (2002) traced the history of rehabilitation services, beginning with the 19th century moral therapists who used structured activity to change behavior. Continuing landmarks included the opening in 1941 of the state-federal vocational rehabilitation system to people with psychiatric disabilities, the development of community mental health centers, the creation of psychosocial rehabilitation centers (such as Fountain House), and the initiation of the federally funded Community Support System in the 1980s.

As the disability rights movement gathered strength throughout the country in the 1980s and 1990s, it also affected the systems providing psychiatric rehabilitation services. Individual empowerment and personal choice helped to propel the development of community-based services and to counteract the myth of the incurability of mental illness. In place of the concept of chronic mental illness came the idea of recovery. According to Anthony and colleagues (2002, p. 31), "Recovery is a deeply personal, unique process of changing one's attitudes, values, feelings, goals, skills, and/or roles. It is a way of living a satisfying, hopeful, and contributing life, with or without limitations caused by the illness. Recovery involves the development of new meaning and purpose in one's life as one grows beyond the catastrophic effects of a mental illness."

The primary interventions in psychiatric rehabilitation are skill development and the identification or creation of environmental supports (Anthony, Cohen, Farkas, & Gagne, 2002). A careful functional assessment serves to identify the individual's strengths and deficits so that a specific plan of services can be developed. The individual is a full partner in the rehabilitation process, exercising choice over direction and speed. Along with individual empowerment, psychiatric rehabilitation principles recognize the importance of relationships in the recovery process. The individual needs to know that trustworthy and caring people are available through good times and difficulties. Services are provided for as long as they are needed and wanted by the individual, and the essential outcomes involve improved residential, educational, and vocational functioning. Another principle of psychiatric rehabilitation is that hope is essential to recovery. Although it cannot substitute for the technologies of rehabilitation and treatment, it is a necessary and complementary contributor to change.

Conclusions

This chapter has summarized a variety of psychotherapeutic and rehabilitative interventions that address some of the issues faced by people with disabilities. The theme of individual control and autonomy is apparent in most of these areas, as is a pragmatic appreciation for tangible outcomes such as the ability to work, to maintain satisfying relationships, and to live independently.

14

Looking Ahead

The previous chapters of this volume have attempted to describe today's realities—sometimes contrasted with those of the past—surrounding the psychological experience of disability, plus the intervention techniques used to resolve some of the problems. This chapter will look to the future and discuss events, trends, and changes that seem necessary or desirable for reducing unproductive psychological suffering and improving the quality of life for people with disabilities.

As this book is going to press, many view the world as an increasingly perilous place, not only for people with disabilities, but for everyone. Within hours of occurrence, graphic accounts of violence from the corners of the globe are brought to our homes. Economic turbulence, earthquakes and hurricanes, wars and rumors of wars form a restless undercurrent beneath the conscious stream of thought we direct to daily activities. Even within the realm of concerns specific to disability, there are some reasons for pessimism. Supreme Court decisions have chipped away at the protection promised under the ADA. Millions of Americans are without health insurance, and unemployment figures for people with disabilities continue to be unacceptably high.

Without sliding to the opposite, Panglossian extreme, however, there are also reasons to believe that developments are unfolding that foreshadow changes and possibly even progress. Among them are a growing respect for diversity in the population of people with disabilities, increased collaboration between and among individuals with disabilities and professional service providers, new developments in medicine and technology, and increased recognition of the spiritual dimensions and needs of people with disabilities.

Diversity

The changing demographics of the United States population have been widely publicized and discussed. The White, Protestant majority of colonial times has evolved into a population that includes people from all corners of the globe. Demographers predict that within a few years people of European heritage will no longer constitute a majority of U.S. citizens but will be outnumbered by people of color, including Native Americans and those with ancestry in Africa, Asia, and Latin America. Rehabilitation providers are increasingly working with clients from diverse backgrounds, and research has suggested that we have not served them with equal effectiveness (Fiest-Price, 1995; Westbrook, 1999a). In addition, the numbers of professionals from racial and ethnic minorities does not match the proportions of clients from these groups, so the professions have not fully benefited from the varied perspectives they might offer.

The 1992 Amendments to the 1973 Rehabilitation Act established the Rehabilitation Cultural Diversity Initiative in recognition of the fact that disproportionately high numbers of people from racial and ethnic minority groups have disabilities. Five socioeconomic factors have been identified that help to account for this disparity. They include employment in physically taxing and dangerous jobs, low income or poverty, lack of health insurance, low educational achievement, and biased assessment procedures (Smart & Smart, 1997). These factors not only help to explain the high incidence of disability but also suggest that professional approaches that seem satisfactory for mainstream customers might not apply equally well to those from special populations.

Traditional psychological theories of personality and counseling were written with little or no regard to cultural issues. There theories, which have been broadly categorized as psychoanalytic, behavioral, and humanistic, have been joined by a "fourth force": multiculturalism. Whereas the earlier theories focused almost exclusively on the individual, multicultural counseling and therapy (MCT) puts emphasis on social and contextual issues and on people within their environments (Ivey, Ivey, & Simek-Morgan, 1997). MCT recognizes that people can only be understood within the context of their culture because culture tells individuals who they are, what goals they should seek, and what strategies are appropriate for achieving them. Different cultures have unique perspectives on family relationships, work, time, independence, and oral (as compared with written) communication, to name a few areas.

American culture places a high value upon individualism, and this acts as a powerful perceptual filter (Westbrook, 1999a). Most Americans believe in equality and would maintain that rehabilitation systems are free of bias. Furthermore, individuals who choose careers in rehabilitation are likely to be among the citizens who most emphatically ascribe to the dignity and equality of all people. Still, the ideology of individualism may serve to obscure our recognition of the fact that effective access to systems relies upon understanding the cultural rules and communicative conventions of the dominant social group (Stanton-Salazar, as cited in Westbrook, 1999). Westbrook also quotes Duarte and Rice (1992) who state that "dominant cultural values related to individualism, self-reliance, and work are evident in rehabilitation legislation, policies, and procedures" (p. 12). As a result, individuals from cultures with alternative priorities may be viewed as non-compliant and prematurely closed from services. Similarly, those individuals with a history of frustrating or discouraging encounters may distrust the system and be reluctant to seek services.

Robert Davila, formerly an official with the Office of Special Education and Rehabilitative Services of the U.S. Department of Education was quoted as saying that "rehabilitation professionals need to learn to recognize the cultural values of minority individuals and to adapt service delivery approaches accordingly" (National Institute on Disability and Rehabilitation Research [NIDRR], 1993). A number of suggestions have been made to aid providers with the process of adaptation (Balcazar, 2001, Westbrook, 1999a, 1999b). Agencies need to have a diverse staff that is able to work collaboratively with customers rather than bestowing services on passive recipients. Bilingual staff, flexible hours, child-care services, and openness to inclusion of family members in the rehabilitation process may also be helpful in reaching diverse communities. Educators and professional organizations are increasingly assuming responsibility for ensuring that providers have some level of skill in working with diverse populations. For example, in 1992 the American Counseling Association delineated multicultural competencies appropriate to its members, and in 2002 the American Psychological Association Council of Representatives approved "Guidelines on Multicultural Education, Training, Research, Practice, and Organizational Change for Psychologists. Accrediting bodies are also requiring attention to multicultural preparation within preservice training programs. It seems that the years of well-intentioned but ignorant practices may be coming to an end.

Aging

The number of older people with disabilities is increasing for two reasons. First, people with disabling conditions that would have led to early death are now surviving for years beyond the onset of the condition. People who sustained spinal cord injury before the availability of antibiotics, for example, seldom lived more than a year or two, and now some are still doing well after three and four decades. Similarly, people with serious head injury seldom survived to live with disability, but improved evacuation and emergency treatment now produce many survivors. HIV/AIDS was originally viewed as an immediate death sentence, but the discovery of increasingly effective medications has transformed it into a chronic disease, and people benefit from services that keep them independent and productive in the community.

Living to older ages following the onset of disability is certainly good news, although the process of aging also may bring increasing functional limitations and secondary conditions. Polio was once considered a stable disability. Following the period of acute infection and rehabilitation, the individual was presumed to plateau and experience no further change. Decades after the epidemics, however, the phenomenon of postpolio syndrome became evident. Muscles that had been weakened by the virus became weaker, and some muscles that had not originally appeared to be affected also showed signs of impairment. The compounding effects of aging on other conditions are also apparent. For example, people with Down syndrome have an increased risk of Alzheimer's dementia. People with spinal cord injury have increased risk of such systemic conditions as diabetes and cardiovascular disease. Research has found (Kemp, 1999) that people with physical disabilities experience the medical problems of aging about 15 years earlier than do people without disabilities. Furthermore, they have three to four times as many additional health problems. Interestingly, however, most people who are aging with a disability also report that life becomes more satisfying over time (Kemp, 1999).

The second reason for the increase in the number of older people with disabilities is that the total number of seniors within the population is growing. The average life span of Americans has been consistently increasing for decades, although the maximum age has not changed greatly. Perhaps with the unlocking of the human genome science will find ways to substantially extend the human life span. For now, the main change is that fewer and fewer people are dying prematurely of infectious diseases, childbirth, and trauma. As a result, greater proportions of the population are living to advanced ages. As many as three-quarters of all people who have lived to 65 years of age or older are alive today (O'Malley, 2002). The implications for disability and rehabilitation are obvious. The term "temporarily able-bodied" is sometimes used to identify anyone without a current disability. It implies, of course, that sooner or later everyone will have disabilities if they live long enough.

About 500,000 older workers leave employment every year because of disabling impairments and about 60% of those between ages 45 and 54 go back to work along with 27% of those age 55–64 (Morrison, 1991). Older workers face a complex array of barriers including discrimination by employers and their own negative attitudes and expectations. They are expected to have obsolete skills and difficulty with learning new ones, to be inflexible, and to have trouble with new technology. When the perceived limitations of age are added to disability, these doubly-disadvantaged workers receive little attention from the rehabilitation system. On the other hand, those who do receive services are more likely to be successful in their efforts to return to work.

Older people constitute a large proportion of the disability community in this country. Approximately 60% of the population of people with disabilities in the U.S. are age 45 or older (Sisco, 1991). The Switzer Seminar recommended that "The vocational rehabilitation system should focus more of its emphasis and efforts toward the older workers with disabilities and develop innovative methods and techniques aimed at promoting independence, personal choice, and dignity for this population" (Perlman & Hansen, 1991, p. 75) They also recommended better training of counselors for this work and more creativity and flexibility in services.

Zola (1991) called for a coalition between the aging and disability communities, maintaining that it is necessitated on both practical and philosophical grounds. The two groups have historically been split, partly because of competition for resources and also because neither group was eager to take on the stigma surrounding the other. Nevertheless, their needs for services that support independence in community living are essentially the same, and together their voices could carry increasing weight. Perhaps a liaison will be facilitated by more positive attitudes resulting from the increasing pride and organization that has occurred within both groups. Nelson (1991) predicted that the baby-boom generation is likely to have a major impact on attitudes toward older workers in the near future. The size of that generation helped to push many of the previous generation into early retirement, but the boomers are not being followed by a large cohort that will have a similar effect upon them. They will care for themselves with favorable legislative changes, and their dominance may make it more acceptable (and, Nelson predicts, even glamorous) to be an older person.

Health Care

The good news about health care is that medical science has made remarkable advances in the treatment of illness and disability, even with some conditions previously thought to be untreatable. Spinal cord injury is a prime example.

Research has demonstrated that neurons in the spinal cord can be helped to regenerate. Many routes toward restoration of function are being tried, including surgical, pharmacological, rehabilitative, regenerative, and remyelinative therapies (Young, 2002). Progress has been enormous since 1995. The key question seems no longer to be whether a cure for spinal cord injury is possible but rather when it will be found.

Delineating the developments in medical research goes beyond the scope of this book. There are astounding developments in many areas of medicine. For example, in pharmacology there are new drugs to treat mental illness. Surgeons can perform prenatal heart surgery on a fetus. Unlocking the human genome raises the hope that cures will be found for any number of genetically linked conditions. In a century medicine has progressed from being primarily supportive of ill and dying patients to a science that produces tangible results in the prevention and treatment of increasing numbers of conditions.

These gains, however, have come at a high price. A look at almost any newspaper or magazine will reveal alarm about the rapidly increasing cost of health care. Employers are reporting annual increases of up to 20% in costs, and state governments are decrying the impact of Medicare and Medicaid costs on their budgets. Consumers are carrying increasing burdens as well, with higher copays and deductibles. Health maintenance organizations (HMOs), which were intended to be the answer to rising health costs, are in trouble as well, with decreasing enrollments and consolidation of plans (O'Malley, 2002).

Dennis O'Malley, president of Craig Hospital, predicts that HMOs are likely to be superceded by insurance plans that cover catastrophic costs and leave responsibility for ordinary prevention and maintenance care to the consumer. He believes that national health policy decisions regarding resource allocations are inevitable because morality and economics are on a collision course. Some form of national health plan is likely inasmuch as the government is already paying about half of all health care costs (O'Malley, 2002).

For people with disabilities, these prospects are threatening. Lives may literally depend upon access to ongoing quality medical care, and in times of shortage there is always the prospect that they will be given the short end of the allocation. One suggested basis for rationing health care is to base decisions on quality-adjusted years of life—in other words, to approve services only for those people who are predicted to live longest at the highest quality of life. The obvious problem is that "outsiders" (including health care professionals who are likely to be the decision makers in such a system) have a significantly lower estimation of the quality of life experienced by people with disabilities than do those people themselves. Similar fears surround the discussion of legalizing assisted suicide. Not Dead Yet was founded by people who suspect that they and others with disabilities may be encouraged to do the world a favor by relinquishing their share of resources for the benefit of those who are younger and healthier. It would be nice to believe that these fears are groundless, but if there is one thing that the disability movement has learned, it is the importance of self-advocacy.

Technology

The development of assistive technology has greatly increased the potential of people with disabilities to live and work in the community. Probably the most potent innovation has been the Internet, with its ability to connect people with information, and with each other. Whether a person needs to identify equipment that will facilitate driving an automobile, or to organize a grassroots campaign on behalf of a legislative proposal, the Internet offers a prime vehicle for accomplishing one's goals.

The computer has made working possible for many people with severe disabilities, offering highly skilled jobs in information processing that demand little, if any, physical capacity. For people who need to work at home, telecommuting may be the answer to avoiding transportation and accessibility hassles. Suggestions for assistive technology solutions can be readily found on line through the Job Accommodation Network (http://janweb.icdi.wvu.edu/) and other Websites.

Inevitably, assistive technology applications will continue to grow and enhance life possibilities for people with disabilities. Medical and counseling services are becoming available in remote areas through telemedicine or telehealth networks (Jerome et al., 2000). Applications are just being created, and in all likelihood they will benefit people in all places and circumstances. Virtual reality is another emerging technology that holds special promise for people whose mobility may be limited by disability. At some point in the future it may be possible to engage a multisensory experience occurring thousands of miles away from the safety and comfort of home. At a more mundane level, perhaps principles of universal design will eventually lead to homes, workplaces, and communities that are accessible to everyone.

New Partnerships

Empowerment of individuals with disabilities has been discussed repeatedly in this book. The enactment of disability rights legislation, especially the

ADA and the creation of a network of Centers for Independent Living provide clear evidence of the growing authority of the disability community. Person-centered planning, and individualized and written plans for educational and vocational rehabilitation services, are also evidence that customers are becoming full partners in decisions about services that affect their lives.

NIDRR's long range plan states that the significance of Rehabilitation research has been enhanced by the combination of the disability rights movement and breakthroughs in biomedical and technological sciences. The agency's activities are being guided by a new understanding of what disability is and how it needs to be addressed. Table 14.1 outlines the distinctions between the "old" and "new" paradigms of disability.

The "old" paradigms resemble the medical model of disability, whereas the "new" paradigms reflect the sociopolitical model of disability that we discussed in Chapter 2 of this book. The significance of a model is that it points to the most important aspects of an issue and suggests the best roads to take in addressing the problems. Clearly, there are times when medical and psychological services are needed in order to help an individual reach the best level of functioning following onset of disability, so the old paradigm has its value in certain times and places. But the new model points out that in the long run, policy makers and researchers need to emphasize the questions of access to the society rather than restricting their attention to individual functioning. The disability rights movement has succeeded in refocusing the lens, and the society has become more enlightened.

Spirituality and Disability

The phenomenon of simultaneous discovery is well-known in science. Scientists, sometimes working on separate continents, produce an important invention or arrive at a major breakthrough at nearly the same moment in time. Similarly, we refer to "an idea whose time has come." After decades of absence or neglect, when the zeitgeist is right for the recognition of a concept, it becomes the focus of writing, research, and application. The relationship of spirituality to physical and psychological health seems to be such a phenomenon. Counselors' and psychologists' recent openness to spirituality issues coincides with a growing interest in the topic within American culture generally, as demonstrated by cover stories in popular magazines (e.g., Gibbs, 2002). Other related developments that have flourished in recent years include multiculturalism in counseling, increased acceptance of qualitative research in psychology, the positive psychology movement, and the popularization of complexity science (more about those later).

TABLE 14.1 Contrast of Paradigms

	"Old" Paradigms	"New" Paradigms
Definition of Disability	An individual is limited by his or her impairment or condition	An individual with an impairment requires an accommodation to perform functions required to carry out life activities
Strategy to Address Disability	Fix the individual, correct the deficit	Remove barriers, create access through accommodation and universal design, promote wellness and health.
Method to Address Disability	Provision of medical, vocational, or psychological rehabilitation services	Provision of supports, e.g., assistive technology, personal assistance services, job coach
Source of Intervention	Professionals, clinicians, and other rehabilitation service providers	Peers, mainstream service providers, consumer information services
Entitlements	Eligibility for benefits based on severity of impairment	Eligibility for accommodations seen as a civil right
Role of Disabled Individual	Object of intervention, patient, beneficiary, research subject	Consumer or customer, empowered peer, research participant, decision maker
Domain of Disability	A medical "problem"	A socioenvironmental issue involving accessibility, accommodations, and equity

Note: From "Contrast of Paradigms," by G. DeJong and B. O'Day, 1999, National Institute on Disability and Rehabilitation Research. Available at http://www.dcddr.org/new/lrp.html. Reprinted with permission of the author.

Psychology emerged as a discipline from philosophy, and much of its early focus concerned consciousness and other subjective matters. The influence of the behaviorists during and after the 1920s, however, led to an increasing emphasis on observable phenomena that could be studied using methods of the physical sciences and a proportional withdrawal of attention from things that could not be seen and measured. Hence, scientific psychology became strongly oriented toward empirical research. The practice of counseling and clinical psychology, of course, by necessity continued to deal with the subjective experience of individuals, but even within that realm certain topics were more acceptable than others.

Spirituality and Religion: Distinctions and Connections

This section will address spirituality and religion, sometimes sliding from one term to the other. We recognize, of course, that they are distinct but related areas. Although it is possible for a person to be highly spiritual without being involved in organized religion (and presumably also possible for one to practice religion in a rote manner with minimal attention to spiritual matters), many people find that religion is the means by which they express their spirituality. For them, spirituality and religion are essentially interchangeable.

Reasons for the Neglect of Spirituality and Religion in Psychosocial Rehabilitation

For many reasons, spiritual matters have rarely been considered during the process of rehabilitation. The medical model of rehabilitation is secular, discarding ancient beliefs that disability is punishment for sinful behavior on the part of individuals or their ancestors, so spiritual issues are considered irrelevant to healing. In addition, counselors may fear offending clients by intruding on intensely personal beliefs. Also, religion has been the source of many negative effects, such as shame and zealotry, in addition to positive effects such as comfort and altruism. Fear of the negative elements may have contributed to counselors' wariness of the area.

Many other reasons contribute to the exclusion of spirituality from rehabilitation services. Most important, perhaps, is that counselors have been relatively unaware of how important these matters are to people dealing with illness and disability (Kilpatrick & McCullough, 1999). A Gallup poll, taken on the eve of the new millennium (Carballo) found that 91% of North Americans have a religious affiliation, and 83% report that God is very important in their lives. Among the believers, 64% see God as a personal being, and most of the rest think of God as a life force or spirit. In addition to this strong base rate of belief, many people become particularly attuned to spiritual matters when they are faced with threat and pain.

It has been suggested that psychologists and counselors are less religious than the general population, and studies indicate that indeed they may be less likely to be involved in organized religion (Kilpatrick & McCullough, 1999) On the other hand, their spiritual interests do not lag. A study of counselors belonging to the American Counseling Association (Kelly, 1995) revealed that almost 90% of respondents have some spiritual orientation, including 70% who indicated a religious affiliation. Kelly also investigated the values held by counselors and found that there was a high level of consensus in support of humanistic values. In particular, they endorsed broad-mindedness and tolerance of others' beliefs, benevolence, and self-direction. On the other hand, they disavowed power as a value, and they were also below normative means on tradition and stimulation. Given the high priority that respondents placed on respecting the diversity of others' values, they may have been particularly reluctant to risk imposing their own views on clients during therapy, and thus avoided the topic altogether

Another reason why spiritual matters typically have been neglected in rehabilitation is that training programs have not prepared psychologists and counselors in this area. They have not been taught how to evaluate or deal with spiritual concerns, and typical interview protocols and psychological tests do not include these domains. Without guidelines or expectations, and with subliminal trepidation about the consequences of exploration, it is easy to see why spirituality would be left out of typical treatment interactions. Some of the methods that could be used to teach about spirituality include case studies, interviews, and readings in the philosophy and literature of diverse cultures (Burke et al., 1999). Coping with loss, aging, and pain are common challenges for people with disabilities, and the spiritual dimensions of any of these could be incorporated into real or composite case studies. Many training programs encourage students to receive counseling for themselves in order to better understand their own motivations, beliefs, and biases, but this effort may not extend to an examination of one's spiritual values. Ironically, when a counselor avoids these matters and does not clearly understand his or her own beliefs, there is increased danger that his or her values may unwittingly influence the counseling process (Burke et al., 1999).

A parallel is apparent between attention to spirituality and to cultural diversity in counseling. For many years, psychological training reflected the dominant culture's assumption of "the melting pot." Counseling theories and methods were presumed to be equally applicable to everyone across the board. The gradual awakening to gender differences and cultural distinctions has produced a raft of recent research and a new sensitivity to the needs of diverse groups. Among the individual differences that may affect a person's response to disability, religious and spiritual beliefs are critically important. As Burke and colleagues noted (1999), the relationship between counselor and client may be jeopardized when the counselor assumes that religion is irrelevant and fails to attend to the unique perspectives of a Jewish, Muslim, Christian, Buddhist, Hindu, or traditional native client. Not only are their practices likely to differ, but their worldviews are almost certainly colored by their faith. In addition, each belief system may be differentially responsive to psychological interventions and each may provide access to unique and beneficial techniques.

Opening the Door to Spirituality and Religion in Rehabilitation

McCarthy (1995) advocated greater openness to spirituality in rehabilitation counseling, stating that "adoption and integration of spiritual perspectives and practices could make rehabilitation more in keeping with its professed ethos. It would reinforce the profession's expressed commitments to: (a) treating the client holistically; (b) maximizing consumer choice and self-responsibility; (c) upholding the dignity and worth of all individuals; and (d) responding to client values" (pp. 91–92). McCarthy's position was echoed by Curtis (1998), who delineated the core values inherent in rehabilitation practice as follows: (1) altruism, which includes individual dignity and worth and the self-actualization process; (2) choice, which includes community participation, integration, least restrictive environment, and mainstreaming normalization; (3) empowerment, which includes independence, self-control, and self-determination; and (4) equality and individualism, which include autonomy, freedom, responsibility, and self-reliance. Values reflect what we hold to be important and, like attitudes, they motivate and guide our actions and choices. These values are reflected in our mission statements and our codes of conduct.

Some other pragmatic reasons argue for the inclusion of spiritual matters in counseling with people who have disabilities. The Joint Commission on Accreditation of Healthcare Organizations (2001) requires that spiritual and religious needs be taken into account in serving patients. Further, individuals may experience services as being more helpful if these needs are addressed. One study (Fitchett, Rybarczyk, DeMarco, & Nicholas, 1999) among medical rehabilitation patients found that people who reported that they had discussed spiritual issues were more likely to describe the counseling as helpful than did those who did not discuss those issues.

The inclusion of religion and spirituality in counseling, however, raises a number of ethical issues. Yarhouse and VanOrman (1999) examined the American Psychological Association's 1992 "Ethical Principles of Psychologists and Code of Conduct" and applied its precepts to work with religious clients. Based upon the principle of competence, psychologists must become knowledgeable about the values and beliefs that affect the reasoning and coping strategies of religious clients. They also need to be aware of the ways in which the beliefs and values of psychological theorists are reflected in theories of personality, because those theories affect the decisions therapists make in counseling. They pointed out the ways in which the values of secular psychology may conflict with the priorities of religious clients, such as the potential conflict between the emphasis that psychology places on the "self" in contrast to religion's frequent focus on the "other" (altruism). Psychologists are more likely to fail to recognize value conflicts when the client is from a cultural or ethnic group whose life view is unfamiliar. Locust (1995) described the many ways in which traditional beliefs of native people may lead to conflict in rehabilitation. For example, religious events and holidays of native people do not appear on our calendar, so an individual may be caught between attending a religious event and keeping an appointment with a rehabilitation counselor or employer.

Integrity, another principle of the APA ethical code, requires psychologists to be attuned to their own beliefs and how these affect their work. Professional responsibility implies that they should be familiar with community resources that could be of help to religious clients, and that they refer individuals whose values present barriers to effective collaboration (Yarhouse & VanOrman, 1999). For example, some individuals may value their spiritual well-being above mental health as typically understood by psychologists, yet the therapist has a responsibility to aid clients in making their own informed life choices.

Yarhouse and VanOrman (1999) made several recommendations for therapists working with religious clients. These included becoming educated about various religious traditions, routinely assessing religious functioning and preferences of clients, and providing services that are congruent with the beliefs and practices of religious clients. Interventions such as the use of prayer, meditation, forgiveness, and the reading or memorization of sacred texts may be useful. They also admonish therapists to be attuned to their own religious values and aware of the values that are inherent in the counseling theories from which they work so that potential conflicts can be recognized. Further, therapists should become knowledgeable about community resources for religious individuals and develop a varied referral network of colleagues from other traditions. Together, these steps can lead to more relevant and effective treatment.

Why Is Spirituality so Important to Human Beings?

Perhaps the most obvious answer to this question is that people have the unique ability to anticipate the future, including their own aging and death. This awareness leads them to ponder the meaning of life, the source of their being, and their relationship to the rest of creation. The desire for spiritual connection is a deep part of the human psyche. McLafferty and Kirylo (2001) noted that outstanding contributors to psychology such as Jung, Frankl, Maslow, and Assagioli agreed that two developmental processes are essential for healthy people. One is the unfolding of individual personality, and the other is the aligning of that personality with a transcendent spiritual center. Vash (1994) noted that "We weaken the effectiveness of our efforts by trying to provide services as if a major aspect of human nature did not exist. Instead of remaining silent, we can learn how to keep our personal opinions under control while we help others deal with their psychospiritual issues" (p. 25).

Spirituality and Health

Given that the vast majority of individuals with severe medical conditions rely on religious coping (Koenig, 1997), and that many individuals have written of the importance of their religious faith in meeting the challenges of disability (e.g., Levy, 1995; Nosek, 1995) one might be led to conclude that believers would consistently show better health and psychological adjustment. In fact, however, research indicates that the relationships are quite mixed and inconsistent (Kilpatrick & McCullough, 1999). Worthington and colleagues (1996) produced a comprehensive summary of empirical research on religion and psychotherapy, which followed his earlier compendium of research conducted between 1974 and 1984. For their recent article they located 148 studies covering such topics as religion and mental health, coping with stress, and religion and counselors. Readers who desire a detailed overview of empirical work in this area may wish to study their article.

One reason for the inconsistent relationships is that different types of religious beliefs and practices may have different effects. Some positive examples include finding meaning in trying experiences, believing that one has intrinsic value to the creator, and having social as well as spiritual support. Byrd (1997) pointed out that participation in a community of faith provides support, acceptance, and caring that cannot be offered by professional agencies. A qualitative study of adults with physical disabilities and parents of children with disabilities (Treloar, 1999) led to the conclusion that religious factors, particularly the individuals' relationship with God, influenced adaptation to disability and stabilized their lives. The spiritual beliefs of the participants enabled them to live with joy and gratitude, despite the challenges of disability. An epidemiological study of 2,812 older adults in Connecticut (Idler & Kasl, 1997, cited in Kilpatrick & McCullough, 1999) found that attending religious services was correlated with fewer interpersonal conflicts and fewer complaints of physical illness. Correlates of religious participation included higher levels of physical activity, higher leisure activity, more close relatives, and higher levels of optimism (Kilpatrick & McCullough, 1999). On the other hand, believing that one's disability is punishment for evil behavior could induce shame and lead a person to succumb to limitations because they seemed to be deserved. Such a belief system would be counterproductive to adjustment. Another example of negative coping includes the belief that one is being abandoned by God (Pargament, 1997). Such beliefs are not unusual. Anderson, Anderson, and Felsenthal (1999) reported that approximately a quarter of the patients they interviewed believed that God was punishing them, and a similar number believed that they were losing purpose in life.

Fitchett and colleagues (1999) suggested a number of mechanisms that may lie behind the mixed correlations between religion and health. First, religion may play a protective role by preventing health problems through avoidance of behaviors such as smoking, and alcohol and recreational drug usage. This should lead to a positive correlation between religion and health. Second, religion may provide consolation to people who are suffering from illness. In this case, the sickest individuals might be expected to rely most on religion, so the correlation between religious feelings and health would be negative. Third, religious practice could be a passive coping strategy that displaces active, problem-oriented coping strategies, and so results in poorer adjustment. The authors conducted a study with people undergoing rehabilitation, predicting that (a) higher levels of spiritual and religious beliefs and practices, (b) higher levels of positive religious coping, and (c) lower levels of negative coping would positively affect their recovery. For the most part, their predictions were not substantiated, although they found that religion might have been consoling to some people who made limited recovery. They found that although correlational data supported their hypotheses, religious variables did not add significantly to a regression equation after physical and psychological variables had been entered. They also found that some forms of negative religious coping may interfere with recovery.

The Challenges of Subjecting Spirituality to Research

The sometimes conflictual or inconclusive results apparent in the research reported to date reflect, in part, the difficulties inherent in studying this subject. Quantitative studies use objective measures and statistical tests to try to identify truths that can be generalized from a sample of participants to the wider population. Measures of spirituality and religion that have traditionally been used include attendance at religious services, participation in other religious activities, private meditation or devotional activities, religious beliefs, and/or positive and negative religious coping.

Perhaps the most ambitious and sophisticated quantitative approach to the study of spirituality was developed by Piedmont (2001) with the creation of the Spiritual Transcendence Scale (STS). He validated it using the Five Factor Model of Personality, an empirically based comprehensive taxonomy of normal personality and individual differences (Costa & McCrae, 1992). The taxonomy includes five major domains: neuroticism, extroversion, openness, agreeableness, and conscientiousness. Piedmont sought to determine whether spiritual variables represent a separate major dimension of personality, distinct from the other five. The STS was subjected to factor analysis and found to have a single primary factor composed of three facet scales: prayer fulfillment, universality (a common bond among all life), and connectedness (a belief that one is part of a greater human reality that cuts across generations and groups). Piedmont concluded that spirituality is, indeed, a major motivational trait that drives behaviors. He believes that because of our awareness of mortality we strive to build an understanding of purpose and the meaning of our lives. Those constructs provide coherence and a reason for living productive lives. They also provide a sense of spiritual transcendence, "the capacity of individuals to stand outside of their immediate sense of time and place and to view life from a larger, more objective perspective. This transcendent perspective is the one in which a person sees a fundamental unity underlying the diverse strivings of nature" (Piedmont, 1999, p. 988).

Qualitative methods represent a way to tap the nuances of spiritual meaning that are unique to individuals. Of the possible approaches to measuring religious and spiritual functioning, the most direct would simply be to ask people to describe how their beliefs and practices might affect the ways they cope with physical problems (Matthews et al., 1998). Matthews and colleagues were particularly concerned about identifying individuals who might blame God or feel they are being punished or feel estranged, characteristics that might indicate a special need for psychological intervention.

Several questions about religion and spirituality were included as part of extensive life story interviews that one of the authors (NC) conducted with 50 people who had lived more than 20 years with spinal cord injury. Following a protocol developed by McAdams (1988) participants were asked to describe their religious beliefs, to indicate the ways in which their beliefs differ from those of other people, and to indicate whether they had changed over the years. The responses were as variable as the individuals themselves. Like the general population, most of the respondents professed belief in God, and most identified with some form of Christianity, but specific responses covered the spectrum of possibilities. Some had a strong and vibrant faith that permeated daily life, others were ambivalent, others apathetic, and a few were adamantly negative. One individual, for example, commented that God is real to him and prayer is wonderful. Another described her belief in the Bible and her personal, hourly relationship with Christ. Another participant said that he believes in a force, a deity, but not organized religions. He added that he was more into spirituality, good and evil, and karma. Someone else said that he believes and prays but avoids going to church because of the hypocrites. Someone else said he had no interest in religion. He believes in Darwin, sees people as primates, and doesn't believe that anyone created the world.

Diversity was also apparent in the relationship between the onset of disability and beliefs. Some said that their views had not changed at all, whereas others said that disability had either weakened or strengthened their faith. For example, one person said that his beliefs were challenged at the time of the injury, and it took a while to reestablish his confidence in God and his connection with the church. Someone else said that she always had a strong faith, and getting injured strengthened it quite a bit. Another said that he was glad that he came to know the truth of God, even though it took a severed spine to make him pay attention. Another person left the church and never felt a need for it afterwards. Still another said that he had become more scientific over the years, so questions of faith aren't as important any more. He then added at bit wistfully, "part of me would like to be wrong."

One additional conclusion that matched other published research is that there was no clear correlation between faith (or lack of it) and quality of life and emotional adjustment. Not that the two were unrelated in the minds of individual respondents. In fact, the opposite was true. People who had strong religious beliefs indicated that it gave them hope and purpose, and helped them to survive. People who professed amorphous spiritual beliefs and those who rejected religion altogether seemed to take their resulting independence as a sign of their positive adjustment.

Complexity Science

Perhaps one reason for the inconsistent findings and the lack of any firm conclusions about relationships between spirituality and disability is that we have not yet developed the research tools that can enable an adequate analysis of the questions we would like to answer. Western science is descended from Greek thought which held that "there are fixed things which change from time to time" (Battram, 1998, p. 13), rather than assuming that change is the constant and natural order of things. The dominant metaphor that science has used to understand the world, at least since the time of Newton, is that of a large machine, often a clock. The metaphor indicates that by investigating all of the parts one can come to understand the whole—that the machine (or the organism) is the sum of its parts. By understanding the parts, it becomes possible to predict and control behavior, and in so doing you have understood and explained the system.

The Newtonian model has been responsible for enormous scientific progress, and its laws have not been revoked. They work spectacularly well for predicting much of the physical and mechanical world. On the other hand, the model does not apply well to living systems because it does not allow for choice, goals, and the idiosyncrasies of perception that result from experience and unique mental models. A new theoretical framework is required to understand these systems. Complexity science (also known as chaos theory) is developing the language, theories, and metaphors to account for such phenomena, ones that depend upon patterns of relationships more than parts. Human beings are complex adaptive systems, and so are weather systems, stock markets, universities, and ecosystems. Such systems consist of multitudes of interconnected agents that seem to function independently according to their own knowledge and interests. As parts of a larger system, however, the agents are interdependent. Because of the linkages between them, their attributes are both cause and effect to the other components in the system.

Complex adaptive systems (also called nonlinear dynamical systems) are constantly experiencing change. Periods of stability are inevitably toppled by internal or environmental disturbances. Stress accumulates, and the system is propelled toward a bifurcation, a choice point. These bifurcations may multiply, leading the system toward a state of disorder and finally into chaos. Chaos in this sense, however, does not mean a hopeless state of confusion and dissipation. Instead, there is within chaos an attractor that serves to maintain boundaries around disordered behavior and that eventually moves the system toward a new stability (Williams & Arrigo, 2002). Outcomes emerge from a process of self-organization, and so it is impossible to predict just what outcomes will occur in these systems (Zimmerman, Lindberg, & Plsek, 2001). The outcomes do not follow in a linear way from the size of the input that the system receives. Very small changes can lead to entirely different and novel outcomes. In any case, the system will be changed; the new stability never will be exactly the same as the old equilibrium (Williams & Arrigo, 2002). It is through the experience of disorder that the system grows and becomes stronger and more flexible.

The process of adjustment to disability may be understood in new ways when seen through the lens of complexity science. In traditional social science research, investigators look for general patterns that apply across samples. Outliers may be discarded as nuisances, and apparently insignificant variables may be disregarded in favor of those that are presumed to have major impact. The principles of complexity science, however, suggest that relatively minor differences in the initial condition of a system may lead to major differences over time (Williams & Arrigo, 2002). Further, the principles of progression from order to disorder and back to order over time, as well as the process self-organization, helps to explain the often observed phenomenon that out of adversity comes growth and strength (Vash, 1994).

With regard to the issue of spirituality and health, the individual elements that may seem to explain one individual's beliefs and practices may lead someone else on quite a different path. Many elements may go into shaping an individual's faith, and there are also emergent elements that cannot be explained by the parts. A complexity science approach would not discard the study of the parts (micro analysis) but would add a holistic analysis to the investigation. Before the availability of powerful computers, such an approach would have been impossible, but it may soon come within reach, allowing us to replace a reductionistic and deterministic search for predictors of behavior with a deeper understanding of human needs and growth.

In addition to opening new windows in the study of individuals and disability, complexity science may provide a theoretical framework for examining the fields of rehabilitation and disability policy. Williams and Arrigo (2002) have written a challenging book that explores the intersection of law and psychology in the mental health system. They propose that many troubling practices such as civil commitment and enforced mental health treatment could be addressed more coherently and often with different results if complexity science were recognized as the theoretical framework for the justice system. Their work is highly recommended as we look ahead to the future of disability and rehabilitation.

In the two decades that have elapsed since publication of the first edition of this book, significant changes have occurred in legislative protection, social attitudes and technology. Taken together, they have improved life with disability for many in western society, but the work is yet unfinished. In the coming decades, continued advocacy and research, enhanced by new tools such as complexity science, may lead us toward deeper understanding of the disability experience and greater capacity for assisting people with disabilities in their struggle for freedom, dignity, and human connectedness.

References

Abledata (2002). *Welcome to ABLEDATA, the premier source for information on assistive technology.* Retrieved July 31, 2002, from http://www.abledata.com

Accessibility (2002). *National Center on Physical Activity & Disability.* Indiana University. Retrieved July 31, 2002, from http://www.ncaonline.org/research/ncpad.htm

Accordino, M. P. (1999). Implications of disability for the family: Implementing behavioral family therapy in rehabilitation education. *Rehabilitation Education, 13*(4), 287–293.

ADAPT. *A Community-based alternative to nursing homes and institutions for people with disabilities.* National ADAPT. Retrieved August 2, 2002, from http://www.adapt.org/casaintr.htm

Aguilera, R. J. (2000). Disability and delight: Staring back at the devotee community, *Sexuality and Disability, 18*(4), 255–261

Allen, K., Finn, M. L., Oddlerez, H., & Willer, B. S. (1994). Family burden following traumatic brain injury. *Rehabilitation Psychology, 39*(1), 29–48.

American Association of Marriage and Family Therapy (AAMFT). (2002). *Who are Marriage and Family Therapists?* Retrieved August 5, 2002, from http://www.aamft.org/faqs/whatis.htm

American Psychiatric Association (1994). *Diagnostic and statistical manual for mental health disorders* (4th ed.). Washington, DC: Author.

Anderson, J. M., Anderson, L. J., & Felsenthal, G. (1999). Pastoral needs and support within an inpatient rehabilitation unit. *Archives of Physical Medicine & Rehabilitation, 74,* 574–578.

Annon, J. S. (1976). *Behavioral treatment of sexual problems: Brief therapy.* Oxford, England: Harper & Row.

Anthony, W., Cohen, M., Farkas, M., & Gagne, C. (2002). *Psychiatric Rehabilitation* (2nd ed.). Boston: Boston University.

Athelstan, G. T., & Crewe, N. M. (1979). Psychological adjustment to spinal cord injury as related to manner of onset of disability. *Rehabilitation Counseling Bulletin, 22,* 311–319.

Bach, G., & Deutch, R. (1970). *Pairing.* New York: Peter H. Wyden.

Balcazar, F. E. (2001, 04/30/02). *Strategies for reaching out to minority individuals with disabilities.* National Center for the Dissemination of Disability Research. Retrieved December 6, 2002, from http://www.ncddr.org/du/researchexchange/v06n02/

Balcazar, F. E., Fawcett, S. B., & Seekins, T. (1991). Teaching people with disabilities to recruit help to attain personal goals. *Rehabilitation Psychology, 36*(1), 31–42.

Balcazar, F. E., Seekins, T., Fawcett, S. B., & Hopkins, B. L. (1990). Empowering people with physical disabilities through advocacy skills training. *American Journal of Community Psychology, 18*(2), 281–296.

Barber, M., Jenkins, R., & Jones, C. (2000). A survivor's group for women who have a learning disability. *British Journal of Developmental Disabilities, 46*(90, Pt. 1), 31–41.

Barker, V. L., & Brunk, B. (1991). The role of a creative arts group in the treatment of clients with traumatic brain injury. *Music Therapy Perspectives, 9*, 26–31.

Barlow, J. H., & Barefoot, J. (1996). Group education for people with arthritis. *Patient Education and Counseling, 27*(3), 257–267.

Battram, A. (1998). *Navigating complexity: The essential guide to complexity theory in business and management.* London: The Industrial Society.

Beck, A. T., Guth, D., Steer, R. A., & Ball, R. (1997). Screening for major depression disorders in medical inpatients with the Beck Depression Inventory for Primary Care. *Behaviour Research and Therapy, 35*(8), 785–791.

Beisser, A. (1979). Denial and affirmation in illness and health. *American Journal of Psychiatry, 136*(8), 1026–1030.

Belanoff, J. K., DeBattista, C., & Schatzberg, A. F. (1998). Adult pharmacology 1: Common usage. In G. P. Koocher, J. C. Norcross, & S. S. I. Hill (Eds.), *Psychologists' desk reference* (pp. 395–400). New York: Oxford University Press.

Benshoof, J. (2000, July 21). *CyberCIL of Arizona: The first virtual center for independent living.* Retrieved August 6, 2002, from http://www.cybercil.com/

Berscheid, E., & Walster, E. (1974). Physical attractiveness. In L. Berkowitz (Ed.), *Advances in experimental social psychology* (Vol. 7, pp. 157–215). New York: Academic Press.

Black, R. B., & Weiss, J. O. (1990). Genetic support groups and social workers as partners. *Health and Social Work, 15*(2), 91–99.

Bodenheimer, C., Kerrigan, A. J., Garber, S. L., & Monga, T. N. (2000). Sexuality in persons with lower extremity amputations. *Disability and Rehabilitation: An International Multidisciplinary Journal, 22*(9), 409–415.

Bolton, B. F. (Ed.). (2001). *Handbook of measurement and evaluation in rehabilitation* (3rd ed.). Gaithersburg, MD: Aspen.

Bontke, C. F., Rattok, J., & Boake, C. (1996). Do patients with mild brain injuries have posttraumatic stress disorder too? *Journal of Head Trauma Rehabilitation, 11*(1), 95–102.

Boyd, T. (2001). *Gym makes working out easy for all.* iCan Online. Retrieved July 31, 2002, from http://www.ican.com/news/fullpage

Bramston, P., & Fogarty, G. (2000). The assessment of emotional distress experienced by people with an intellectual disability: A study of different methodologies. *Research in Developmental Disabilities, 21*(6), 487–500.

Brewin, C. R. (1989). Cognitive change processes in psychotherapy. *Psychological Review, 96*(3), 379–394.

Bridges, W. (1994). *Job shift: How to prosper in a workplace without jobs.* Reading, MA: Addison-Wesley.

Brinded, P. M. J. (1998). A case of acquittal following confession in a police videotaped interview. *Psychiatry, Psychology and Law, 5*(1), 133–138.

Brown, S. (1999). *Peer counseling: Advocacy-oriented peer support.* Retrieved August 6, 2002, from http://www.ilru.org/ilnet/files/reading/peer1.html

Brown, S. A., & Hanis, C. L. (1995). A community-based, culturally sensitive education and group-support intervention for Mexican Americans with NIDDM: A pilot study of efficacy. *The Diabetes Educator, 21*(3), 203–210.

Bruce, M. L. (2000). Depression and disability. In G. M. Williamson & D. R. Shaffer (Eds.), *Physical illness and depression in older adults: A handbook of theory, research, and practice* (pp. 11–29). New York: Kluwer Academic/Plenum Publishers.

Buck, F. M. (1993). Parenting by fathers with physical disabilities. In F. P. Haseltine, S. S. Cole, et al. (Eds.), *Reproductive issues for persons with physical disabilities* (pp. 163–185). Baltimore: Paul H. Brookes.

Buck, F. M., & Hohmann, G. W. (1983). Parental disability and children's adjustment. *Annual Review of Rehabilitation, 3*, 203–241.

Buckelew, S. P., et al. (1994). Self-efficacy and pain behavior among subjects with fibromyalgia. *Pain, 59*(3), 377–384.

Buckelew, S. P., Conway, R., Parker, J., Deuser, W. E., Read, J., Witty, T. E., Hewett, J. E., Minor, M., Johnson, J. C., Van Male, L., McIntosh, M. J., Nigh, M., & Kay, D. R. (1998). Biofeedback/relaxation training and exercise interventions for fibromyalgia: A prospective trial. *Arthritis Care and Research, 11*(3), 196–209.

Buckelew, S. P., Huyser, B., Hewett, J. E., Parker, J. C., et al. (1996). Self-efficacy predicting outcome among fibromyalgia subjects. *Arthritis Care and Research, 9*(2), 97–104.

Bulman, R., & Wortman, C. B. (1977). Attributions of blame and coping in the "real world". Severe accident victims respond to their lot. *Journal of Personality and Social Psychology, 35*, 351–363.

Burke, M. T., Hackney, H., Hudson, P., Miranti, J., Watts, G. A., & Epp, L. (1999). Spirituality, religion, and CACREP curriculum standards. *Journal of Counseling and Development, 77*(3), 251–257.

Byrd, E. K. (1997). Concepts related to inclusion of the spiritual component in services to persons with disability and chronic illness. *Journal of Applied Rehabilitation Counseling, 28*(4), 26–29.

Carballo, M. *Gallup International Millennium Survey: Religion in the world at the end of the millennium.* Gallup de la Argentina. Retrieved June 10, 2002, from http://www.gallup-international.com/

Carson, A. J., Ringbauer, B., MacKenzie, L., Warlow, C., & Sharpe, M. (2000). Neurological disease, emotional disorder, and disability: They are related: A study of 300 consecutive new referrals to a neurology outpatient department. *Journal of Neurology, Neurosurgery and Psychiatry, 68*(2), 202–206.

Centers for Disease Control (1998, 4/14/2001). Disabilities. Conference proceedings of National Conference on Disability and Health: Building Bridges for Science and Consumers. National Center on Birth Defects and Developmental Disabilities. Retrieved July 15, 2002, from http://www.cdc.gov/ncbddd/dh/publications/

Centers for Disease Control (2001, September, 6). Prevention. Healthy people with disabilities: HP 2010 data on disparities. Retrieved July, 15, 2002, from http://www.cdc.gov/ncbddd/fact/hpfs2.htm

Chaisson, R. E., Keruly, J. C., McAvinue, S., Gallant, J. E., & Moore, R. D. (1996). Effects of an incentive and education program on return rates for PPD test reading in patients with HIV infection. *Journal of Acquired Immune Deficiency Syndromes and Human Retrovirology, 11*(5), 455–459.

Chambless, D. L. (1998). Empirically validated treatments. In G. P. Koocher, J. C. Norcross, & S. S. I. Hill (Eds.), *Psychologists' desk reference* (pp. 209–219). New York: Oxford University Press.

Chiodo, A., Cole, T. M., Finkel, S., Jacobson, R., & Stockford, J. (2001). *A health promotion workshop for persons with spinal cord injury: Participants' manual.* Ann Arbor, MI: University of Michigan Health System.

Chwalisz, K. (1996). The perceived stress model of caregiver burden: Evidence from spouses of persons with brain injuries. *Rehabilitation Psychology, 41*(2), 91–114.

Chwalisz, K., & Vaux, A. (2000). Social support and adjustment to disability. In R. G. Frank & T. R. Elliott (Eds.), *Handbook of rehabilitation psychology* (pp. 537–552). Washington, DC: American Psychological Association.

Clare, I. C. H., & Gudjonsson, G. H. (1995). The vulnerability of suspects with intellectual disabilities during police interviews: A review and experimental study of decision-making. *Mental Handicap Research, 8*(2), 110–128.

Cole, S. S. (1991). Facing the challenges of sexual abuse in persons with disabilities. In R. P. Marinelli & A. E. Dell Orto (Eds.), *The psychological & social impact of disability* (3rd ed., pp. 223–235). New York: Springer Publishing.

Commission on Rehabilitation Counselor Certification (CORC). (2001). *Professional Code of Ethics for Rehabilitation Counselors.* Retrieved August 6, 2002, from http://www.crccertification.com/code.html

Connell, C., & Berkowitz, H. (1976). *Rehabilitation for the disabled family in stress.* Research prepared for the California State Department of Rehabilitation at Los Angeles, Los Angeles, CA.

Corbett, J. (1999). Disability arts: Developing survival strategies. In P. Retish & S. Reiter (Eds.), *Adults with disabilities: International perspectives in the community* (pp. 171–181). Mahwah, NJ: Lawrence Erlbaum Associates.

Corker, M. (2001). "Isn't that what girls do?": Disabled young people construct (homo) sexuality in situated social practice. *Educational and Child Psychology, 18*(1), 89–107.

Cornish, E. (Ed.) (1982). *Communication tomorrow: The coming of the information society.* Bethesda, MD: World Future Society.

Costa, P. T. J., & McCrae, R. R. (1992). *NEO-PI-R professional manual.* Odessa, FL: Psychological Assessment Resources.

Cousins, N. (1979). *Anatomy of an illness.* New York: Norton.

Cox, B. J. (1999). Predictors of depression in adults with cerebral palsy: A biopsychosocial model. *Dissertation Abstracts, 60*(4-B), 1847.

Coyne, J. C., Thompson, R., Palmer, S. C., Kagee, A., & Maunsell, E. (2000). Should we screen for depression? Caveats and potential pitfalls. *Applied and Preventive Psychology, 9*, 101–121.

Crewe, N. M. (1996). Gains and losses due to spinal cord injury: Views across 20 years. *Topics in Spinal Cord Injury, 2*(2), 47–58.

Crewe, N. M., & Athelstan, G. T. (1981). Functional assessment in vocational rehabilitation: A systematic approach to diagnosis and goal setting. *Archives of Physical Medicine & Rehabilitation, 62,* 299–305.

Crewe, N. M., & Athelstan, G. T. (1984). *Functional assessment inventory manual.* Monomonie, WI: The University of Wisconsin-Stout.

Crumbaugh, J. (1977). The Seeking of Noetic Goals Test (SONG): A complementary scale to the Purpose of Life Test (PIL). *Journal of Clinical Psychology, 33*(3), 900–907.

Cullum, C. M., & Thompson, L. L. (1997). Neuropsychological diagnosis and outcome in mild traumatic brain injury. *Applied Neuropsychology, 41*(1), 6–16.

Curtis, R. S. (1998). Values and valuing in rehabilitation. *Journal of Rehabilitation, 64*(1), 42–47.

Cushman, L. A., & Scherer, M. J. (Eds.). (1995). *Psychological assessment in medical rehabilitation*. Washington, DC: American Psychological Association.

Dana, R. H. (2000). An assessment-intervention model for research and practice with multicultural populations. In R. H. Dana (Ed.), *Handbook of cross cultural and multicultural personality assessment. Personality and clinical psychology series* (pp. 5–16), Mahwah, NJ: Lawrence Erlbaum Associates.

Danseco, E. R. (1997). Parental beliefs on childhood disability: Insights on culture, child development and intervention. *International Journal of Disability, Development and Education, 44*(1), 41–52.

Dawes, R. M., Faust, D., & Meehl, P. E. (1993). Statistical prediction versus clinical prediction: Improving what works. In G. Keren & C. Lewis (Eds.), *A handbook for data analysis in the behavioral sciences: Methodological issues* (pp. 351–367). Hillsdale, NJ: Lawrence Erlbaum Associates, Inc.

DeJong, G., & O'Day, B. (1999, 2/22/2002). *Contrast of Paradigms*. National Institute on Disability and Rehabilitation Research. Retrieved December 5, 2002, from http://www.dcddr.org/new/lrp.html

Dersh, J. J. (2000). A comprehensive evaluation of psychopathology in chronic musculoskeletal pain disability patients. *Dissertation Abstracts, 61*(6-B), 3273.

Design, E. W. (2002, July 3). *Through the Looking Glass Website*. Retrieved July 19, 2002, from http://www.lookingglass.org

Diaz Olavarrieta, C., Cummings, J. L., Velazquez, J., & Garcia de al Cadena, C. (1999). Neuropsychiatric manifestations of multiple sclerosis. *Journal of Neuropsychiatry and Clinical Neurosciences, 11*(1), 51–57.

Dimenet (2000). *Virtual Center for Independent Living*. Retrieved August 6, 2002, from http://www.virtualcil.com

Doherty, W. J., McDaniel, S. H., & Hepworth, J. (1994). Medical family therapy: An emerging arena for family therapy. *Journal of Family Therapy, 16*(1), 31–46.

Donohue, J., & Gebhard, P. (1995). The Kinsey Institute/Indiana University report on sexuality and spinal cord injury. *Sexuality and Disability, 13*(1), 7–85.

Duarte, J. A., & Rice, B. D. (1992). *Cultural diversity in rehabilitation*. Fayetteville, AR: Arkansas Research & Training Center in Vocational Rehabilitation.

Dupont, S. (1996). Sexual function and ways of coping in patients with multiple sclerosis and their partners. *Sexual and Marital Therapy, 11*(4), 359–372.

e-bility (2002a). *Louise Sauvage: My Story*. e-bility, Inclusive IT. Retrieved July 31, 2002, from http://www.e-bility.com/articles/sauvage.shtml

e-bility (2002b). *The sky is the limit!* e-bility Inclusive IT. Retrieved July 31, 2002, from the World Wide Web: http://www.e-bility.com/articles/skydiving.shtml

Edworthy, S. M., & Devins, G. M. (1999). Improving medication adherence through patient education distinguishing between appropriate and inappropriate utilization: Patient education study group. *Journal of Rheumatology, 26*(8), 1793–1801.

Ehlers-Flint, M. L. (2001). Perceptions of parenting and social supports of mothers with cognitive disabilities (Doctoral dissertation). *Parenting with a Disability, 9*(1), 8.

Eisenmann, R. (1995). Cruel treatment of learning disabled, emotionally disturbed prisoners: The dilemma of a humanistic psychologist in an inhumane setting. *International Journal of Adolescence and Youth, 5*(3), 189–194.

Elliott, T. R., & Frank, R. G. (1996). Depression following spinal cord injury. *Archives of Physical Medicine & Rehabilitation, 77*, 816–823.

Elliott, T. R., Shewchuk, R. M., & Richards, J. S. (2001). Family caregiver social problem-solving abilities and adjustment during the initial year of the caregiving role. *Journal of Counseling Psychology, 48*(2), 223–232.

Ellis, A. (1997). Using Rational Emotive Behavior Therapy techniques to cope with disability. *Professional Psychology: Research and Practice, 28*(1), 17–22.

Elman, R. A. (2001). Mainstreaming immobility: Disability pornography and its challenge to two movements. In C. M. Rezetti, J. L. Edleson, & R. K. Bergen (Eds.), *Sourcebook on violence against women* (pp. 193–207). Thousand Oaks, CA: Sage Publications.

Enders, A., & Hall, M. (Eds.). (1990). *Assistive technology sourcebook*. Washington, DC: Resna Press.

Erikson, D., & Erikson, L. (1992). Knowledge of sexuality in adolescents with spina bifida. *Canadian Journal of Human Sexuality, 1*(4), 195–199.

Feuerstein, P. B. (1995). Individuals with disabilities in families and society: An empowerment approach. In M. A. Blotzer & R. Ruth (Eds.), *Sometimes you just want to feel like a human being: Case studies of empowering psychotherapy with people with disabilities* (pp. 107–119). Baltimore, MD: Paul H. Brookes.

Fiest-Price, S. (1995). African Americans with disabilities and equity in vocational rehabilitation services: One state's review. *Rehabilitation Counseling Bulletin, 39*(2), 119–129.

Fitchett, G., Rybarczyk, B., DeMarco, G. A., & Nicholas, J. J. (1999). The role of religion in medical rehabilitation outcomes: A longitudinal study. *Rehabilitation Psychology, 44*(4), 333–353.

Fow, N. R., & Rockey, L. S. (1995). A preliminary conceptualization of the influence of personality and psychological development on group therapy with spinal cord patients. *Journal of Applied Rehabilitation Counseling, 26*(1), 30–32.

Frankl, V. (1970). *The will to meaning: Foundations and applications of logotherapy.* New York: Plume Books.

Freundlich, M. (1998). The Americans with Disabilities Act: What adoption agencies need to know. *Bridges*(Fall), 3–5.

Frey, W. D., & Nieuwenjuijsen, R. R. (1990). The Ertomis Assessment Method: An innovative job placement strategy. In M. Berkowitz (Ed.), *Forging linkages: Modifying disability benefit programs to encourage employment* (pp. 121–156). New York: Rehabilitation International.

Fromm, E. (1956). *The art of loving.* New York: Harper & Row.

Furey, E. M., & Niesen, J. J. (1994). Sexual abuse of adults with mental retardation by other consumers. *Sexuality and Disability, 12*(4), 285–295.

Gervin, A. P. (1991). Music therapy compensatory technique utilizing song lyrics during dressing to promote independence in the patient with a brain injury. *Music Therapy Perspectives, 9*, 87–90.

Gibbs, N. (2002, July 1). Apocalypse Now. *Time, 160,* 40–48.

Gill, C. J. (1996). Dating and relationship issues. In D. M. Krotoski, M. A. Nosek, & M. A. Turk (Eds.), *Women with physical disabilities* (pp. 117–124). Baltimore: Paul H. Brookes.

Goffman, E. (1961). *Asylums.* Hawthorne, NY: Aldine.

Gold, D. (1996). Attempts to create friendship in the lives of students with disabilities: The case of 'circles of friends'. *Dissertation Abstracts International Section A: Humanities and Social Sciences.* Aug.; Vol. 57(2-A) 0638.

Gonzales, L. (1999). Secondary conditions cause burden. *Window on Wellness, (Summer)*, 22–23.

Gonzalez, S., Steinglass, P., & Reiss, D. (1987). *Family-centered interventions for people with chronic disabilities.* Washington, DC: George Washington University.

Granger, C. V., & Hamilton, B. B. (1992). UDS report: The Uniform Data System for Medical Rehabilitation report for first admissions for 1990. *American Journal of Physical Medicine and Rehabilitation, 71*, 108–113.

Grayson, D. A., Mackinnon, A., Jorm, A. F., Creasey, H., & Broe, G. A. (2000). Item bias in the Center for Epidemiologic Studies Depression Scale: Effects of physical disorders and disability in an elderly community sample. *Journals of Gerontology: Series B: Psychological Sciences and Social Sciences, 55B*(5), 273–282.

Griffin, K. W., Friend, R., Kaell, A. T., Bennett, R. S., & Wadhwa, N. K. (1999). Negative affect and physical symptom reporting: A test of explanatory models in two chronically ill populations. *Psychology and Health, 14*(2), 295–307.

Griss, B. (2000). *Urgent action needed: Olmstead victory dismantled by disastrous Rodriguez court decision, threatening future of community-based services.* Justice for All. Retrieved August 1, 2002, from http://www.jfanow.org/cgi/getli.pl?1227

Grove, W. M., Zald, D. H., Lebow, B. S., Snitz, B. E., & Nelson, C. (2000). Clinical versus mechanical prediction: A meta-analysis. *Psychological Assessment, 12*(1), 19–30.

Gurland, B., Katz, S., & Pine, Z. M. (2000). Complex unity and tolerable uncertainty: Relationships of physical disorder and depression. In G. M. Williamson, D. R. Shaffer, & P. A. Parmelee (Eds.), *Physical illness and depression in older adults: A handbook of theory, research, and practice* (pp. 311–330). Dordrecht, Netherlands: Kluwer Academic Publishers.

Guth, P. E. (2000). The effects of depression in head injured adults as related to educational level, gender, and activity level. *Dissertation Abstracts, 61*(4–B), 1803.

Gwin, L. (2002). ADAPT stops traffic in D.C: Wins MiCASSA talks with budget keepers, labor leaders. *Mouth Magazine, 72*, 4.

Hall, C. S., Lindzey, G., & Campbell, J. B. (1998). *Theories of personality* (4th ed.). New York: John Wiley & Sons, Inc.

Hampton, N. Z. (2000). Self-efficacy and quality of life in people with spinal cord injuries in China. *Rehabilitation Counseling Bulletin, 43*(2), 66–74.

Hanson, R. D. (2000). Personal, familial, and social predictors of burden in HIV/AIDS informal caregivers (immune deficiency). *Dissertation Abstracts International— Section A (Humanities Social Sciences), 61*(5-A), 2055.

Harkin, T. (2001). *Congressional Record on MiCASSA: Introduction 8/1/01.* Retrieved August 2, 2002, from http://www.ncil.org/micassa1298.htm

Hayman, B. (1975). *Man in Search of Meaning.* Term paper prepared for the United States International University at San Diego, California.

Heinemann, A. W., Goranson, N., Ginsburg, K., & Schnoll, S. (1989). Alcohol use and activity patterns following spinal cord injury. *Rehabilitation Psychology, 34*(3), 191–205.

Heinrich, R. K., & Tate, D. G. (1996). Latent variable structure of the Brief Symptom Inventory in a sample of persons with spinal cord injuries. *Rehabilitation Psychology, 41*(2), 131–147.

Herbert, J. T. (1989). Assessing the need for family therapy: A primer for rehabilitation counselors. *Journal of Rehabilitation, 55*, 45–51.

Herbert, J. T. (1998). Therapeutic effects of participating in an adventure therapy program. *Rehabilitation Counseling Bulletin, 41*(3), 201–216.

Hilyer, K. (1997). Redesigning vocational evaluation for career development. In R. Fry (Ed.), *The issues papers. Eighth national forum on issues in vocational assessment* (pp. 111–116). Menomonie, WI: University of Wisconsin-Stout.

Holmbeck, G. N., Johnson, S. Z., Wills, K. E., McKernon, W., Rose, B., Erklin, S., & Kemper, T. (2002). Observed and perceived parental overprotection in relation to psychosocial adjustment in preadolescents with a physical disability: The mediational role of behavioral autonomy. *Journal of Consulting and Clinical Psychology, 70*(1), 96–110.

Huebner, R. A., & Thomas, K. R. (1995). The relationship between attachment, psychopathology, and childhood disability. *Rehabilitation Psychology, 40*(2), 111–124.

Imparato, A. J. (2000). *Top ten reasons to renew the pledge.* Justice for All. Retrieved August 1, 2002, from http://www.jfanow.org/cgi/getli.pl?1065

Ivey, A. E., Ivey, M. B., & Simek-Morgan, L. (Eds.) (1997). *Counseling and psychotherapy: A multicultural perspective* (4th ed.). Boston: Allyn and Bacon.

Jackson, A., & Haverkamp, B. E. (1991). Family response to traumatic brain injury. *Counselling Psychology Quarterly, 4*(4), 355–366.

Jensen, A., & Silverstein, R. (2000). *Improvements to the SSDI and SSI Work Incentives and Expanded Availability of Health Care Services to Workers with Disabilities under the Ticket to Work and Work Incentives Improvement Act of 1999.* Law, Health Policy & Disability Center. Retrieved July 25, 2002, from http://www.its.uiowa.edu/law/lhpdc/rrtc/

Jerome, L. W., DeLeon, P. H., James, L. C., Folen, R., Earles, J., & Gedney, J. J. (2000). The coming of age of telecommunications in psychological research and practice. *American Psychologist, 55*(4), 407–421.

Joint Commission on Accreditation of Healthcare Organizations (2001). *2001–2002 Comprehensive accreditation manual for behavioral health care* (pp. PE1–PE54). Chicago: Author.

Jung, C. (1929). The problems of modern psychotherapy. In E. A. Read (Ed.), *The collected works of C. G. Jung* (Vol. 16). Princeton, NJ: Princeton University Press.

Kabat-Zinn, J. (1991). *Full catastrophe living: Using the wisdom of your body and mind to face stress, pain and illness.* New York: Dell Publishing.

Kammerer-Quayle, B. (2002). Image and behavioral skills training for people with facial difference and disability. In M. G. Brodwin, F. Tellez, & S. K. Brodwin (Eds.), *Medical, psychosocial, and vocational aspects of disability* (2nd ed., pp. 95–106). Athens, GA: Elliott & Fitzpatrick.

Kanner, A. M., & Nieto, J. C. R. (1999). Depressive disorders in epilepsy. *Neurology, 53*(5, Supplement 2), S26–S32.

Kaye, H. S. (1998). *Is the status of people with disabilities improving?: Disability statistics abstract #21.* Washington, DC: U.S. Department of Education.

Kelly, E. W. J. (1995). Counselor values: A national survey. *Journal of Counseling and Development, 73*(6), 648–653.

Kemp, B. J. (1999, April). Aging with a disability: What's been learned? *New Mobility,* 28–34.

Kemp, B. J., Kahan, J. S., Krause, J. S., Adkins, R. H., & Nava, G. (2002). *A naturalistic study of treating depression with psychotherapy and medicine in persons with long-term spinal cord injury.* Unpublished manuscript.

Kemp, B. J., Krause, J. S., & Adkins, R. A. (1999). Depressive symptomatology among African-American, Latino, and Caucasian participants with spinal cord injury. *Rehabilitation Psychology, 44*, 235–247.

Kemp, B. J., & Vash, C. (1971). Productivity after injury in a sample of spinal cord injured persons: A pilot study. *Journal of Chronic Diseases, 24*(2), 259–275.

Kerr, N. (1977). Understanding the process of adjustment to disability. In J. Stubbins (Ed.), *Psychosocial aspects of disability.* Baltimore, MD: University Park.

Kerr, S. (2000). The application of the Americans with Disabilities Act to the termination of the parental rights of individuals with mental disabilities. *Journal of Contemporary Health Law and Policy, 16*(Summer), 387–426.

Kettl, P., et al. (1991). Female sexuality after spinal cord injury. *Sexuality and Disability, 9*(4), 287–295.

Keyes, K., Jr. (1975). *Handbook to higher consciousness.* Berkeley, CA: Living Love.

Kiernan, W. (2000). Where we are now: Perspectives on employment of persons with mental retardation. *Focus on Autism and Other Developmental Disabilities, 15*(2), 90–96.

Kilpatrick, S. D., & McCullough, M. E. (1999). Religion and spirituality in rehabilitation psychology. *Rehabilitation Psychology, 44*(4), 388–402.

King, C., & Kennedy, P. (1999). Coping effectiveness training for people with spinal cord injury: Preliminary results of a controlled trial. *British Journal of Clinical Psychology, 38*(1), 5–14.

Kirk, J. (1999). Indices of depression among individuals with physical disabilities. *Dissertation Abstracts, 60*(5-B), 2346.

Kirshbaum, M. (1995). Serving families with disability issues: Through the Looking Glass. *Marriage and Family Review, 21*(1–2), 9–28.

Kirshbaum, M. (1996). Mothers with physical disabilities. In D. M. Krotoski, M. A. Nosek, & M. A. Turk (Eds.), *Women with physical disabilities* (pp. 125–134). Baltimore: Paul H. Brookes.

Knox, R., & Jutai, J. (1996). Music-based rehabilitation of attention following brain injury. *Canadian Journal of Rehabilitation, 9*(3), 169–181.

Koenig, H. G. (1997). Use of religion by patients with severe medical illness. *Mind/Body Medicine, 2*, 31–36.

Kostyk, D., Fuchs, D., Tabisz, E., & Jacyk, W. R. (1993). Combining professional and self-help group intervention: Collaboration in co-leadership. *Social Work with Groups, 16*(3), 111–123.

Krause, J. S., & Crewe, N. M. (1991). Chronologic age, time since injury, and time of measurement: Effect on adjustment after spinal cord injury. *Archives of Physical Medicine & Rehabilitation, 72*(2), 91–100.

Krause, J. S., Kemp, B. J., & Coker, J. L. (2000). Depression after spinal cord injury: Relation to gender, ethnicity, aging, and socioeconomic indicators. *Archives of Physical Medicine & Rehabilitation, 81*, 1099–1109.

Krauss, H. H., Godfrey, C., Kirk, J., & Eisenberg, D. M. (1998). Alternative health care: Its use by individuals with physical disabilities. *Archives of Physical Medicine & Rehabilitation, 79*(11), 1440–1447.

Kutner, B. (1977). Milieu therapy. In R. P. Marinelli & A. E. Dell Orto (Eds.), *The psychological and social impact of physical disability* (pp. 334–341). New York: Springer Publishing.

Lasky, R. G., Dell Orto, A. E., & Marinelli, R. P. (1977). Structured existential therapy: A group approach to rehabilitation. In R. P. Marinelli & A. E. Dell Orto (Eds.), *The psychological and social impact of physical disability* (1st ed., pp. 319–333). New York: Springer Publishing.

Lawrence, R. H., Tennstedt, S. L., & Assmann, S. F. (1998). Quality of the caregiver-care recipient relationship: Does it offset negative consequences of caregiving for family caregivers? *Psychology and Aging, 13*(1), 150–158.

Leahy, M. J. (1997). Qualified providers of rehabilitation counseling services. In D. R. Maki & T. F. Riggar (Eds.), *Rehabilitation counseling profession and practice* (pp. 95–110). New York: Springer Publishing.

Lenze, E. J., Rogers, J. C., Martire, L. M., Mulsant, B. H., & Rollman, B. L. (2001). The association of late-life depression and anxiety with physical disability: A review of the literature and prospectus for future research. *American Journal of Geriatric Psychiatry, 9*(2), 113–135.

Leong, E. T. L. (1996). Toward an integrative model for cross-cultural counseling and psychotherapy. *Applied & Preventative Psychology, 5*, 189–209.

Levin, J. B., Lofland, K. R., Cassisi, J. E., Poreh, A. M., & Blonsky, E. R. (1996). The relationship between self-efficacy and disability in chronic low back pain patients. *International Journal of Rehabilitation and Health, 2*(1), 19–28.

Levy, M. (1995). To stand on holy ground: A Jewish spiritual perspective on disability. *Rehabilitation Education, 9*(2–3), 163–170.

Lewin, K. (1935). *A dynamic theory of personality.* New York: McGraw Hill.

Lifchez, R. (1987). *Rethinking architecture: Design students and physically disabled people.* Berkeley: University of California Press.

Llewellyn, G., & McConnell, D. (2002). Mothers with learning difficulties and their support networks. *Journal of Intellectual Disability Research, 46*(1), 17–34.

Locust, C. (1995). The impact of differing belief systems between Native Americans and their rehabilitation service providers. *Rehabilitation Education, 9*(2–3), 205–215.

Longmore, P. K. (1999). *Disability policy and politics, considering consumer influences.* National Rehabilitation Association. Retrieved August 1, 2002, from http://www.mswitzer.org/sem99/papers/longmore.html

Lubin, J. (2002). *Disability travel and recreation resources.* Retrieved July 31, 2002, from http://www.makoa.org/travel.htm

Luce, G. (1979). *Your second life.* New York: Delacorte/Seymour Lawrence.

Malgady, R. G. (1996). The question of cultural bias in assessment and diagnosis of ethnic minority clients: Let's reject the null hypothesis. *Professional Psychology: Research and Practice, 27*(1), 73–77.

Marinelli, R. P., & Dell Orto, A. E. (1999). *The psychological and social impact of disability* (4th ed.). New York: Springer Publishing.

Marshall, C. A., Johnson, M. J., & Johnson, S. R. (1996). Responding to the needs of American Indians with disabilities through rehabilitation counselor education. *Rehabilitation Education, 10*(2 & 3), 185–199.

Martz, E., & Cook, D. W. (2001). Physical impairments as risk factors for the development of posttraumatic stress disorder. *Rehabilitation Counseling Bulletin, 44*(4), 217–221.

Maslow, A. (1965). *Eupsychian management*. Homewood, IL: Richard Irwin.

Maslow, A., & Mittleman, B. (1951). *Principles of abnormal psychology: The dynamics of psychic illness* (Revised ed.). New York: Harper.

Masserman, J. (1955). *The practice of dynamic psychiatry*. Philadelphia: W. B. Saunders.

Mastroyannopoulou, K., Stallard, P., Lewis, M., & Lenton, S. (1997). The impact of childhood non-malignant life-threatening illness on parents: Gender differences and predictors of parental adjustment. *Journal of Child Psychology and Psychiatry and Allied Disciplines, 38*(7), 823–829.

Mathews, R. M., Mathews, S. A., & Pittman, J. L. (1985). Peer counseling: Consumer involvement in independent living programs. *Rehabilitation Counseling Bulletin, 28*(7), 161–166.

Matthews, D. A., McCullough, M. E., Larson, D. B., Koenig, H. G., Swyers, J. P., & Milano, M. G. (1998). Religious commitment and health status. *Archives of Family Medicine, 7*, 118–124.

Mayerson, A. (1992). *The history of the ADA: A movement perspective*. Disability Rights Education and Defense Fund. Retrieved August 1, 2002, from http://www.dredf.org/articles/adahist.html

McAdams, D. P. (1988). *Power, intimacy, and the life story: Personological inquiries into identity*. New York: Guilford Press.

McAfee, J. K., & Musso, S. L. (1995). Training police officers about persons with disabilities: A 50-state analysis. *Remedial and Special Education, 16*(1), 53–63.

McAllan, L. C., & Ditillo, D. (1994). Addressing the needs of lesbian and gay clients with disabilities. *Journal of Applied Rehabilitation Counseling, 25*(1), 26–35.

McCarthy, H. (1995). Integrating spirituality into rehabilitation in a technocratic society. *Rehabilitation Education, 9*(2–3), 87–95.

McCarthy, M. (1998). Whose body is it anyway? Pressures and control for women with learning disabilities. *Disability and Society, 13*(4), 557–574.

McDaniel, M. F. (1991). Enhancing the psychological adjustment of visually impaired adults through cognitive group therapy. *Dissertation Abstracts Intl.* Sept. Vol. 52 (3-B): 1728.

McLafferty, C. L., & Kirylo, J. D. (2001). Spirituality and positive psychology. *American Psychologist, 56*(1), 84–85.

McNeil, J. E., & Greenwood, R. (1996). Can PTSD occur with amnesia for the precipitating event? *Cognitive Neuropsychiatry, 1*(3), 239–246.

Meade, C. (2002). *Sexuality and disability*. Sexuality Information & Education Council of the United States. Retrieved July 22, 2002, from http://www.siecus.org/pubs/biblio/bibs0009.html

Medlar, T. M. (1993). Sexual counseling and traumatic brain injury. *Sexuality and Disability, 11*(1), 57–71.

Meyer, G. J., Finn, S. E., Eyde, L. D., Kay, G. G., Moreland, K. L., Dies, R. R., Eisman, E. J., Kubiszyn, T. W., & Read, G. M. (2001). Psychological testing and psychological assessment: A review of evidence and issues. *American Psychologist, 56*(2), 128–165.

Monga, T. N., Tan, G., Ostermann, H. J., Monga, U., & Grabois, M. (1998). Sexuality and sexual adjustment of patients with chronic pain. *Disability and Rehabilitation: An International Multidisciplinary Journal, 20*(9), 317–329.

Moos, R. H., & Shaeffer, J. A. (1984). The crisis of physical illness: An overview and conceptual approach. In R. H. Moos (Ed.), *Coping with physical illness 2: New perspectives*. New York: Plenum Press.

Morrison, J. (1995). *DSM-IV Made Easy*. New York: Guilford Press.

Morrison, M. H. (1991). Employment of older workers with a disability: Attitudes and legal issues. In L. G. Perlman & C. E. Hansen (Eds.), *Aging, disability and the nation's productivity* (pp. 27–32). Reston, VA: National Rehabilitation Association.

Moss, K., Ullman, M., Starrett, B. E., Burris, S., & Johnsen, M. C. (1999). Outcomes of employment discrimination charges filed under the Americans with Disabilities Act. *Psychiatric Services, 50*(8), 1028–1035.

National Institute of Mental Health (NIMH). (1980). *Announcement of community support system strategy development and implementation grants*. Rockville, MD: Author.

National Institute of Mental Health (NIMH). (1999, October 5). *Facts about post-traumatic stress disorder*. Retrieved June 25, 2002, from http://www.nimh.nih.gov/anxiety/ptsdfacts.cfm

National Institute on Disability and Rehabilitation Research (NIDRR). (1993). Culturally sensitive rehabilitation. *Rehab Brief, 15*(8), 1–4.

Nayak, S., Wheeler, B. L., Shiflett, S. C., & Agostinelli, S. (2000). Effect of music therapy on mood and social interaction among individuals with acute traumatic brain injury and stroke. *Rehabilitation Psychology, 45*(3), 274–283.

Neath, J., Bellini, J., & Bolton, B. (1997). Dimensions of the Functional Assessment Inventory for five disability groups. *Rehabilitation Psychology, 42*(3), 183–207.

Nelson, J. (1991). Response to Malcolm Morrison. In L. G. Perlman & C. E. Hansen (Eds.), *Aging, disability and the nation's productivity* (p. 35). Reston, VA: National Rehabilitation Association.

Nesbitt, J. (1979). Recreation and careers in recreation for disabled people. *American Rehabilitation, 5*(1).

Nester, M. A. (1993). Psychometric testing and reasonable accommodation for persons with disabilities. *Rehabilitation Psychology, 38*, 75–84.

Nester, M. A., & Colberg, M. (1984). The effects of negation mode, syllogistic invalidity, and linguistic medium on the psychometric properties of deductive reasoning tests. *Applied Psychological Measurement, 8*(1), 71–79.

Nosek, M. A. (1995). The defining light of vedanta: Personal reflections on spirituality and disability. *Rehabilitation Education, 9*(2–3), 171–182.

Nosek, M. A. (1996). Sexual abuse of women with physical disabilities. In D. M. Krotoski, M. A. Nosek, & M. A. Turk (Eds.), *Women with physical disabilities* (pp. 153–173). Baltimore: Paul H. Brookes.

Nosek, M. A., Howland, C., Rintala, D. H., Young, M. E., & Chanpong, G. F. (2001). National study of women with physical disabilities: Final report. *Sexuality and Disability, 19*(1), 5–40.

Olkin, R. (1999). *What psychotherapists should know about disability.* New York: The Guilford Press.

O'Malley, D. J. (2002). *The changing health care system and implications for the rehabilitation industry.* Paper presented at the American Association of Spinal Cord Injury Psychologists and Social Workers, Las Vegas, Nevada.

O'Toole, C. J. (2000). The view from below: Developing a knowledge base about an unknown population. *Sexuality and Disability, 18*(3), 207–224.

O'Toole, C. J., & Bregante, J. L. (1992). Lesbians with disabilities. *Sexuality and Disability, 10*(3), 163–172.

Ott, R. J. (2002). *Never Surrender.* Retrieved July 31, 2002, from http://www.certain victory.com/rjo-story.html/

Pancsofar, E. L., & Steere, D. E. (1997). The C.A.P.A.B.L.E. process: Critical dimensions of community-based assessment. *Journal of Vocational Rehabilitation, 8*(1), 99–108.

Pargament, K. I. (1997). *The psychology of religion and coping: Theory, research, practice.* New York: Guilford Press.

Pendergrass, S., Nosek, M. A., & Holcomb, J. D. (2001). Design and evaluation of an internet site to educate women with disabilities on reproductive health care. *Sexuality and Disability, 19*(1), 71–83.

Penninx, B. W. J. H., Leveille, S., Ferrucci, L., van Eijk, J. T. M., & Guralnik, J. M. (1999). Exploring the effect of depression on physical disability: Longitudinal evidence from the established populations for epidemiologic studies of the elderly. *American Journal of Public Health, 89*(9), 1346–1352.

Perlman, L. G., & Hansen, C. E. (Eds.) (1991). *Aging, disability and the nation's productivity.* Reston, VA: National Rehabilitation Association.

Perske, R. (1997). Prisoners with mental disabilities in 1692 Salem and today. *Mental Retardation, 35*(4), 315–317.

Pfeiffer, D. (1999). Eugenics and disability discrimination. In R. P. Marinelli & A. E. Dell Orto (Eds.), *The psychological and social impact of disability* (4th ed., pp. 12–31). New York: Springer Publishing.

Piedmont, R. L. (1999). Does spirituality represent the sixth factor of personality? Spiritual transcendence and the Five Factor Model. *Journal of Personality, 67*(6), 985–1013.

Piedmont, R. L. (2001). Spiritual transcendence and the scientific study of spirituality. *Journal of Rehabilitation, 67*(1), 4–14.

Quittner, A. L., & DiGirolamo, A. M. (1998). Family adaptation to disability and illness. In R. T. Ammerman & J. V. Campo (Eds.), *Handbook of pediatric psychology and psychiatry: Disease, injury, and illness* (Vol. 2, pp. 70–102). Needham Heights, MA: Allyn & Bacon, Inc.

Rabkin, J. G., Wagner, G. J., & DelBene, M. (2000). Resilience and distress among amyotrophic lateral sclerosis patients and caregivers. *Psychosomatic Medicine, 62*(2), 271–279.

Radloff, L. S. (1977). The CES-D scale: A self-report depression scale for research in the general population. *Applied Psychological Measurement, 1*, 385–401.

Rama, S., Ballentine, R., & Ajaya, S. (1976). *Yoga and psychotherapy: The evolution of consciousness.* Glenview, IL: Himalayan Institute.

Raspberry, W. (1989, January 6). New name a search for acceptance. *Lansing State Journal,* p. 6A.

Redford, D., & Whitaker-Lee, P. (1999). *Peer mentor volunteers: Empowering people for a change.* Houston: The Institute for Rehabilitation and Research. Retrieved August 6, 2002, from http://www.lsi.ukans.edu/apps/riil/review.asp?694

Regenold, M., Sherman, M. F., & Fenzel, M. (1999). Getting back to work: Self-efficacy as a predictor of employment outcome. *Psychiatric Rehabilitation Journal, 22*(4), 361–367.

Reidy, K., & Caplan, B. (1994). Causal factors in spinal cord injury: Patients' evolving perceptions and associations with depression. *Archives of Physical Medicine & Rehabilitation, 75*(8), 837–842.

Reiss, D., & Oliveri, M. E. (1987). *Developing a clear image of the family.* Washington, DC: The Rehabilitation Research and Training Center, George Washington University.

Richter, C. (1958). On the phenomenon of sudden death in animals and man. In C. F. Reed, I. E. Alexander, & S. S. Tomkins (Eds.), *Psychopathology: A source book.* Cambridge, MA: Harvard University Press.

Rintala, D. H., Howland, C. A., Nosek, M. A., Bennet, J. L., & Young, M. E. (1997). Dating issues for women with physical disabilities. *Sexuality and Disability, 15*(4), 219–242.

Roberts, E. (1977). Mealtimes in an institution: A disabled person's experiences. In E. A. Perske (Ed.), *Mealtimes for severely and profoundly handicapped persons: New concepts and attitudes.* Baltimore: University Park.

Rolland, J. S. (1994). In sickness and in health: The impact of illness on couples' relationships. *Journal of Marital and Family Therapy, 20*(4), 327–347.

Rolland, J. S. (1999). Parental illness and disability: A family systems framework. *Journal of Family Therapy, 21*(3), 242–266.

Rothbaum, B. O., Hodges, L. F., Ready, D., Graap, K., & Alarcon, R. D. (2001). Virtual reality exposure therapy for Vietnam veterans with posttraumatic stress disorder. *Journal of Clinical Psychiatry, 62*(8), 617–622.

Roy-Byrne, P. P., & Katon, W. (2000). Anxiety management in the medical setting: Rationale, barriers to diagnosis and treatment, and proposed solutions. In D. I. Mostofsky & D. H. Barlow (Eds.), *The management of stress and anxiety in medical disorders* (pp. 1–14). Boston: Allyn and Bacon.

Rybarczyk, B., Szymanski, L., & Nicholas, J. J. (2000). Limb amputation. In R. G. Frank & T. R. Elliott (Eds.), *Handbook of rehabilitation psychology* (pp. 29–47). Washington, DC: American Psychological Association.

Saad, S. C. (1997). Disability and the lesbian, gay man, or bisexual individual. In M. L. Sipsky & C. J. Alexander (Eds.), *Sexual function in people with disability and chronic illness: A health professional's guide* (pp. 413–427). Gaithersburg, MD: Aspen Publishing.

Saarijaervi, S., Rytoekoski, U., & Alanen, E. (1991). A controlled study of couple therapy in chronic low back pain patients: No improvement of disability. *Journal of Psychosomatic Research, 35*(6), 671–677.

Salmon, G., & Abell, S. (1996). Group therapy for adults with learning disability: Use of active techniques. *Psychiatric Bulletin, 20*(4), 221–223.

Saxton, M. (1983). Peer counseling. In N. M. Crewe & I. K. Zola (Eds.), *Independent living for physically disabled people* (pp. 171–186). San Francisco: Jossey-Bass.

Sbordone, R. J. (1999). Post-traumatic stress disorder: An overview and its relationship to closed head injuries. *Neurorehabilitation, 13*(2), 69–78.

Schrag, A., Jahanshahi, M., & Quinn, N. P. (2001). What contributes to depression in Parkinson's disease? *Psychological Medicine, 31*(1), 65–73.

Schulz, R., & Quittner, A. L. (1998). Caregiving for children and adults with chronic conditions: Introduction to the special issue. *Health Psychology, 17*(2), 107–111.

Scotch, R. K. (1999). *Disability Policy: An Overview*. National Rehabilitation Association. Retrieved August 1, 2002, from http://www.mswitzer.org/sem99/papers/

Scroggin, C., Kosciulek, J. F., Sweiven, K. A., & Enright, M. S. (1999). Impact of situational assessment on the career self-efficacy of people with disabilities. *Vocational Evaluation and Work Adjustment Journal, 32*(2), 97–107.

Seekins, T., Mathews, R. M., & Fawcett, S. B. (1984). Enhancing leadership skills for community self-help organizations through behavioral instruction. *Journal of Community Psychology, 12*(2), 155–163.

Segal, M. E., & Schall, R. R. (1996). Life satisfaction and caregiving stress for individuals with stroke and their primary caregivers. *Rehabilitation Psychology, 41*(4), 303–320.

Seligman, M. E. P. (1975). *Helplessness: On depression, development, and death*. San Francisco: W. H. Freeman.

Seligman, M. E. P., & Csikszentmihalyi, M. (2000). Positive psychology: An introduction. *American Psychologist, 55*(1), 5–14.

Seligman, M., & Darling, R. B. (1997). *Ordinary families, special children: A systems approach to childhood disability* (2nd ed.). New York: The Guilford Press.

Shapiro, J. P. (1993). *No pity*. New York: Times Books.

Shewchuk, R. M., Richards, J. S., & Elliott, T. R. (1998). Dynamic processes in health outcomes among caregivers of patients with spinal cord injuries. *Health Psychology, 17*(2), 125–129.

Shnek, Z. M., Foley, F. W., LaRocca, N. G., Smith, C. R., & Halper, J. (1995). Psychological predictors of depression in multiple sclerosis. *Journal of Neurologic Rehabilitation, 9*(1), 15–23.

Shushan, R. (1974). *Assessment and reduction of deficits in the physical appearance of mentally retarded people*. Los Angeles: University of California.

Shuttlesworth, R. P. (2000). The search for sexual intimacy for men with cerebral palsy. *Sexuality and Disability, 18*(4), 263–282.

Singer, G. H. S., & Powers, L. E. (Eds.) (1993). *Families, disability, and empowerment: Active coping skills and strategies for family interventions*. Baltimore: Paul H. Brookes.

Sipski, M. L. (1993). The impact of spinal cord trauma on female sexual function. In F. P. Haseltine, S. S. Cole, & D. B. Gray (Eds.), *Reproductive issues for persons with physical disabilities* (pp. 209–220). Baltimore: Paul H. Brookes.

Sisco, K. (1991). Employment of the older worker with a disability: An overview. In L. G. Perlman & C. E. Hansen (Eds.), *Aging, disability and the nation's productivity* (pp. 11–15). Reston, VA: National Rehabilitation Association.

Smart, J. F., & Smart, D. W. (1997). The racial/ethnic demography of disability. *Journal of Rehabilitation, 63*(4), 9–15.

Smith, S. J., & Young, C. A. (2000). The role of affect on the perception of disability in multiple sclerosis. *Clinical Rehabilitation, 14*(1), 50–54.

Sobsey, D., & Mansell, S. (1994). An international perspective on patterns of sexual assault and abuse of people with disabilities. *International Journal of Adolescent Medicine and Health, 7*(2), 153–178.

Social Security Administration Office of Disability. (2002, July 24). Disability. *Social Security Online Disability Programs.* Retrieved July 24, 2002, from http://www.ssa.gov/disability/

Soondergaard, B., Davidsen, F., Kirkeby, B., Rasmussen, M., & Hey, H. (1992). The economics of an intensive education programme for asthmatic patients: A prospective controlled trial. *Pharmacoeconomics, 1*(3), 207–212.

Special Olympics (2002). *About Special Olympics.* Retrieved July 31, 2002, 2002, from http://www.specialolympics.org/

Stein, P. N., Gordon, W. A., Hibbard, M. R., & Sliwinski, M. J. (1992). An examination of depression in the spouses of stroke patients. *Rehabilitation Psychology, 37*(2), 121–130.

Stenager, E., Stenager, E. N., & Jensen, K. (1994). Sexual problems in multiple sclerosis. *International Journal of Adolescent Medicine and Health, 7*(2), 95–105.

Stude, E. W. B. (2002). Drug abuse. In M. G. Brodwin, F. Tellez, & S. K. Brodwin (Eds.), *Medical, psychosocial and vocational aspects of disability* (2nd ed., pp. 27–39). Athens, GA: Elliott & Fitzpatrick.

Swartz, D. B. (1993). A comparative study of sex knowledge among hearing and deaf college freshmen. *Sexuality and Disability, 11*(2), 120–147.

Swartz-Kulstad, J. L., & Martin, W. E. J. (1999). Impact of culture and context on psychosocial adaptation: The cultural and contextual guide process. *Journal of Counseling and Development, 77*, 281–293.

Szollos, A. A., & McCabe, M. P. (1995). The sexuality of people with mild intellectual disability: Perceptions of clients and caregivers. *Australia and New Zealand Journal of Developmental Disabilities, 20*(3), 205–222.

Tate, D. G., & Forchheimer, M. B. (1998). Enhancing community reintegration following inpatient rehabilitation for persons with spinal cord injury. *Topics in Spinal Cord Injury, 4*(1), 42–55.

Tate, D. G., Forchheimer, M. B., & Roller, A. (1998). Changes in lifestyle: The effects of participation in a wellness program. *Archives of Physical Medicine & Rehabilitation, 79*(10), 1333.

Taub, D. E., Blinde, E. M., & Greer, K. R. (1999). Stigma management through participation in sport and physical activity: Experiences of male college students with physical disabilities. *Human Relations, 52*(11), 1469–1484.

Thackeray, B. (2000). *Harris Poll: Hopeful signs of progress.* Justice for All. Retrieved August 1, 2002, from http://www.jfanow.org/cgi/getli.pl?1114

Thierry, J. M. (1998). Promoting the health and wellness of women with disabilities. *Journal of Women's Health, 7*(5), 505–507.

Thomas, S. W. (1999). Vocational evaluation in the 21st century: Diversification and independence. *Journal of Rehabilitation, 65*(1), 10–15.

Toffler, A. (1980). *The third wave.* New York: William Morrow.

Toseland, R. W., Rossiter, C. M., & Labrecque, M. S. (1989). The effectiveness of peer-led and professionally led groups to support family caregivers. *Gerontologist, 29*(4), 465–471.

Toseland, R. W., Rossiter, C. M., Peak, T., & Hill, P. (1990). Therapeutic processes in peer led and professionally led support groups for caregivers. *International Journal of Group Psychotherapy, 40*(3), 279–303.

Toseland, R. W., & Smith, G. C. (1990). Effectiveness of individual counseling by professional and peer helpers for family caregivers of the elderly. *Psychology and Aging, 5*(2), 256–263.

Treloar, L. L. (1999). Perceptions of spiritual beliefs, response to disability, and the church. *Dissertation Abstracts Intl. Section A—Humanities and Social Sciences, 60*(2-A), 0562.

Trieschmann, R. B. (1995). The energy model: A new approach to rehabilitation. *Rehabilitation Education, 9*(2–3), 217–227.

Trieschmann, R. B. (2001). Spirituality and energy medicine. *Journal of Rehabilitation, 67*(1), 26–32.

U.S. Department of Education. (2001). *Percentage distribution of disabled persons 6 to 21 years old receiving education services for the disabled, by age group and educational environment: United States and outlying areas: 1998–99.* Retrieved September 18, 2002, from http://nces.ed.gov//pubs2002/digest2001

U.S. Department of Labor. (1991). *Dictionary of occupational titles* (4th ed.). Washington, DC: U.S. Government Printing Office.

U.S. Paralympics (2002). *About U.S. Paralympics* Retrieved July 21, 2002, from http://www.usparalmpics.org

Vash, C. (1975). The psychology of disability. *Rehabilitation Psychology, 22*(3).

Vash, C. (1976). *Psychological growth and acknowledgment of disability.* Paper presented at the Wright Institute Training Seminar: Psychological Aspects of Disability, San Francisco, CA.

Vash, C. (1977). *Re-focusing psychological services in vocational rehabilitation.* Paper presented at the American Psychological Association, San Francisco, CA.

Vash, C. (1977). *Rights of people with disabilities.* Paper presented to the Annual Convention of the Occupational Therapy Association of California (p. 446), Costa Mesa, CA.

Vash, C. (1978b). *Avocational Rehabilitation.* Keynote address presented at the Horizons West Therapeutic Recreation Conference on April 15, 1978 at the Handicapped Recreation Center, San Francisco.

Vash, C. (1980). Sheltered industrial employment. In E. A. Pan (Ed.), *Annual Review of Rehabilitation* (Vol. 1, pp. 80–120). New York: Springer Publishing.

Vash, C. L. (1994). *Personality and adversity: Psychospiritual aspects of rehabilitation.* New York: Springer Publishing.

Vaux, A. (1988). *Social support: Theory, research, and intervention.* New York: Praeger Publishers.

Wallander, J. L., & Venters, T. L. (1995). Perceived role restriction and adjustment of mothers of children with chronic physical disability. *Journal of Pediatric Psychology, 20*(5), 619–632.

Warden, D. L., Labbate, L. A., Salazar, A. M., Nelson, R., Sheley, E., Staudenmeier, J. & Martin, E. (1997). Posttraumatic stress disorder in patients with traumatic brain injury and amnesia for the event. *Journal of Neuropsychiatry and Clinical Neurosciences, 9*(1), 18–22.

Warschausky, S., Kay, J. B., & Kewman, D. G. (2001). Hierarchical linear modeling of FIM growth characteristics following SCI. *Archives of Physical Medicine & Rehabilitation, 82*(3), 329–334.

Watson, A. L., Franklin, M. E., Ingram, M. A., & Eilenberg, L. B. (1998). Alcohol and other drug abuse among persons with disabilities. *Journal of Applied Rehabilitation Counseling, 29*(2), 22–39.

Weigartz, P. S. (2000). Depression in patients with complex partial seizures. *Dissertation Abstracts, 60*(9-B), 4916.

Weingardt, K. R., Hsu, J., & Dunn, M. E. (2001). Brief screening for psychological and substance abuse disorders in veterans with long-term spinal cord injury. *Rehabilitation Psychology, 46*(3), 271–278.

Westbrook, J. T. (1999a, 04/30/02). *Disability, diversity and dissemination: A review of the literature on topics related to increasing the utilization of rehabilitation research outcomes among diverse consumer groups: Part 1: Theoretical Framework.* National Center for the Dissemination of Disability Research. Retrieved December 6, 2002, from http://www.ncddr.org/du/researchexchange/v04n01/

Westbrook, J. T. (1999b, 08/16/99). *Disability, diversity and dissemination: A review of the literature on topics related to increasing the utilization of rehabilitation research outcomes among diverse consumer groups: Part 2: Applying the concepts to research and dissemination and utilization.* National Center on Dissemination of Disability Research. Retrieved December 9, 2002, from http://222.ncddr.org/researchexchange/v04n02/systems.html

Westbrook, M. T., & Legge, V. (1993). Health practitioners' perceptions of family attitudes toward children with disabilities: A comparison of six communities in a multicultural society. *Rehabilitation Psychology, 38*(3), 177–185.

Whyte, A. S., & Niven, C. A. (2001). Psychological distress in amputees with phantom limb pain. *Journal of Pain and Symptom Management, 22*(5), 938–946.

Williams, C. R., & Arrigo, B. A. (2002). *Law, psychology, and justice.* Albany: State University of New York Press.

Wingerson, N. W., & Wineman, N. M. (2000). The mental health, self-efficacy, and satisfaction outcomes of a community counseling demonstration project for multiple sclerosis patients. *Journal of Applied Rehabilitation Counseling, 31*(2), 11–17.

Wolkstein, E. (Ed.). (2002). *Second national conference on substance abuse and coexisting disabilities.* Dayton, OH: Wright State University.

Worthington, E. L. Jr., Kurusu, T. A., McCollough, M. E., & Sandage, S. J. (1996). Empirical research on religion and psychotherapeutic processes and outcomes: A 10-year review and research prospectus. *Psychological Bulletin, 119*(3), 448–487.

Wright, B. A. (1983). *Physical Disability—A Psychosocial Approach* (2nd ed.). New York: Harper & Row.

Wright, J. C., & Telford, R. (1996). Psychological problems following minor head injury: A prospective study. *British Journal of Clinical Psychology, 35*(3), 399–412.

Wyeth, D. (personal communications, June 29, 2000).

Yarhouse, M. A., & VanOrman, B. T. (1999). When psychologists work with religious clients: Applications of the general principles of ethical conduct. *Professional Psychology: Research and Practice, 30*(6), 557–562.

Young, W. (2002). *Past, present, and future spinal cord injury research.* Paper presented at the American Association of Spinal Cord Injury Psychologists and Social Workers, Las Vegas, Nevada.

Zasler, N. D. (1993). Sexuality issues after traumatic brain injury: Clinical and research perspectives. In F. P. Haseltine, S. S. Cole, & D. B. Gray (Eds.), *Reproductive issues for persons with physical disabilities* (pp. 229–237). Baltimore: Paul H. Brookes.

Zimmerman, B., Lindberg, C., & Plsek, P. (2001). *Edgeware: Insights from complexity science for health care leaders* (2nd ed.). Irving, TX: VHA Inc.

Zola, I. K. (1991). Aging and disability: Toward a unified agenda. In R. P. Marinelli & A. E. Dell Orto (Eds.), *The psychological & social impact of disability* (3rd ed., pp. 289–294). New York: Springer Publishing.

Zola, I. K. (1991). Communication barriers between "the able-bodied" and "the handicapped." In R. P. Marinelli & A. E. Dell Orto (Eds.), *The psychological and social impact of disability* (3rd ed., pp. 157–164). New York: Springer Publishing.

Zuckerman, M. E. A. (1978). Sensation seeking in England and America: Cross cultural age and sex comparison. *Journal of Consulting and Clinical Psychology, 46*(1), 139–149.

Index

⑤ *Springer Publishing Company*

The Psychological and Social Impact of Disability, *4th Edition*

Robert P. Marinelli, EdD, CRC,
and Arthur E. Dell Orto, PhD, CRC

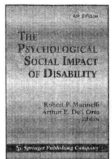

"This book addresses many of the issues that can help to create a better understanding, awareness, and appreciation of people with disabilities."
—American Journal of Nursing

Formatted to include thought-provoking study questions and disability awareness exercises, this text is recommended for students in rehabilitation counseling and physical therapy education programs as well as professionals in rehabilitation, psychology, and social work. Carefully selected articles and personal narratives capture the unique aspects of the psychological and social effects of disability.

Contents:

- The Political Implications of Disability Definitions and Data, *H. Hahn*
- Helping Families Manage Severe Mental Illness, *K. Mueser*
- Disability and Value Change: An Overview and Reanalysis of Acceptance of Loss Theory, *Kelly C. M-H. Keany and R. L. Glueckauf*
- Castification of People with Disabilities: Potential Disempowering Aspects of Classification in Disability Services, *E. M. Szymanski and H. T. Trueba*
- Sexuality, Disability, and Reproductive Issues Through the Lifespan, *S. S. Cole and T. M. Cole*
- Applying Beck's Cognitive Therapy to Livneh's Model of Adaptation to Disability, *J. Stewart*
- The Family Experience of Mental Illness: Implications for Intervention, *D. T. Marsh and D. L. Johnson*
- Dual Diagnosis of Mental Health and Substance Abuse: Contemporary Challenges for Rehabilitation, *S. Kelley and J. Benshoff*

1999   488pp   0-8261-2213-2   hardcover

536 Broadway, New York, NY 10012 • **Order On-Line: www.springerpub.com**